# Gynaecology

by Ten Teachers

# Gynaecology

## by Ten Teachers

under the direction of

## Stanley G. Clayton

Edited by
**Stanley G. Clayton**
**T. L. T. Lewis**
**G.D. Pinker**

## Fourteenth edition

Edward Arnold
A division of Hodder & Stoughton
LONDON MELBOURNE AUCKLAND

© 1985 Edward Arnold (Publishers) Ltd

First published in Great Britain 1919

| | | | |
|---|---|---|---|
| First edition | 1919 | Eighth edition | 1949 |
| Reprinted | 1919 | Ninth edition | 1953 |
| Second edition | 1921 | Reprinted | 1956 |
| Reprinted | 1922 | Tenth edition | 1959 |
| Third edition | 1924 | Reprinted | 1960 |
| Reprinted | 1926 | Eleventh edition | 1964 |
| Fourth edition | 1930 | Twelfth edition | 1971 |
| Reprinted | 1932, 1933 | (renamed *Gynaecology*) | |
| Fifth edition | 1934 | Reprinted | 1976, 1978 |
| Reprinted | 1935 | Thirteenth edition | 1980 |
| Sixth edition | 1938 | First published in paperback | 1981 |
| Reprinted | 1939 | Reprinted | 1981, 1982 |
| Seventh edition | 1942 | Fourteenth edition | 1985 |
| Reprinted | 1943, 1944 | Reprinted | 1987, 1989 |

*British Library Cataloguing in Publication Data*

Gynaecology. – 14th ed.
  1. Gynaecology
  I. Clayton, *Sir* Stanley George
  II. Lewis, Thomas Loftus Townshend
  III. Pinker, George Douglas
  618.1       RG101

ISBN 0-7131-4460-2

Whilst the advice and information in this book is believed to be true and accurate at the date of going to press, neither the author nor the publisher can accept any legal responsibility or liability for any errors or omissions that may be made.

Typeset in IBM 10pt Press Roman by A Tek-Art, Croydon, Surrey. Printed and bound in Great Britain for Edward Arnold, the educational, academic and medical division of Hodder and Stoughton Limited, 41 Bedford Square, London WC1B 3DQ by Butler & Tanner Ltd, Frome and London.

# List of contributors

## Director

Sir Stanley Clayton, MD, MS (Lond), FRCP, FRCS, FRCOG.
Emeritus Professor of Obstetrics and Gynaecology, University of London: Honorary Consulting Surgeon, King's College Hospital, Queen Charlotte's Hospital and Chelsea Hospital for Women.

## Contributors

J. Michael Brudenell, MB, BS (Lond), FRCS, FRCOG.
Obstetric and Gynaecological Surgeon, King's College Hospital; Gynaecological Surgeon, Queen Victoria Hospital, East Grinstead.

Geoffrey V.P. Chamberlain, MD (Lond), FRCS, FRCOG.
Professor of Obstetrics and Gynaecology, St. George's Hospital Medical School.

Denys V.I. Fairweather, MD (St. Andrew's), FRCOG.
Professor of Obstetrics and Gynaecology, School of Medicine, University College London.

John C. Hartgill, FRCS (Ed), FRCOG.
Obstetric and Gynaecological Surgeon, The London Hospital.

Joseph M. Holmes, MD (Lond), FRCOG.
Obstetric and Gynaecological Surgeon, University College Hospital.

Thomas L.T. Lewis, CBE, MB, B.Chir (Cantab), FRCS, FRCOG.
Emeritus Obstetric and Gynaecological Surgeon, Guy's Hospital, Queen Charlotte's Hospital and Chelsea Hospital for Women.

George D. Pinker, CVO, MB, BS (Lond), FRCS (Ed), FRCOG.
Obstetric and Gynaecological Surgeon, St. Mary's Hospital; Gynaecological Surgeon, Samaritan Hospital; Honorary Consultant Surgeon, Royal Women's Hospital, Melbourne.

David W.T. Roberts, MA, M.Chir (Cantab), FRCS, FRCOG.
Obstetric and Gynaecological Surgeon, St. Mary's Hospital and the Middlesex Hospital.

Marcus E. Setchell, MA, MB, B.Chir (Cantab), FRCS, FRCS (Ed), FRCOG.
Obstetric and Gynaecological Surgeon, St. Bartholomew's Hospital.

Ronald W. Taylor, MD (Liverpool), FRCOG.
Professor of Obstetrics and Gynaecology, St. Thomas's Hospital Medical School.

The chapter on Psychosexual Disorders has been written by invitation by:

Dr Margaret E. Christie-Brown, MB, BS (Lond).
Consultant Psychotherapist, Queen Charlotte's Hospital and Chelsea Hospital for Women.

# Preface

This book was first published with the title *Diseases of Women by Ten Teachers* in 1919, so that in this edition we complete 66 years of service to students and practitioners. Throughout these years all the contributors have been active teachers and examiners in the London Medical Schools, and we hope that this edition will continue to reflect the long and proud tradition of practical clinical teaching in London.

We have attempted to give a broad but comprehensive description of the physiology, pathology, diagnosis and treatment of gynaecological disorders. While the book will probably be of greatest value to undergraduate students it may also serve as a basic text, to which more specialized reading can be added, for those who are already qualified and are starting postgraduate work.

In the preface to the preceding edition we remarked on the changing pattern of gynaecological practice, with the increasing use of scientific methods of investigation, more time given to the promotion and control of fertility, and extensive use of hormones in treatment. These changes have continued with even greater speed and this will be evident in the text; every chapter has been thoroughly revised and many sections have been rewritten.

We are grateful to Dr John McEwan of King's College Hospital for his helpful comments on the chapter on contraception, to Dr R.J. Whittle of St Bartholomew's Hospital for advice about radiotherapy, to Mr J.A. Jordan of the Birmingham and Midland Hospital for Women for colposcopic photographs, and to Mrs Audrey Besterman for her expert help with many new figures.

London, 1984

SGC
TLTL
GDP

# Contents

# 1

# Anatomy of the pelvic organs

Knowledge of anatomy assists in gynaecological diagnosis and is essential for gynaecological surgery. Some of the details in this chapter are included for reference rather than for memorization, but the student may well revise his anatomical knowledge before proceeding.

## The external genitalia

### The vulva

**The mons pubis** is composed of fibro-fatty tissue which covers the bodies of the pubic bones. Inferiorly it divides to become continuous with the labium majus of each side. The skin that covers it bears pubic hair, the upper limit of which is usually horizontal.

**The labia majora** are two folds of skin and subcutaneous fat which merge posteriorly into the perineum where they are joined together by the fourchette. The skin covering them contains sebaceous and sweat glands, and a few specialized apocrine glands, from which a tumour known as a hidradenoma (p. 143) may arise. The lateral aspects of the labia majora bear hair follicles. In the deepest part of each labium is a core of fatty tissue continuous with that of the inguinal canal, and the fibres of the round ligament terminate here. During development a diverticulum of the peritoneal cavity, the *processus vaginalis,* accompanies the round ligament into the inguinal canal. It usually disappears, but may persist as the canal of Nuck.

**The labia minora** are two thin folds of skin which lie between the labia majora. Anteriorly they divide into two parts, the upper of which unite over the clitoris to form the prepuce, and the lower of which unite to form the frenulum. The skin of the labia minora bears no hair follicles, although sebaceous glands and a few sweat glands are present. The labia minora are very sensitive and contain some erectile tissue.

**The clitoris** consists of the glans, the body and two crura which diverge posteriorly to be attached to the descending rami of the pubic bones. The glans is covered with modified skin containing many nerve endings. The body and the crura are composed of erectile tissue. The ischiocavernosus muscles surround the crura and by their contraction produce erection of the clitoris.

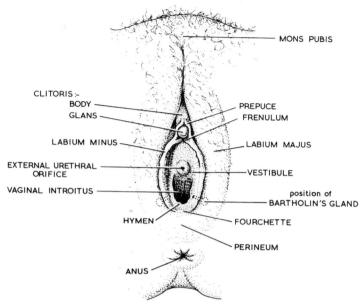

**Fig. 1.1**  The vulva.

The **vestibule** is bounded anterolaterally by the labia minora and posteriorly by the fourchette. Into the vestibule open the urethra, the ducts of Bartholin's glands and the vagina.

The **vestibular bulbs** are two oblong masses of erectile tissue which lie on either side of the vaginal entrance from the vestibule.

**Bartholin's glands (vestibular glands)** are two small racemose glands situated on either side of the vaginal orifice deep to the posterior ends of the labia minora. During sexual excitation they secrete thin mucus which serves as a lubricant. The duct on each side opens in the groove between the labium minus and the hymen. Each duct is about 0.5 cm long, and unless it is inflamed the orifice cannot usually be seen. The gland cannot be palpated unless it is pathologically enlarged by inflammation or, very rarely, by new growth.

The **hymen** is a membrane composed of connective tissue and covered by stratified squamous epithelium on both aspects. It is perforated centrally, the opening varying in size from a pin-hole to one that admits two fingers. The hymen is partially ruptured at the first coitus and further disrupted during childbirth. Any tags remaining after rupture are known as carunculae myrtiformes.

The **superficial perineal muscles** lie superficial to the urogenital diaphragm, and are illustrated in Fig. 1.11.

# The internal reproductive organs

## The vagina

The vagina is a muscular canal lined by stratified squamous epithelium which leads from the uterus to the vulva. Its length averages 10 cm. The anterior and posterior walls are normally in apposition. The vagina meets the anteverted uterus at a right angle. The cervix projects into the vaginal vault, which is described as having four fornices — anterior, posterior and two lateral. The posterior vaginal wall is longer than the anterior wall, so that the posterior fornix is deeper than the anterior. The vaginal walls are rugose with transverse folds.

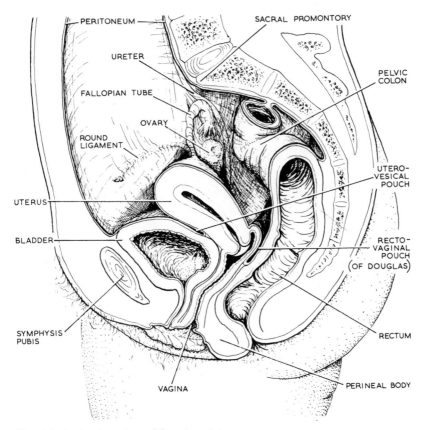

**Fig. 1.2** Sagittal section of female pelvis.

The vagina is normally kept moist by the secretion of the uterine and cervical glands, and by a watery transudate through its epithelial lining; it has no glands. During the reproductive period of life the stratified squamous epithelium is thick and contains glycogen from the influence of oestrogens, but before puberty and after the menopause it is devoid of glycogen. After puberty Döderlein's bacillus appears in the vagina and produces lactic acid by its action on the glycogen in the epithelial cells, so that the vaginal secretion has a pH of about 4. The acid reaction persists until the menopause and restricts the growth of pathogenic organisms.

Laterally the vagina is supported by the strong *cardinal ligaments* (transverse cervical ligaments) which form a sling extending from the side walls of the pelvis to the vaginal vault and supravaginal cervix. The vagina is also supported in its middle third by the medial edges of the levator ani muscles, from which fibres are given off to blend with the muscular coat of the vagina.

Posteriorly the lower part of the vagina is supported by the *perineal body,* which is formed by decussating fibres of the levator ani muscles and of the superficial perineal muscles. In its middle third the vagina is separated from the rectum by only a thin rectovaginal septum of fascia. The recto-vaginal pouch lies immediately behind the upper third of the vagina, where the peritoneum is reflected from the rectum over the posterior vaginal fornix to reach the supravaginal cervix and the body of the uterus.

## The uterus

The uterus has thick muscular walls which surround a small cavity lined by endometrium. In shape it resembles a pear flattened from before back-wards. In adult life it weighs about 70 g and is about 7.5 cm long, with walls about 2 cm thick. It consists of two unequal parts: an upper corpus, or body, which is about 5 cm long; and a lower cervix, or neck, which is about 2.5 cm long. In the child the cervix forms about two-thirds of the total length of the uterus, and the body but one-third, whereas in the adult these proportions are reversed. In old age the uterus shrinks, the muscular walls atrophy and the vaginal portion of the cervix becomes almost flat.

### Corpus uteri

The cavity of the uterus is triangular with the base uppermost, and the apex at the junction with the cervix where it is narrowed to form the internal os. At the upper angles are the openings of the Fallopian tubes. The walls of the cavity are normally in contact. The part of the body of the uterus which is above the points of entrance of the Fallopian tubes is known as the *fundus.*

The plain muscle fibres of the uterine wall are arranged in three layers. The outer longitudinal and inner circular layers are thin; in the thick middle layer the muscle bundles decussate. The uterus is extremely vascular and nearly half the bulk of the middle layer is taken up by blood vessels.

The cavity is lined with columnar epithelium, the *endometrium.* In the infant the uterine lining consists of a single layer of cubical epithelium set on a thin layer of cellular connective tissue stroma. During childhood numerous glands develop; they are of simple tubular type reaching from

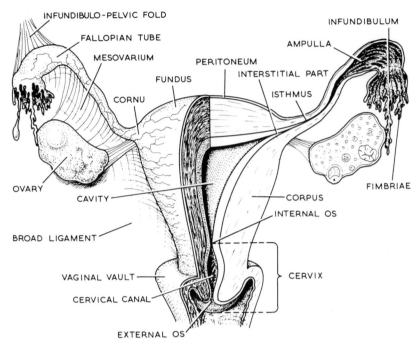

INFUNDIBULO-PELVIC FOLD

FALLOPIAN TUBE

MESOVARIUM

FUNDUS

CORNU

OVARY

CAVITY

BROAD LIGAMENT

VAGINAL VAULT

CERVICAL CANAL

EXTERNAL OS

PERITONEUM

INFUNDIBULUM

AMPULLA

INTERSTITIAL PART

ISTHMUS

FIMBRIAE

CORPUS

INTERNAL OS

CERVIX

**Fig. 1.3** Uterus, tubes and ovaries from behind.

the surface down to the muscle fibres. The endometrium remains at this stage of development until puberty. From that time until the menopause the endometrium undergoes cyclical changes known as the menstrual cycle, which are described in the next chapter. After the menopause the endometrium atrophies and becomes a thin layer containing a few residual glands, which tend to lie obliquely.

### Cervix uteri

The cervix is cylindrical in shape and continuous above with the body of the uterus. It is described in two parts — supravaginal and vaginal. The vaginal part projects below into the vault of the vagina.

The cervical canal is spindle shaped, being constricted above at the internal os and below at the external os, where it opens into the vagina. In women who have not borne children the external os is circular, but after labour it has the form of a transverse slit. The vaginal surface of the cervix is covered with squamous epithelium which extends to the margin of the external os.

The wall of the cervix consists of fibromuscular tissue. The canal is lined by mucous membrane with a median vertical ridge from which transverse folds radiate on both the anterior and posterior surfaces; this arrangement is called the arbor vitae.

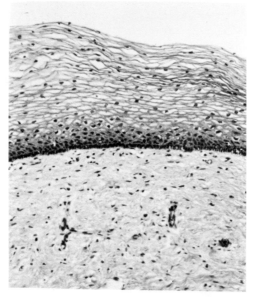

**Fig. 1.4**  Normal ectocervical epithelium.

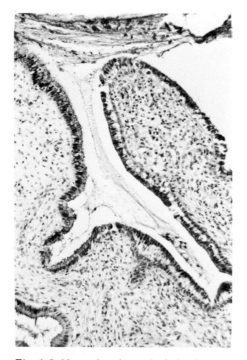

**Fig. 1.5**  Normal endocervical gland.

The cervical epithelium is of tall columnar type, ciliated on the folds but not in the furrows. The nuclei of the cells are basal. The glands are racemose and branch deeply into the fibromuscular stroma. There is an abrupt change at the external os from the columnar to the squamous type of epithelium, and it is at this transformation zone that carcinoma is particularly liable to arise.

### Relations
In most women the uterus is anteverted, that is to say the long axis of the uterus is directed forwards. The body of the uterus is also bent forwards on the cervix (anteflexed). The opposite condition of retroversion with retroflexion is found in about 20 per cent of normal women.

The body of the uterus is completely covered with peritoneum except for a narrow area on each side where the peritoneum sweeps away laterally to form the broad ligament. Posteriorly the peritoneum passes downwards from the uterine body to cover the posterior surface of the supravaginal cervix and the upper third of the posterior vaginal wall. This peritoneum forms the anterior boundary of the rectovaginal pouch of Douglas. The entrance to the pouch is bounded laterally by two peritoneal folds which reach from the posterolateral aspects of the cervix in front to the third piece of the sacrum behind. These uterosacral folds lie on either side of the rectum and cover the uterosacral ligaments.

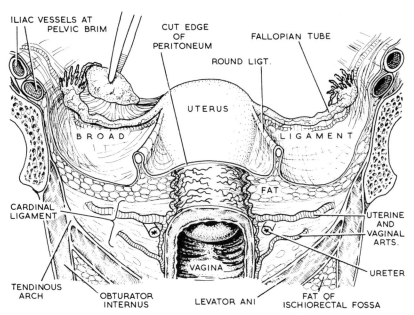

**Fig. 1.6** Coronal section of female pelvis, viewed from in front.

Anteriorly the uterus is covered with peritoneum only as far down as the level of the internal os; below this the peritoneum is reflected onto the bladder, forming the uterovesical pouch. The supravaginal cervix is below this peritoneal reflection, and is only separated from the bladder by a thin layer of connective tissue. On either side the peritoneum is deflected to form the broad ligaments.

The uterine artery passes inwards to reach the uterus at about the level of the internal os. At this point the ureter passes forwards to cross below the artery at a distance of about 2 cm from the side of the cervix.

## The Fallopian tubes (uterine tubes)

The Fallopian tube on either side extends outwards from the uterine cornu to end near the ovary. At the abdominal ostium the tube opens into the peritoneal cavity, which is therefore in communication with the exterior of the body, via the uterus and vagina. The tubes are oviducts which convey the ova from the Graafian follicles to the uterus.

The Fallopian tube runs in the upper margin of the broad ligament, part of which, known as the *mesosalpinx,* encloses it, so that the tube is completely covered with peritoneum except for a narrow strip along its inferior aspect. Each tube is about 10 cm long and is described in four parts; (1) the interstitial portion, (2) the isthmus, (3) the ampulla and (4) the infundibulum or fimbrial portion.

The *interstitial portion* lies within the wall of the uterus, while the *isthmus* is the narrow portion adjoining the uterus, and this passes into the widest and longest portion, the *ampulla.* This in turn terminates in the fimbriated extremity known as the *infundibulum,* where the funnel-shaped opening of the tube into the peritoneal cavity is surrounded by finger-like processes called fimbriae, into which the muscle coat does not extend. Their inner surfaces are covered by ciliated epithelium similar to that lining the tube itself. One of these fimbriae is longer than the others and extends to, and partly embraces, the ovary.

The muscle fibres of the wall of the tube are arranged in an inner circular and an outer longitudinal layer. The tubal epithelium forms a number of branched folds or plicae which run longitudinally; the lumen of the ampulla is almost filled with these folds. The folds have a cellular stroma, but at their bases the epithelium is only separated from the muscle by a very scanty amount of stroma. There is no submucosa and there are no glands. The epithelial cells are cilated; most of the cilia act in the direction of the uterus. Changes occur in the tubal epithelium during the menstrual cycle, but are less evident than in the endometrium, and there is no exfoliation.

## The ovaries

The ovaries are two almond-shaped solid organs, measuring about 3.5 cm in length, 2 cm in depth and 1 cm in thickness.

In the child the ovaries are small structures about 1.5 cm long, with smooth surfaces. In the months preceding puberty the ovaries increase in size to that of the adult. This considerable increase in size is brought about not only by proliferation of the stroma cells, but also by commencing maturation of the ovarian follicles, which is described in detail later. The mature and actively functioning ovary contains numerous Graafian (ovarian) follicles which vary in size from microscopical dimensions up to about 2 cm in diameter. The cyclical changes which occur in the follicles during the menstrual cycle are described below. After the menopause no active follicles are present and the ovary becomes a small shrunken structure with a wrinkled surface.

The position of the ovary varies considerably, but it usually lies against the peritoneum of the lateral pelvic wall in the ovarian fossa, bounded above by the external iliac vein, and behind by the ureter where it runs downwards and forwards in front of the internal iliac artery. The ovary is not covered with peritoneum; it is attached at its hilum to the posterior surface of the broad ligament. The most lateral part of the broad ligament is called the infundibulopelvic fold, and this supports the outer pole of the ovary. The inner pole is suspended from the cornu of the uterus by the ovarian ligament; this is continuous with the round ligament which is also attached to the cornu below the Fallopian tube.

**Microscopical structure**
The ovary consists chiefly of stroma, composed of spindle-shaped connective tissue cells. It is covered by a layer of cubical cells, continuous at the hilum with the peritoneum forming the mesovarium. These lie on a dense layer of connective tissue, the *tunica albuginea*. The Graafian follicles are interspersed throughout the stroma, and some of them may be seen bulging at the surface. They vary in size according to their stage of development. Each primordial follicle contains an oöcyte (ovum). Between puberty and the menopause some of the primordial follicles mature and form ripe follicles, one or more of which rupture at about day 14 of each menstrual cycle. The ripe follicle which ruptures to discharge its oöcyte is converted into a *corpus luteum,* which eventually retrogresses and becomes a fibrous *corpus albicans.* For every follicle which ruptures and discharges its oöcyte a number of other follicles start to ripen, but they do not rupture and are described as atretic follicles.

The primordial follicle consists of a large central cell, the oöcyte, which is surrounded by a single layer of flattened cells. As the follicle matures these cells proliferate to form a number of layers of cells surrounding the oöcyte, called the *membrana granulosa*. After a time, fluid is secreted between some of the granulosa cells so as to form a follicle. The oöcyte is displaced to one side of the follicle, and the part of the membrana granulosa which surrounds it and attaches it to the side of the follicle is known as the cumulus oöphorus (discus proligerus).

While these changes are taking place the stromal cells surrounding the follicle also proliferate to form the theca. This consists of two layers: the

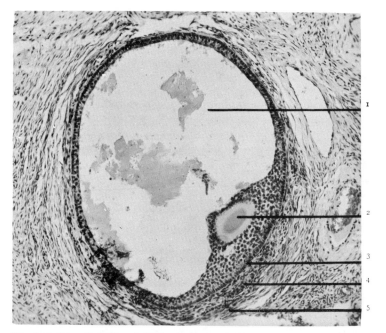

**Fig. 1.7**  Ripe Graafian follicle: 1, liquor folliculi; 2, oöcyte; 3, granulosa cells; 4, theca interna; 5, theca externa.

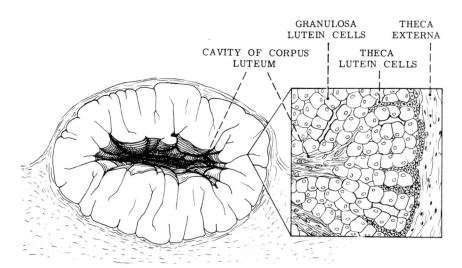

**Fig. 1.8**  Corpus luteum.

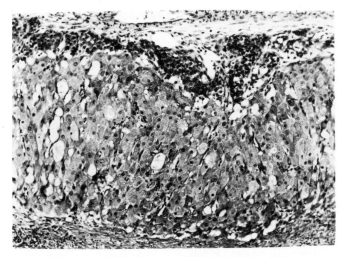

**Fig. 1.9** Microscopical section of corpus luteum. The cavity is below and the dark theca-lutein cells are seen above the large granulosa-lutein cells.

inner *theca interna* is vascular with a rich capillary network; the outer *theca externa* is mainly fibrous.

During maturation the Graafian follicle gradually enlarges and reaches the surface of the ovary. At about day 14 of the menstrual cycle the follicle ruptures, and the oöcyte with some of the granulosa cells still attached to it is discharged into the peritoneal cavity.

After rupture and escape of the oöcyte and liquor folliculi the Graafian follicle collapses. The cells of the theca interna become enlarged, and their cytoplasm contains lipoid; they are now called *theca-lutein cells*. Enlargement of the granulosa cells with accumulation of lipoid quickly follows, and these cells are now called *granulosa-lutein cells*. Blood vessels from the theca interna grow in to vascularize the lutein layer, and there is sometimes slight bleeding into the cavity of the now fully formed corpus luteum. The granulosa-lutein and theca-lutein layers become infolded into the cavity, giving a characteristic pleated appearance, with a bright yellow colour. The corpus luteum may be about 1 cm in diameter.

If conception occurs in the particular cycle, the corpus luteum continues to grow, reaching its maximum size at about the 12th week of pregnancy, but otherwise it begins to degenerate just before the next menstruation. All its elements retrogress and it is gradually organized by ingrowing fibroblasts and converted into a structureless hyaline mass known as the corpus albicans.

# The bladder, urethra and ureter

## The bladder

The average capacity of the bladder is 400 ml. The bladder is lined with transitional epithelium. The involuntary muscle of its wall is arranged in an inner longitudinal layer, a middle circular layer and an outer longitudinal layer.

The ureters open into the base of the bladder after running medially for about 1 cm through the vesical wall. The urethra leaves the bladder in front of the ureteric orifices; the triangular area lying between the ureteric orifices and the internal meatus is known as the trigone. At the internal meatus the middle layer of vesical muscle forms anterior and posterior loops round the neck of the bladder, some of the fibres of the loops being continuous with the circular muscle of the urethra.

The base of the bladder is related to the cervix, with only a thin layer of connective tissue intervening. Below it is separated from the anterior vaginal wall by the pubocervical fascia, which stretches from the pubis to the cervix.

## The urethra

The female urethra is about 3.5 cm long, and it has a slight posterior angulation at the junction of its lower and middle thirds. It is lined with transitional epithelium. The smooth muscle of its wall is arranged in outer longitudinal and inner circular layers. As the urethra passes through the two layers of the urogenital diaphragm (triangular ligament) it is embraced by the striated fibres of the deep transverse perineal muscle (compressor urethrae), and some of the striated fibres form loops on the urethra. Between the muscular coat and the epithelium is a plexus of veins. There are a number of tubular mucous glands and, in the lower part, a number of crypts, which occasionally become infected.

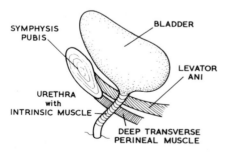

SYMPHYSIS PUBIS

BLADDER

LEVATOR ANI

URETHRA with INTRINSIC MUSCLE

DEEP TRANSVERSE PERINEAL MUSCLE

**Fig. 1.10** Diagram to show the muscles concerned in the control of micturition.

In its upper two-thirds the urethra is separated from the symphysis by loose connective tissue, but in its lower third it is attached to the pubic ramus on each side by strong bands of fibrous tissue called the pubo-urethral ligaments. Posteriorly it is related to the anterior vaginal wall, to which it is firmly attached in its lower two-thirds. The upper part of the urethra is mobile, but the lower part is relatively fixed.

Medial fibres of the pubococcygeus portion of the levator ani muscles are inserted into the urethra and vaginal wall, and when they contract they pull the anterior vaginal wall forwards and the upper part of the urethra with it, forming an angle of about 100° between the posterior wall of the urethra and the bladder base. On voluntary voiding of urine the base of the bladder and the upper part of the urethra descend and this posterior angle disappears, so that the base of the bladder and the posterior wall of the urethra come to lie in a straight line. It was formerly claimed that absence of this posterior angle was the cause of stress incontinence (see p. 334) but this has not been substantiated.

## The ureter

As the ureter crosses the brim of the pelvis it lies in front of the bifurcation of the common iliac artery. It runs downwards and forwards on the lateral wall of the pelvis to reach the pelvic floor, and then passes inwards and forwards attached to the peritoneum of the back of the broad ligament, to pass beneath the uterine artery. It next passes forwards through a fibrous tunnel, the ureteric canal, in the upper part of the cardinal ligament. It finally runs close to the lateral vaginal fornix to enter the trigone of the bladder.

Its blood supply is derived from small branches of the ovarian artery, from a small vessel arising from near the iliac bifurcation, from a branch of the uterine artery where it crosses it, and from small branches of the vesical arteries.

Because of its close relationship to the cervix, to the vault of the vagina and to the uterine artery, the ureter may be damaged during hysterectomy. Apart from being cut or tied, in radical procedures it may undergo necrosis because of interference with its blood supply. The ureter may be displaced upwards by fibromyomata or cysts which are growing between the layers of the broad ligament and may suffer injury if its position is not noticed at operation.

## The rectum

The rectum extends from the level of the third sacral vertebra to a point about 2.5 cm in front of the coccyx, where it passes through the pelvic floor to become continuous with the anal canal. Its direction follows the curve of the sacrum and it is about 11 cm in length.

In its upper third its front and sides are covered by the peritoneum of the rectovaginal pouch; in its middle third only the front is covered by peritoneum. In the lower third there is no peritoneal covering and the rectum is separated from the posterior wall of the vagina by the recto-vaginal fascial septum. Lateral to the rectum are the two uterosacral ligaments, beside which run some of the lymphatics draining the cervix and vagina.

# Pelvic muscles, ligaments and fasciae

## The pelvic diaphragm

The pelvic diaphragm is formed by the levatores ani muscles.

### Levatores ani muscles

Each is a broad, flat muscle, the fibres of which pass downwards and inwards. Together with its fellow of the opposite side, the two muscles constitute the pelvic diaphragm. The muscle arises by a linear origin from: (1) the lower part of the body of the os pubis, (2) from the internal sur-face of the parietal pelvic fascia along the 'white line' (arcus tendineus) and (3) from the pelvic surface of the ischial spine. It is inserted into: (1) the pre-anal raphé and the central point of the perineum where the muscle meets its fellow of the opposite side, (2) the wall of the anal canal, where the fibres blend with the deep external sphincter muscle, (3) the postanal or anococcygeal raphé, where again it meets its fellow of the opposite side, and (4) the lower part of the coccyx (Fig. 1.12). The muscle is described in two parts; the pubococcygeus arises from the pubic bone and the anterior part of the arcus tendineus, while the iliococcygeus arises from the posterior part of the arcus and the ischial spine.

The medial borders of the pubococcygeus muscles pass on either side from the pubic bone to the pre-anal raphé. They thus embrace the vagina, and on contraction have some sphincteric action. The nerve supply is from the third and fourth sacral nerves.

The muscles support the pelvic and abdominal viscera, including the bladder. The most medial part of each muscle is described as the pubo-coccygeal portion. The medial edge of this passes beneath the bladder and lateral to the urethra, into which some of its fibres are inserted. Together with fibres from the opposite muscle they form a loop which maintains the angle between the posterior aspect of the urethra and the bladder base. During micturition this loop relaxes to allow the bladder neck and upper urethra to open and descend.

**The urogenital diaphragm (triangular ligament)** lies below the levator ani muscles and consists of two layers of pelvic fascia which fill the gap between the descending pubic rami. The deep transverse perineal muscle (compressor urethrae) lies between the two layers, and the diaphragm is pierced by the urethra and vagina.

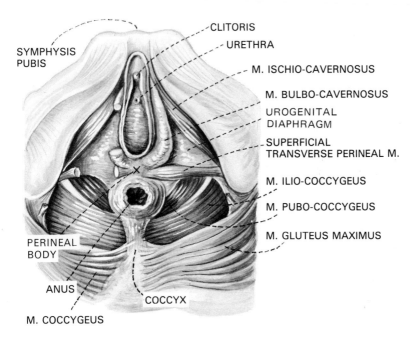

**Fig. 1.11** Pelvic floor from below.

### The perineal body

This is the pyramidal mass of muscular tissue which lies between the anal canal and the lower third of the vagina. Its apex is at the lower end of the rectovaginal septum at the point where the rectum and posterior vaginal walls come into contact. Its base is covered with skin and extends from the fourchette to the anus. It is the point of insertion of the superficial perineal muscles, and is bounded above by the levatores ani muscles where they come into contact in the midline between the posterior vaginal wall and the rectum.

### The pelvic peritoneum

The peritoneum is reflected from the lateral borders of the uterus to form on either side a double fold of peritoneum known as the *broad ligament.* This is not a 'ligament' but a peritoneal fold, and it does not support the uterus. The Fallopian tube runs in the upper free edge of the broad ligament as far as the point at which the tube opens into the peritoneal cavity; the part of the broad ligament which is lateral to the opening is called the

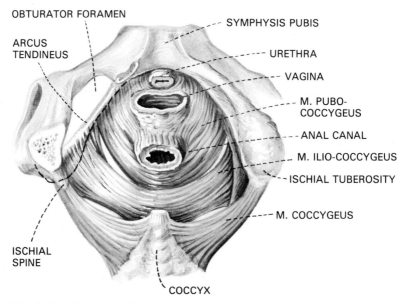

OBTURATOR FORAMEN

SYMPHYSIS PUBIS

ARCUS
TENDINEUS

URETHRA

VAGINA

M. PUBO-
COCCYGEUS

ANAL CANAL

M. ILIO-COCCYGEUS

ISCHIAL TUBEROSITY

M. COCCYGEUS

ISCHIAL
SPINE

COCCYX

**Fig. 1.12**  Pelvic floor from below; deeper dissection.

*infundibulopelvic fold,* and in it the ovarian vessels and nerves pass from the side wall of the pelvis to lie between the two layers of the broad ligament. The portion of the broad ligament which lies above the ovary is known as the mesosalpinx, and between its layers are to be seen any Wolffian remnants which may be present (see p. 75). Below the ovary the base of the broad ligament widens out and contains a considerable amount of loose connective tissue, called the *parametrium.* The ureter is attached to the posterior leaf of the broad ligament at this point.

The ovary is attached to the posterior layer of the broad ligament by a short mesentery (*mesovarium*) through which the ovarian vessels and nerves enter the hilum.

The *rectovaginal pouch* has already been described (p. 6). It will be noted that while the vagina does not have any peritoneal covering in front, behind it is in contact with the rectovaginal pouch for about 2 cm, where the vagina is separated from the abdominal cavity only by the peritoneum and thin fascia. The peritoneal cavity can be opened by posterior colpotomy at this point.

### The ovarian ligament and round ligament

The ovarian ligament lies beneath the posterior layer of the broad ligament and passes from the medial pole of the ovary to the uterus just below the point of entry of the Fallopian tube.

The round ligament is the continuation of the same structure and runs forwards under the anterior leaf of peritoneum to enter the inguinal canal, ending in the subcutaneous tissue of the labium majus. Together, the ovarian and round ligaments are homologous with the gubernaculum testis of the male. The round ligament is seldom tense enough to prevent the uterus from becoming retroverted; it has no other supporting function.

## The pelvic fascia and pelvic cellular tissue

Connective tissue fills the irregular spaces between the various pelvic organs. Much of it is loose cellular tissue, but in some places it is condensed to form strong ligaments which contain some smooth muscle fibres, and it forms the fascial sheaths which invest the various viscera. The pelvic arteries, veins, lymphatics and nerves, and the ureters run in it.

The cellular tissue is continuous above with the extraperitoneal tissue of the abdominal wall, but below it is cut off from the ischiorectal fossa by the pelvic fascia and the levator ani muscles. There is a considerable collection of cellular tissue in the wide base of the broad ligament and at the side of the cervix and vagina, spoken of as the *parametrium.*

The pelvic fascia may be regarded as a specialized part of this connective tissue. Anatomists describe parietal and visceral components. The *parietal pelvic fascia* lines the wall of the pelvic cavity, covering the obturator internus and pyramidalis muscles. There is a thickened 'white line' (the arcus tendineus) on the side wall of the pelvis from which the levator ani muscle arises and where the cardinal ligament gains its lateral attachment. Where the parietal pelvic fascia encounters bone, as in the pubic region, it blends with the periosteum. It also forms the upper layer of the urogenital diaphragm (triangular ligament).

Each viscus has a fascial investment, which is dense in the case of the vagina and cervix and at the base of the bladder, but is tenuous or absent over the body of the uterus and the dome of the bladder. Various processes of the *visceral pelvic fascia* pass inwards from the peripheral layer of parietal pelvic fascia. From the point of view of the gynaecologist, certain parts of the visceral fascia are of particular importance, as follows.

The essential support of the uterus and vaginal vault is provided by the *cardinal ligaments* (transverse cervical ligaments). These are two strong fan-shaped fibromuscular expansions which pass from the cervix and vaginal vault to the side wall of the pelvis on either side (see Fig. 10.2).

The *uterosacral ligaments* run from the cervix and vaginal vault to the sacrum. In the erect position they are almost vertical in direction and support the cervix.

The bladder is supported laterally by condensations of the vesical pelvic fascia on each side, and there is also a sheet of *pubocervical fascia* which lies beneath it anteriorly.

# Arteries supplying the pelvic organs

## The ovarian artery

Because the ovary develops on the posterior abdominal wall and later migrates down into the pelvis it derives its blood supply directly from the abdominal aorta. The ovarian artery arises from the aorta just below the renal artery and runs downwards on the anterior surface of the psoas muscle to the pelvic brim where it crosses in front of the ureter, and then passes into the infundibulopelvic fold of the broad ligament. The artery divides into branches which supply the ovary and tube and then run on to reach the uterus, where they anastomose with the terminal branches of the uterine artery.

## The internal iliac (hypogastric) artery

This is a short vessel about 2 cm in length which begins at the bifurcation of the common iliac artery in front of the sacroiliac joint. It soon divides into anterior and posterior divisions; the branches which supply the pelvic viscera are all from the anterior division.

**The uterine artery** provides the main blood supply to the uterus. The artery first runs downwards on the lateral wall of the pelvis, running in the same direction as the ureter. It then turns inwards and forwards, lying in the base of the broad ligament. By this change of direction the artery crosses above the ureter at a distance of about 2 cm from the uterus at the level of the internal os. On reaching the wall of the uterus the artery turns upwards to run tortuously to the upper part of the uterus where it anastomoses with the ovarian artery. In this part of its course it sends many branches into the substance of the uterus.

The artery supplies a branch to the ureter as it crosses it, and shortly afterwards another branch is given off to supply the cervix and upper vagina.

**The vaginal artery** is another branch of the internal iliac artery which runs at a lower level to supply the vagina.

**The vesical arteries** are variable in number. They supply the bladder and terminal ureter. One usually runs in the roof of the ureteric canal.

**The middle haemorrhoidal artery** often arises in common with the lowest vesical artery.

**The pudendal artery** is another branch of the internal iliac artery. It leaves the pelvic cavity through the sciatic foramen and, after winding round the ischial spine, enters the ischiorectal fossa where it gives off the inferior haemorrhoidal artery. It terminates in branches which supply the perineal and vulval structures, including the erectile tissue of the vestibular bulbs and clitoris.

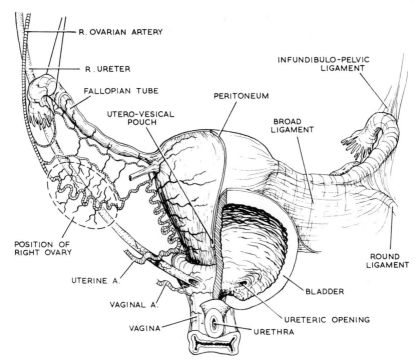

R. OVARIAN ARTERY

R. URETER

FALLOPIAN TUBE

UTERO-VESICAL POUCH

PERITONEUM

INFUNDIBULO-PELVIC LIGAMENT

BROAD LIGAMENT

POSITION OF RIGHT OVARY

ROUND LIGAMENT

UTERINE A.

VAGINAL A.

VAGINA

BLADDER

URETERIC OPENING

URETHRA

**Fig. 1.13** Anterior view of the uterus, tubes and ovaries and blood supply.

## The superior haemorrhoidal artery

This artery is the continuation of the inferior mesenteric artery and descends in the base of the pelvic mesocolon. It divides into two branches which run on either side of the rectum and supply numerous branches to it.

# The pelvic veins

The veins around the bladder, uterus, vagina and rectum form plexuses which intercommunicate freely.

Venous drainage from the uterine, vaginal and vesical plexuses is chiefly into the internal iliac veins.

Venous drainage from the rectal plexus is via the superior haemorrhoidal veins to the inferior mesenteric veins, and the middle and inferior haemorrhoidal veins to the internal pudendal veins and so to the iliac veins.

The ovarian veins on each side begin in the pampiniform plexus which lies between the layers of the broad ligament. There are at first two veins on each side which accompany the corresponding ovarian artery. Higher up the vein becomes single; that on the right ends in the inferior vena cava and that on the left in the left renal vein.

## The pelvic lymphatics

Lymph draining from the lower extremities and the vulval and perineal regions is all filtered through the inguinal and superficial femoral nodes before continuing along the deep pathways on the side wall of the pelvis. One deep chain passes upwards lateral to the major blood vessels, forming in turn the external iliac, common iliac and para-aortic groups of nodes. Medially another chain of vessels passes from the deep femoral nodes through the femoral canal to the obturator and internal iliac groups of nodes. The last nodes are interspersed among the origins of the branches of the internal iliac artery, receiving lymph directly from the organs supplied by this artery, including the upper vagina, cervix and body of the uterus. From the internal iliac and common iliac nodes afferent vessels pass up the para-aortic chains, and finally all the lymphatic drainage from the legs and pelvis flows into the lumbar lymphatic trunks and the cisterna chyli at the level of the second lumbar vertebra. From here all the lymph is carried by the thoracic duct through the thorax, with no intervening nodes, to empty into the junction of the left subclavian and internal jugular veins. Tumour cells which penetrate or bypass the pelvic and para-aortic nodes are rapidly disseminated via the great veins at the root of the neck.

The lymphatic vessels from individual parts of the genital tract drain into this system of pelvic lymph nodes in the following manner.

The *vulva and the perineum* medial to the labiocrural skin folds contain superficial lymphatics which pass upwards towards the mons pubis and then curve laterally to the superficial inguinal and femoral nodes. Drainage from these is through the fossa ovalis into the deep femoral nodes. The largest of these, lying in the upper part of the femoral canal, is known as the node of Cloquet.

*Vagina.* The lymphatics of the lower third follow the vulval drainage to the superficial inguinal nodes, whereas those from the upper two-thirds pass upwards to join the lymphatic vessels of the cervix.

*Cervix.* The lymphatics pass either laterally in the base of the broad ligament or posteriorly along the uterosacral ligaments to reach the side wall of the pelvis. Most of the vessels drain to the internal iliac, obturator and external iliac nodes, but vessels also pass directly to the common iliac and lower para-aortic nodes, so that radical surgery for carcinoma of the cervix should include removal of all these node groups on both sides of the pelvis.

*Corpus uteri.* Nearly all the lymphatic vessels join those leaving the cervix and therefore reach similar groups of nodes. A few vessels at the fundus follow the ovarian channels, and there is an inconstant pathway along the round ligament to the inguinal nodes.

The *ovary and Fallopian tube* have a plexus of vessels which drain along the infundibulopelvic fold to the para-aortic nodes on both sides of the midline. On the left these are around the left renal pedicle, whilst on the right there may be only one node intervening before the lymph flows into

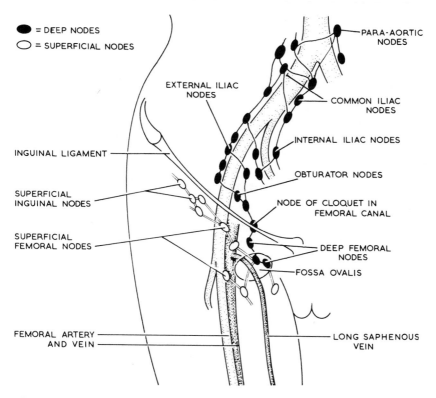

**Fig. 1.14** Diagram to show inguinal, femoral and iliac lymphatic nodes.

the thoracic duct, thus accounting for the rapid early spread of metastatic carcinoma to distant sites such as the lungs.

*Bladder and urethra.* The drainage is to the iliac nodes, whilst the lymphatics of the lower part of the urethra follow those of the vulva.

*Rectum.* The lymphatics from the lower anal canal drain to the superficial inguinal nodes, and the remainder of the rectal drainage follows pararectal channels accompanying the blood vessels to both the internal iliac nodes (middle haemorrhoidal artery) and the para-aortic nodes at the origin of the inferior mesenteric artery.

## Nerves of the pelvis

### Nerve supply of the vulva and perineum

The *pudendal nerve* arises from the second, third and fourth sacral nerves. As it passes along the outer wall of the ischiorectal fossa it gives off an inferior haemorrhoidal branch, and divides into the perineal nerve and the dorsal nerve of the clitoris. The perineal nerve gives the sensory supply to the vulva; it also innervates the anterior part of the external anal sphincter and levator ani, and the superficial perineal muscles. The dorsal nerve of the clitoris is sensory.

Sensory fibres from the mons and labia also pass in the *ilio-inguinal* and *genitofemoral nerves* to the first lumbar root. The *posterior femoral cutaneous nerve* carries sensation from the perineum to the small sciatic nerve, and thus to the first, second and third sacral nerves.

The main nerve supply of the levator ani muscles comes from the third and fourth sacral nerves.

## Nerve supply of the pelvic viscera

To describe what can be seen on dissection of the extensive autonomic nerve supply of the pelvic organs is one thing — to determine the physiological functions of the various parts of the system is another.

Nerve fibres of the pre-aortic plexus of the sympathetic nervous system are continuous with those of the *superior hypogastric plexus,* which lies in front of the last lumbar vertebra and is wrongly called the 'presacral nerve'. Below, the superior hypogastric plexus divides, and on each side its fibres are continuous with fibres passing beside the rectum to join the *uterovaginal plexus* (inferior hypogastric plexus, or plexus of Frankenhäuser). This plexus lies in the loose cellular tissue posterolateral to the cervix below the uterosacral folds of peritoneum. Parasympathetic fibres from the second, third and fourth sacral nerves join the uterovaginal plexus. Fibres from (or to) the bladder, uterus, vagina and rectum join the plexus. The uterovaginal plexus contains a few ganglion cells, so it is likely that a few motor nerves have their relay stations there and then pass onwards with the blood vessels to the viscera.

The ovary is not innervated by the nerves already described, but from the *ovarian plexus* which surrounds the ovarian vessels and joins the pre-aortic plexus high up.

This description has avoided any conjecture as to the particular function of the sympathetic and parasympathetic nerves, and no opinion has been expressed as to whether the various nerves carry sensory or motor impulses. Clinical facts are few. It is evident that afferent sensory impulses are carried in the superior hypogastric plexus. If this is divided at the operation of 'presacral neurectomy', pain from the bladder and uterus can be blocked. Apart from a transient pelvic hyperaemia there is no change in the motor function of either bladder or uterus. At an ordinary hysterectomy the uterovaginal plexus is not disturbed, but after a more extensive Wertheim operation there may be painless atony and distension of the bladder, which is attributed to loss of bladder sensation because the sacral connections of the uterovaginal plexus have been divided.

So much for the sensory side. The motor effects are far less certain. Stimulation of the cut lower end of the hypogastric plexus seems to have

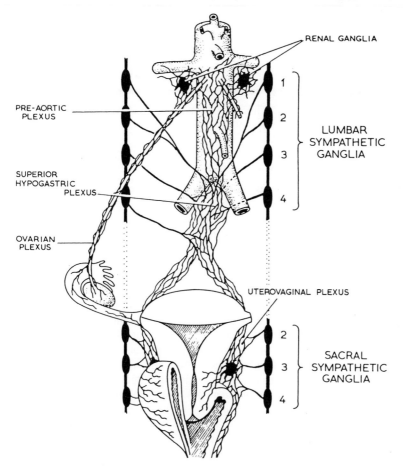

RENAL GANGLIA

PRE-AORTIC
PLEXUS

SUPERIOR
HYPOGASTRIC
PLEXUS

OVARIAN
PLEXUS

1
2
3
4

LUMBAR
SYMPATHETIC
GANGLIA

UTEROVAGINAL PLEXUS

2
3
4

SACRAL
SYMPATHETIC
GANGLIA

**Fig. 1.15** Diagram to show nerve supply of pelvic organs.

no effect on the bladder or the uterus. Although it has been stated that the parasympathetic nerves are excitatory to the musculature of the body of the uterus and inhibitory to that of the cervix, and that the sympathetic has the opposite effect, there is not general agreement about this.

The myometrium contains both $\alpha$ and $\beta$ adrenergic receptors and also cholinergic receptors. In the non-pregnant uterus the balance of their action is uncertain, but during pregnancy strong stimulation of $\beta$ receptors with $\beta$ mimetic drugs such as isoxsuprine will inhibit myometrial activity.

# 2

# Development of the female pelvic organs

## The internal genitalia

The genital organs begin to differentiate and become identifiable in the fifth week of intra-uterine life when the embryo is approximately 10 mm long. At this stage the primitive gut is suspended from the dorsal aspect of the coelomic cavity in the midline by mesentery, and this is flanked on either side by a longitudinal ridge, covered by coelomic epithelium. This is produced by the mesonephros; the Wolffian (mesonephric) duct lies on the lateral side of it (Fig. 2.1).

The coelomic epithelium on the medial side of the mesonephros proliferates into several layers, and cords of cells (the medullary cords) extend into the underlying mesoderm, which also increases considerably to form a prominent swelling on the medial side of the mesonephros, called the genital ridge. This is the future ovary. The germ cells which eventually give rise to the ova migrate from the wall of the yolk sac into the genital ridge.

At the same time a groove of coelomic epithelium becomes invaginated into the lateral side of the mesonephros, and from this groove a solid core of cells extends in a caudal direction, running close to the lateral side of the Wolffian duct. Later this core canalizes, but retains its communication anteriorly with the coelom; this is the Müllerian or paramesonephric duct, which will form the Fallopian tubes, uterus and upper vagina. The anterior open end will become the ostium, and around this the fimbriae later develop (Fig. 2.2).

The Müllerian and Wolffian ducts are suspended from the dorsal body wall by a broad mesentery. In the pelvic region the free edges of this genital mesentery incline medially, meet and fuse together in the midline to form a septum between the hind-gut, which later forms the rectum, and the urogenital sinus, which will form the bladder and urethra. In this septum the Müllerian ducts pass medially across the front of the Wolffian ducts, and also meet and fuse in the midline. They then turn caudally again as a single, solid rod of cells, and extend caudally until they make contact with the urogenital sinus; they produce a prominent elevation in its posterior wall – the Müllerian tubercle (Fig. 2.3).

This rod of cells regresses, and a solid cord of epithelial cells derived from the urogenital sinus grows upward in its place, extending as far as the cervix. The central cells of this cord break down to form the lumen of the vagina. The hymen marks the site from which this upward growth of sinus

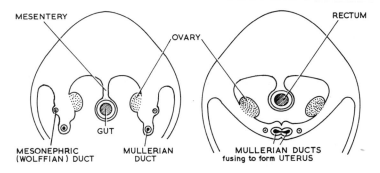

**Fig. 2.1** Diagrams to show steps in the formation of the broad ligament.

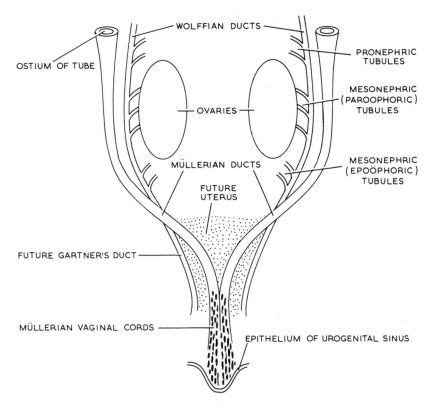

**Fig. 2.2** Diagram of Müllerian and Wolffian systems.

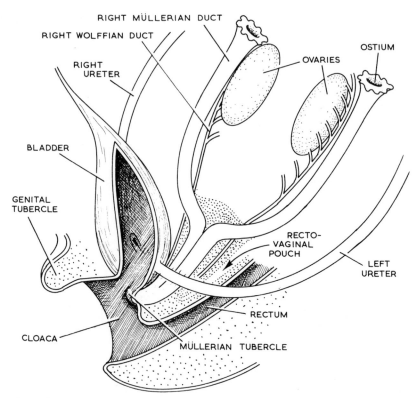

**Fig. 2.3** Diagram to show formation of female pelvic organs. It is emphasized that this is a diagram, not a representation of the actual appearance of the structures.

cells began. The surrounding mesoderm of the genital septum gives rise to the musculature of both the vagina and the uterus.

The ovary and the upper part of the Müllerian duct, which becomes the Fallopian tube, develop in the upper part of the coelom, and receive their blood supply from the corresponding segment of the aorta. During fetal life the ovary and Fallopian tube gradually descend into the pelvis, and the blood vessels lengthen accordingly.

The mesonephros degenerates almost completely, but a few tubules may persist in the broad ligament, where they give rise to cysts in adult life (see p. 75). In the male the Wolffian duct forms the vas deferens, but it degenerates in the female fetus. It can sometimes still be traced in the adult female, when it is known as Gartner's duct. This runs medially through the broad ligament and down the side of the vagina, where cysts may form in it.

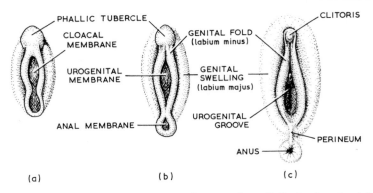

PHALLIC TUBERCLE
CLOACAL MEMBRANE
UROGENITAL MEMBRANE
ANAL MEMBRANE

CLITORIS
GENITAL FOLD (labium minus)
GENITAL SWELLING (labium majus)
UROGENITAL GROOVE
PERINEUM
ANUS

(a)          (b)          (c)

**Fig. 2.4** Stages in development of external genitalia in female. (a), at 7 weeks; (b), at 10 weeks; (c), at 12 weeks.

The ovary, like the testis, has a gubernaculum; this extends from the inferior pole of the ovary to the internal inguinal ring. In addition, it becomes incorporated into the uterine wall at the point of entry of the Fallopian tube. It persists in the adult as the ovarian ligament and the round ligament of the uterus.

## The external genitalia

The urogenital sinus — which forms the bladder, urethra and vestibule — develops as a ventral diverticulum from the hind-gut. At first the urogenital sinus and the hind-gut open into a common cavity, the cloaca, which at this stage is separated from the exterior by the cloacal membrane. Later this sinus is completely separated from the hind-gut by a septum of meso-derm which divides the cloacal membrane into a posterior part which temporarily closes the future anus, and an anterior part, the urogenital membrane.

In front of this membrane arises a midline tubercle, the phallic tubercle. On either side two ridges develop, the inner called the genital folds and the outer the genital swellings. Eventually the phallic tubercle forms the clitoris; the inner genital folds form the labia minora, and the frenulum and prepuce of the clitoris; while the outer genital swellings give rise to the labia majora. Finally, the urogenital membrane disappears, so that the vestibule communicates with the exterior through the vulva.

# 3

# The menstrual cycle

Throughout the childbearing years of a woman's life rhythmic changes concerned with the process of reproduction take place in a monthly cycle involving the hypothalamus, the pituitary gland, the ovaries, the endometrium and the secondary sex organs. The periodicity is inherent in the hypothalamus, which controls the menstrual cycle through the hormones of the anterior pituitary and the ovaries.

Menstruation is the most striking outward manifestation of the cycle, but elaborate changes are taking place in the ovaries and endometrium, and indeed in the whole body, throughout the cycle. After a menstrual period the endometrium proliferates in preparation for the reception of a fertilized ovum. If the ovum embeds in the endometrium, that proliferates further to become the decidua of pregnancy. Should conception not occur the endometrium undergoes necrosis and disintegrates. Menstruation is therefore the outward sign of the end of an abortive cycle and the optimistic commencement of the next.

## The control of ovarian hormone production

Although the length of the normal cycle may vary from woman to woman and from time to time in a particular woman, for clarity we will describe a cycle of 28 days, taking the first day of menstruation as day 1.

The hypothalamus, acting through the anterior lobe of the pituitary gland, controls the output of oestrogen and progesterone by the ovaries. The part of the hypothalamus most directly concerned is the median eminence, but this ill-defined concentration of small ganglion cells is influenced by other parts of the central nervous system. From the hypothalamus a decapeptide *gonadotrophin-releasing hormone* passes by the hypophyseal portal veins to the anterior lobe of the pituitary gland, where it causes the release of two gonadotrophic hormones, which are proteins of high molecular weight. These are *follicle-stimulating hormone* (FSH) and *luteinizing hormone* (LH).

It was at first thought that there were two releasing hormones, FSH-RH for FSH and LH-RH for LH, but it is probable that there is only one, simply termed GnRH. This is released in pulses, and in turn the pituitary gland releases FSH and LH in a pulsatile manner.

Follicle-stimulating hormone brings about the development of Graafian follicles within the ovary. Each follicle consists of a maturing ovum, with surrounding granulosa cells and theca interna cells derived from the ovarian stroma. These granulosa and theca cells produce oestradiol in gradually increasing amounts as the follicle matures. At about day 12 of the cycle there is a sudden surge in the output of luteinizing hormone lasting about 36 hours, and a lesser rise in the output of FSH. The LH surge brings about ovulation on about day 14.

In the early part of the cycle up to 50 follicles start to mature, but normally only one dominant follicle matures fully and ovulates while the others retrogress; we do not know how this selection is brought about.

When the ovum has been released from the follicle there is a temporary fall in the oestrogen level, and the FSH and LH levels are reduced. The granulosa and theca cells of the empty follicle become swollen and take up fat. The whole structure of the follicle takes on a yellow colour and is therefore known as the corpus luteum. The corpus luteum secretes increasing amounts of progesterone and also of oestradiol, so that the oestrogen level rises again. If the ovum is not fertilized, the corpus luteum degenerates in the last week of the cycle into a hyaline body known as the corpus albicans. The levels of oestrogen and progesterone fall, that ovarian cycle ends and menstruation occurs.

The level of LH in the blood is fairly constant except during the pre-ovulatory surge. The level of FSH starts to rise *before* menstruation, falls a little during the first half of the cycle, and then shows another transient rise just before ovulation (see Fig. 3.1). This premenstrual rise in FSH stimulates the development of Graafian follicles and one dominant follicle eventually ovulates. As the follicle develops it secretes increasing amounts of oestrogen.

It is believed that a *moderate* rise in oestrogen level inhibits the output of FSH (by negative feedback), probably by inhibition of the output of GnRH, and this would explain the fall in FSH level that occurs in the first half of the cycle and also after ovulation. On the other hand, a *large* rise in oestrogen level stimulates the output of GnRH (by positive feedback), thus accounting for the surge of LH and FSH that causes ovulation.

It is not known whether LH has any inhibiting effect on the hypothalamic output of gonadotrophin-releasing hormone or on the pituitary gland.

If the ovum released should be fertilized, the developing trophoblast around the embryo produces chorionic gonadotrophin. This replaces the pituitary gonadotrophins which are depressed by the circulating oestrogen and progesterone, and the corpus luteum goes on functioning for 3 or 4 months until the placenta is mature enough to produce the large amounts of both steroids on which the continuation of the pregnancy depends.

Many outside influences play upon the hypothalamic – pituitary – ovarian axis. The cerebral cortex can exert a profound influence, exemplified by amenorrhoea due to emotional disturbances. Other endocrine glands, notably the thyroid and adrenals, affect ovarian function, and their malfunction may disturb the whole pattern of sex hormone production. Even nutrition and the nebulous 'general health' can have important effects.

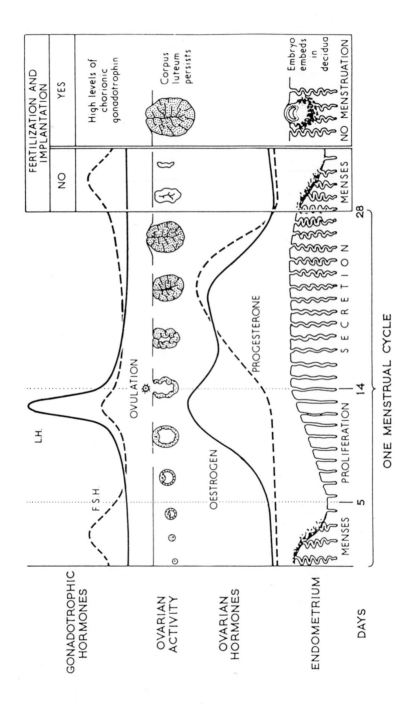

**Fig. 3.1** Diagram to show events in the menstrual cycle and early pregnancy.

In some animals the pituitary is stimulated by oestrogen from the developing follicle to produce a third hormone, *luteotrophin,* which appears to be identical with prolactin, and is necessary for the maintenance and function of the corpus luteum. In women this does not seem to be the case, although abnormally high levels will inhibit ovulation (see p. 261).

Before the onset of menstrual periods, the development of the secondary sex characteristics associated with puberty is brought about by oestrogen secreted by ovarian follicles which do not reach full maturity and there-fore do not ovulate. This is achieved by means of the cyclical elaboration of subthreshold concentrations of FSH and LH by the pituitary gland.

It is believed that all the primordial follicles are already present in the ovary by the 20th week of fetal life. They remain quiescent until puberty, and only a selected few reach complete maturity at the rate of one a month for the duration of the childbearing years. It has been estimated that there are about 250 000 primordial follicles in the ovaries at birth, and many of them degenerate before puberty. Several follicles begin to mature in each menstrual cycle, but normally only one reaches full maturity; the remainder degenerate.

## The endometrial cycle

Cyclical changes in the histological structure of the endometrium are caused by the action of the ovarian hormones. Two anatomical divisions of the endometrium become evident during the cycle. Next to the uterine muscle is the *stratum basalis,* which does not undergo cyclical disintegration during menstruation, and from which the endometrium regenerates after the period. Superficial to the basal layer is the functional layer; cyclical changes occur in all the structures of this layer — in the glands, the stroma and the blood vessels. It is subdivided into the deeper *stratum spongiosum* and the superficial *stratum compactum.* The changes in the functional layer are continuous, but may conveniently be described in two phases: the follicular phase precedes ovulation, and the luteal phase follows it.

*Follicular phase*
After menstruation only the stratum basalis is left. Soon, low cubical surface epithelium grows out from the stumps of the glands to cover the denuded surface. Under the influence of oestrogen from the ripening follicle, the cells of the surface epithelium and those in the glands become taller and more columnar. The glands, which are at first straight, narrow and tubular, gradually elongate and widen, becoming slightly tortuous as they do so. The stromal cells hypertrophy and develop a mantle of cyto-plasm around their nuclei. Two types of blood vessels are seen in the endometrium: short straight arterioles in the basal layer, and long coiled arterioles which grow up into the functional layer during the follicular phase.

*Luteal phase*

After ovulation the corpus luteum secretes both oestrogen and progesterone, and these bring about progestational changes in the endometrium. Endometrial cells contain specific receptors for progesterone, which are induced by oestrogens, therefore progesterone can only act on endometrium which has been primed by oestrogen. The cells of the glandular epithelium show specific changes. Early in this phase their nuclei become pushed towards the lumina of the glands by subnuclear vacuoles containing glycogen. Later the secretion is passed out of the cells into the lumina of the glands which become filled with debris containing mucus and glycogen, and the cell nuclei take up their former positions near the basement membrane. The glands become extremely tortuous and their epithelium projects into their lumina to give a scalloped appearance. Hypertrophy of the stroma cells continues until they resemble the decidual cells of pregnancy. Near the surface in the stratum compactum the stromal cells are closely packed, and the necks of the glands are straight. The deeper stratum spongiosum is almost entirely composed of convoluted glands and elaborately coiled arterioles, with comparatively few stromal cells.

*Menstruation*

Towards the end of the cycle the concentrations of oestrogen and progesterone fall. There is rapid shrinkage of the thickness of the endometrium with leucocytic infiltration. Many of the arterioles show intense vasoconstriction, and some of the coiled arterioles become kinked as the endometrium shrinks so that there is stasis of blood flow in them. From time to time some of the arterioles relax, and bleeding occurs through the necrosed walls of vessels in the functional layer of the endometrium, which leads to its disintegration. The basal layer is not involved in these changes and it is not shed with the rest of the endometrium; it is from this layer that regeneration takes place. The blood which is shed with fragments of endometrium clots in the uterine cavity, but the coagulum is dissolved by plasmin before it is discharged through the cervix, unless the rate of bleeding is very rapid.

The endometrium, and to a less extent the myometrium, is able to synthesize *prostaglandins* from arachidonic acid by the action of the enzyme cyclo-oxygenase, especially during the luteal phase of the cycle. Endometrial production of prostaglandins depends on the levels of oestrogen and progesterone, but details of this still need elucidation.

It is likely that the arteriolar contraction and endometrial necrosis which has been described in the preceding section is caused by prostaglandins. Excessive bleeding from the disintegrating endometrium is prevented by continuing vasoconstriction, myometrial contraction, and by local aggregation of platelets with deposition of fibrin around them. Different prostaglandins have different actions (see p. 240), but in normal menstruation it is probable that $PGF_{2\alpha}$ has the dominant effect.

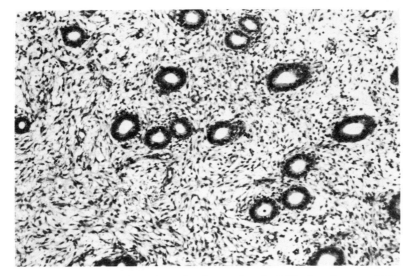

**Fig. 3.2** Microscopical section of endometrium in follicular phase. × 100

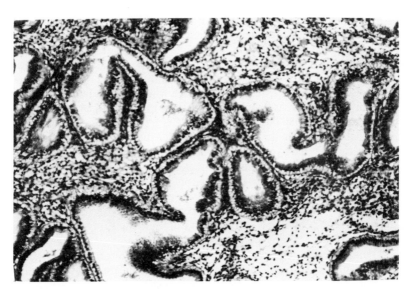

**Fig. 3.3** Microscopical section of endometrium in luteal phase. × 100

## Anovular cycles

In the case of women who are taking the combined oral contraceptive pill, and in some spontaneous cycles, ovulation does not occur but periodic bleeding takes place. Because of inhibition of the pituitary by rising concentration of oestrogen the secretion of FSH is reduced, the oestrogen concentration then falls, regression of the endometrium takes place with vasoconstriction and necrosis, and withdrawal bleeding occurs in the same way as in normal menstruation. The endometrium shows no luteal changes, and it is not so completely denuded as in normal menstruation.

# Clinical features of menstruation

Menstruation begins (the menarche) at puberty, which normally occurs between the ages of 11 and 15 years, and continues throughout the childbearing period of life, ending at the menopause which usually occurs between the ages of 47 and 53.

The menstrual cycle averages 28 days and as a rule follows a regular rhythm, but variations of between 21 and 35 days may be accepted as normal. Irregular and infrequent cycles may occur for a few months after puberty.

Each menstrual period lasts on average 4 to 5 days, but the duration of the flow and the amount of blood lost vary considerably in different women. It is impossible to define a standard of normal loss; while the average loss over the whole period may be 40 ml (ranging from 20 to 80 ml) an increase or prolongation of the usual loss for an individual is of more significance than the actual amount. The menstrual flow consists of partially haemolysed blood, mucus and cellular debris. It is usually scanty and viscid at first, later becoming bright red, and finally brown towards the end of the period. Small clots and fragments of endometrium may be seen, but large clots are only passed when the bleeding is excessive. Normally blood clot is dissolved by plasmin as it is formed in the cavity of the uterus, so that the lochia remains fluid. If the bleeding is heavy the blood passes through the cervix and clots in the vagina, and there is not time for the enzyme to act on any clot which is formed in the uterus itself.

During menstruation uterine contractions cause slight dilatation of the cervical canal and expel the menstrual products. The contractions help to control the loss of blood. Menstruation, especially in younger and nulliparous women is not infrequently accompanied by painful uterine contractions. Such pain, if it is sufficient to call for medical advice, is described as dysmenorrhoea, and is discussed on p. 246.

Premonitory symptoms, such as pelvic discomfort and backache, soreness of the breasts, headache and general malaise, may sometimes precede the period. There may be a gain of weight of 1 kg or more because of retention of water and sodium chloride. If these symptoms are sufficient to make the patient seek medical help, they are referred to as the premenstrual tension syndrome. Treatment is described on p. 249.

## Menstrual hygiene

It is particularly important that girls should be taught to regard menstruation as a normal healthy function. Unless they suffer from severe pain, women should continue their normal occupations; moderate exercise and normal bowel action are helpful in dispelling pelvic congestion. A daily bath should on no account be discontinued. Sanitary towels or vaginal tampons of sterilized compressed absorbent material are used. The choice of protection is a personal one. Sanitary towels are usually more appropriate in the first few months after the menarche while the girl is becoming used to menstruation, but many girls soon find the tampons more comfortable and convenient. They need to be changed more frequently than external pads, and may not be effective if there is abnormally heavy loss. If the presence of a tampon in the vagina is forgotten it will soon cause a most offensive discharge.

**Toxic shock syndrome** is a very rare complication of the use of tampons. During the period there is high fever, syncope and an erythematous skin rash. The syndrome has been attributed to proliferation of a strain of *Staphylococcus aureus* that produces an enterotoxin. The syndrome is so rare that it would be unreasonable to advise against the use of tampons.

# 4

# The sex hormones

We now review the physiological actions of the natural sex hormones. In gynaecological treatment many synthetic compounds are used; these are described in Chapter 27 (p. 251), and some details of chemistry are postponed for consideration in that chapter.

## Gonadotrophin-releasing hormone (GnRH)

The neurosecretory cells of the medial basal hypothalamus secrete releasing hormones for most of the anterior pituitary trophic hormones, and also a hormone that inhibits the release of prolactin. The action of gonadotrophin-releasing hormone has been described in the previous chapter.

## The pituitary hormones

Hormones secreted by the pituitary gland which are related to gynaecological work include:
1. Gonadotrophins of the anterior pituitary gland:
    (a) follicle-stimulating hormone (FSH);
    (b) luteinizing hormone (LH).
2. Prolactin of the anterior pituitary gland.
3. Oxytocic factor of the posterior pituitary gland.

## Pituitary gonadotrophic hormones

The gonadotrophic hormones control the functions of the gonad in both sexes. FSH and LH are secreted by the basophil cells of the anterior pituitary, whereas prolactin is secreted by the acidophil cells. It is still not possible to obtain an extract from the pituitary consisting of pure FSH or LH, and it is therefore not possible to do more than compare the gonadotrophic activity of any body fluid with that of an arbitrary standard preparation. The international reference preparation of human gonadotrophic derived from menopausal urine is commonly used (IRP.HMG). This is said to contain 40 i.u. of FSH per mg, and 4 i.u. of LH per mg.

Biological methods of assay of FSH and LH were formerly used, but it is now possible to make reliable estimations of the blood levels of these hormones by radioimmunoassay. The difficulties remain that there are no chemically pure preparations of FSH and LH that can be used as standards, and also that cross-reactions between these hormones occur.

FSH controls maturation of the ovarian follicle and then, in combination with LH, causes ovulation. FSH begins to be secreted towards the end of the *previous* cycle, and rises to a peak in concentration at about day 5 of the cycle under consideration, then the concentration falls slightly before rising to a second peak at about day 12 (see Fig. 3.1). FSH and LH are released in pulses, in response to pulses of GnRH.

LH is responsible, with FSH, for ovulation and the subsequent formation of the corpus luteum. LH concentration begins to rise at the beginning of the cycle and reaches a peak at about day 12. The surge of secretion of the gonadotrophic hormones at this time is the trigger for ovulation about 36 hours later. If conception occurs, LH secretion continues until chorionic gonadotrophin takes over the luteotrophic function.

The blood of women at the time of the menopause contains greatly increased amounts of gonadotrophins, as a result of the fall in level of oestrogen which would otherwise inhibit its production.

## Chorionic gonadotrophin

Although this hormone is not secreted by the pituitary gland but by the chorionic tissue of the placenta, it is mentioned here because its actions are similar to those of LH. Its function is to sustain the corpus luteum until the placental secretion of hormones is well established. Human chorionic gonadotrophin (hCG) can be assayed by immunological methods. The level in blood and urine reaches its highest point in normal pregnancy between the 8th and 12th weeks. Abnormally high levels occur in multiple pregnancy, and with hydatidiform mole and choriocarcinoma. Details of the immunological tests for pregnancy are given in 'Obstetrics by Ten Teachers'.

## Prolactin

This anterior pituitary hormone is responsible for the initiation and maintenance of lactation after the breasts have been under the previous influence of oestrogen and progesterone. It is a polypeptide which is secreted in a pulsatile manner by specialized anterior pituitary cells (lactotrophs). Unlike the release of other anterior pituitary hormones, that of prolactin is inhibited, not stimulated, by a hypothalamic factor, dopamine. During lactation prolactin levels rise after stimulation of the nipple, when dopamine levels fall.

Prolactin may be involved in the control of ovulation, and may be an agent which prevents further ovulation once fertilization of the oöcyte has occurred. When prolactin levels are raised ovulation ceases.

The normal prolactin level in plasma varies widely between 100 and 800 m.i.u./ℓ. There is diurnal variation, and the level rises with stress or emotional factors. Hyperprolactinaemia may occur with pituitary adenomata (see p. 233).

## Oxytocin

The posterior lobe of the pituitary gland secretes oxytocin, which causes strong contraction of the smooth muscle of the uterus. The sensitivity of the muscle to oxytocin increases in late pregnancy.

## The ovarian hormones

The ovaries secrete oestrogens and progesterone.

### Oestrogens

Oestrogens are secreted by the granulosa and theca cells of the ovarian follicles, and subsequently by the same cells after they have been luteinized to form the corpus luteum. Oestrogens are also secreted in smaller quantities by the suprarenal cortex.

During pregnancy the fetal suprarenal cortex and liver are concerned in the formation of large amounts of oestrogens (as oestriol) which are transferred by the placenta to the maternal blood, and then excreted in the urine.

The ovary produces *oestradiol 17β* from cholesterol and progesterone. Oestradiol undergoes degradation, chiefly to *oestrone* and *oestriol*. In clinical practice only these three 'classic' oestrogens are usually considered, although at least 16 other oestrogens are found in small quantities in human urine. The chemical structure of the oestrogens is given in Chapter 27 (p. 251).

Oestrogens are conjugated in the liver with glycuronic acid, and to a less extent with sulphuric acid, before they are excreted in the urine. About 70 per cent of the production of oestrogens is dealt with in this way. The remainder is excreted in the faeces. There is much recycling of oestrogens from the gut. They reach the intestine in the bile, and the conjugated compounds are broken down by micro-organisms and then reabsorbed as active hormones. Any disturbance of liver function or of the intestinal flora can upset this process and alter the menstrual cycle temporarily.

The urinary excretion of oestrogens can be measured by chemical methods. The total daily excretion of oestrogens, chiefly as oestrone and oestriol, is about 50 μg on day 7 of the menstrual cycle, rising to about 120 μg at the time of ovulation. After a slight fall the excretion rises again to 100 μg in the premenstrual phase, and falls off fairly rapidly before menstruation. Plasma oestrogen levels can be measured by radioimmunoassay.

### *Physiological actions*

*The secondary sexual characteristics.* The alterations in physical appearance which take place at the time of puberty and herald sexual maturity are due to the secretion of small amounts of oestrogens. Hypertrophy of the breasts, the appearance of pubic and axillary hair, secretion of the apocrine glands, changes in the voice and appearance of the face and figure with the deposition of fat on the hips and thighs are examples of secondary sexual characteristics.

*Actions on the uterus, Fallopian tubes and vagina* (1) The hypertrophy of the uterus, Fallopian tubes and lower genital tract which takes place at puberty, and the hypertrophy and increased vascularity in pregnancy are due to oestrogen secretion. Diminished secretion after the menopause results in atrophic changes in these organs.

(2) Oestrogen also controls the monthly proliferative phase of the endometrium. Withdrawal of oestrogen is responsible for menstruation.

(3) The motility of the Fallopian tubes is increased by oestrogen.

(4) The cervical glands respond to circulating oestrogen by secreting an abundance of clear alkaline mucus, which protects spermatozoa from the vaginal acidity. This is most evident at the time of ovulation, when the blood concentration of oestrogen is highest.

(5) Oestrogen causes proliferation of the epithelial cells of the vagina with increase in the thickness of the superficial stratified layers and a great increase in their glycogen content. This is converted by Döderlein's bacilli into lactic acid, so that the vaginal pH is low and resistance to pathogenic micro-organisms is increased.

*Inhibition of pituitary activity.* See p. 29.

*Action on the breasts.* Oestrogens bring about proliferation of the duct system. For alveolar development, progesterone is also needed.

*Actions during pregnancy.* In pregnancy very large amounts of oestrogen are secreted. The fetal adrenal cortex plays a part in synthesis; the placenta does not have all the enzymes necessary to complete the synthesis of oestrogens. The daily excretion of oestrogens in the urine (chiefly as oestriol) rises throughout pregnancy from the non-pregnant maximum of about 0.12 mg to between 10 and 50 mg at term. It is not surprising therefore that there are widespread physiological effects. The hypertrophy and hyperaemia of the uterus and breasts have been mentioned. The high blood levels of steroids in pregnancy cause retention of water and salt. (The same effect is seen to a smaller degree in the premenstrual phase of the menstrual cycle.)

**Progesterone**

Progesterone is the hormone secreted (together with oestradiol) by the corpus luteum. It is responsible for the luteal phase of the menstrual cycle.

Progesterone is converted in the liver to pregnanediol and other metabolites which are excreted in the bile and in the urine. Pregnanediol is biologically inert, but its concentration in the urine can be estimated by chemical methods as a rough index of progesterone activity. It is now more usual to measure the blood progesterone level by radioimmunoassay. A blood concentration of 15 nmol/l or more is taken as confirmation that ovulation has occurred in a particular cycle.

The chemistry of progesterone and of some of the many synthetic progestogens is described on p. 255.

*Physiological actions*

*Action on the endometrium.* The luteal phase of the endometrial cycle is due to the action of progesterone, but this will only occur if the endometrium has previously been primed by the action of oestrogens.

The part played by progesterone in bringing about menstruation is not certain. The blood concentration of progesterone in a normal cycle falls at the same time as that of oestrogen, but some women bleed regularly each month, in a way clinically indistinguishable from normal menstruation, without ever ovulating, forming a corpus luteum or secreting any progesterone. However, in such anovular cycles the degree of endometrial disintegration may be less than in normal cycles.

*Actions during pregnancy*

(1) Progesterone prepares the endometrium for reception of the fertilized ovum by stimulating decidual reaction.

(2) The pattern of spontaneous rhythmic uterine contractions changes in the luteal phase of the menstrual cycle from small frequent contractions to infrequent but stronger contractions. This may explain why spasmodic dysmenorrhoea occurs only in the presence of a corpus luteum, that is to say in ovular cycles.

(3) Progesterone secretion is essential for the maintenance of pregnancy. Early in gestation this is the function of the corpus luteum, but after about the 12th week the chorionic tissue of the placenta takes over the production.

(4) Progesterone causes growth of the alveolar tissue of the breast, provided that there has been previous oestrogenic action.

## Prostaglandins

Although these are locally produced and therefore not strictly to be described as hormones, they play an important part in the menstrual cycle (see p. 240).

## Androgens in gynaecology

Androgens are metabolic precursors of oestrogens, and they are found in small amounts in the blood and urine of normal women. They are secreted by the suprarenal cortex and the stromal cells of the ovary. The part they play in normal female physiology is probably slight, although they may have some effect on libido. In cases of oestrogen deficiency, acne and hypertrichosis may be manifestations of androgenic activity.

Adrenal virilism, or the *adrenogenital syndrome,* may be caused in adults by hyperplasia or a tumour of the suprarenal cortex, when the 17-oxosteroid excretion in the urine is increased. In the fetus and child *adrenal pseudohermaphroditism* may occur because of a metabolic disorder of the cortex (see p. 66).

Testosterone is secreted by a rare ovarian tumour, the *androblastoma* (see p. 207), and testosterone levels are increased in *polycystic ovary syndrome* (see p. 195).

# 5

# Puberty and the menopause

## Puberty

The onset of menstruation (the menarche) should be regarded as the culmination of a transitional stage in a girl's development. The term puberty refers not only to the complete functioning of the hormonal cycle for the first time but also to the gradual changes in the secondary sexual characteristics which precede the menarche.

In girls the earliest sign of puberty is enlargement of the breast buds, which most frequently occurs at the age of 11 years, with a range from 9 to 13 years. Pubic hair usually appears a year later, and at this time there is a spurt of growth, so that for a time girls may be taller than boys of comparable age, but after that females grow less rapidly than males because of earlier epiphyseal closure. The mean age of the menarche is 13 years, with a range from 11 to 15 years.

Deposition of subcutaneous fat provides the rounded female contour. The mons pubis and labia majora increase in size, with the appearance of pubic and axillary hair. The infantile uterus enlarges, and the bony pelvis acquires female characteristics. Adolescent interest in boys may be accompanied by shyness and fluctuating moods, but how far this is the result of educational and social stress rather than endocrine changes is hard to tell.

The age of onset of menstruation may be modified by heredity, nutrition or environment, and appears to be falling in Britain. Sexual maturity often occurs earlier in tropical countries, but this is a racial characteristic and not an effect of the climate.

During childhood rhythmic discharges of GnRH occur but with low amplitude. At puberty the amplitude of the discharges increases, so that FSH and LH are produced and in turn the level of oestrogens rises. The secretion of oestrogens begins about 3 years before the menarche. Early cycles may be anovular, with no formation of corpora lutea and therefore no production of progesterone.

### Precocious menstruation

The onset of menstruation has been recorded even before the age of 4 years, and the case of Lima Medina who became pregnant at the age of 5 is well attested.

The majority of cases of precocious puberty are of the primary or 'constitutional' type. No other abnormality is found, and in other respects the child develops normally, except that breast development and the growth of the pelvic bones may be advanced, whereas the epiphyses of the long bones may fuse early, causing a slight reduction in stature.

However, all cases of precocious puberty require careful investigation to exclude any underlying disease of the endocrine system. A granulosa cell tumour of the ovary, or very rarely a malignant teratoma, may secrete sufficient oestrogens to cause uterine bleeding, enlargement of the breasts and growth of pubic hair. Such a tumour can usually be felt on pelvic examination under anaesthesia, and seen at laparoscopy.

Very rarely, pathological lesions in the region of the hypothalamus or pituitary gland may cause sexual precocity. This event has been recorded in cases of encephalitis, of hydrocephalus and of tumours in the region of the third ventricle and pineal body.

In males hyperplasia or a neoplasm of the suprarenal cortex will cause precocious puberty. In the female the abnormal androgens will cause hirsutes, growth of the clitoris and premature muscular development, but not uterine bleeding.

Children with 'constitutional' precocious puberty may be treated with synthetic analogues of gonadotrophin-releasing hormone. If these analogues are administered continuously and for a prolonged time they bind to the pituitary receptors so that they become unresponsive to GnRH, and the output of gonadotrophins and of ovarian hormones falls.

### Delayed puberty

Delay in the onset of menstruation occasionally occurs, and the menarche may be as late as 17 years. Amenorrhoea persisting after this time is usually accompanied by hypoplasia of the genital tract. Investigation should be started at or before this age if the periods do not appear.

### Menorrhagia of puberty

Excessive blood loss sometimes occurs in early cycles. Anovular cycles are very frequent at this age, and puberty menorrhagia is due to excessive secretion of oestrogen without progesterone. The periods may be heavy and fairly regular, or continuous bleeding may occur from endometrial hyperplasia (see p. 241). In most cases the condition improves spontaneously in a few cycles as ovulation is established, and reassurance of the child and her mother is all that is needed.

If the bleeding is heavy, norethisterone 5 mg twice daily by mouth may be given for 21 days; after a few days withdrawal bleeding will occur, and another course can then be started. Two or three courses should suffice. Alternatively, the combined oral contraceptive containing oestrogen and progesterone may be given for two or three cycles.

# The menopause

The termination of the reproductive period of life in a woman is marked by the cessation of the menstrual periods and is known as the menopause.

The word climacteric is sometimes used to describe the 'change of life'.

Menstruation generally ceases between the ages of 47 and 52. Sometimes the menopause is delayed up to the age of 55 or even later; sometimes it occurs at 40 or even earlier. An early puberty tends to be followed by a late menopause, while a late onset of menstruation is often followed by an early cessation. The times of puberty and the menopause are to some extent a racial characteristic. In a few women the periods stop abruptly; more often the loss gradually diminishes, or a period now and then is missed until they finally cease. Anovular cycles are more frequent as the menopause approaches. Fertility is therefore diminished, and pregnancy is exceedingly rare after the age of 50.

At the time of the menopause few Graafian follicles can be found in the ovaries, which shrink in size. The ovarian production of oestrogen ceases and the pituitary gland, liberated from negative feeback (see p. 28), produces gonadotrophic hormones in excess. In some women oestrogens are still found, probably from the suprarenal cortex or by conversion of androgens in fat tissues.

After the menopause there is gradual atrophy of the genital organs. The uterus diminishes in size, and the endometrium becomes thin and atrophic. The vaginal wall becomes thin and smooth with a fall in the acidity of the secretion, and the fornices become shallow around a small cervix. The labia are flatter and the growth of pubic hair is diminished. The ligaments and fascia which support the uterus atrophy, and prolapse may become evident if there has been previous damage during childbirth. Atrophic endometritis, atrophic vaginitis and atrophic changes in the vulva may occur.

## Climacteric symptoms

While the menopause may occur without any symptoms other than the cessation of menstruation, it is not infrequently associated with other symptoms, of which the commonest is the occurrence of hot flushes. There is flushing of the face and neck, often with sweating. The flushes are very variable in duration and frequency; they may only be momentary, or they may last for up to 15 minutes and recur many times a day. When they are severe they cause discomfort and embarrassment. During a flush there is a rise in peripheral blood flow (as measured in the arm) and a rise in pulse rate, but no change in blood pressure.

The cause of flushes is uncertain. There is a fall in the level of circulating oestrogens, and a temporary rise in the level of gonadotrophins, both FSH and LH. It was found that flushes are checked by administering oestrogens or testosterone. Because of these facts it was suggested that flushes were caused by the rise in gonadotrophin levels. However, women with and without flushes have similar gonadotrophin levels, and in cases in which oestrogens control the flushes the gonadotrophin levels do not fall. Moreover, flushes do not occur when gonadotrophins are given to induce ovulation, and they have been reported in women after hypophysectomy. All these facts have thrown doubt on the theory that flushes are caused by gonadotrophins.

Flushes are particularly severe if there is an abrupt change in hormone balance, for example after bilateral oöphorectomy in a young woman, and they can even occur in men after orchidectomy.

Some women gain weight at about the time of the menopause. There is no evidence that this is due to endocrine changes of the pituitary or ovaries; it is more likely to be the result of a lower level of general activity. On the other hand, osteoporosis has been attributed to oestrogen deficiency, and claims are made that it can be prevented by giving oestrogens. The loss of calcium from bone causes a tendency to fractures with relatively slight trauma, especially of the wrist and femur.

Atrophic changes in the vulva may cause discomfort and dyspareunia (see p. 101). The reduction in vaginal acidity may allow organisms to survive there and cause vaginitis (see p. 112) or endometritis (see p. 119), but it should be emphasized that these events occur in only a small number of women.

Other symptoms such as headache, insomnia and depression may be attributed to the menopause, but there is not much evidence that these symptoms are of endocrine origin; it is more likely that they are of emotional origin, perhaps associated with the passing of an important phase of life, sometimes with fear of loss of sexual attractiveness, or loss of an identifiable role in the family as children grow up and leave home.

It has already been stated that the periods may cease suddenly or gradually diminish at the menopause. Although excessive or irregular loss is not uncommon at about the time of the menopause this must never be accepted as normal or 'just the change'. In every such case the possibility of malignant disease must be considered, and full examination with endometrial biopsy is essential.

## Management

The majority of women soon adjust to their new situation, especially if they have the understanding and support of their husband and family, but in others one or more of their problems will be severe enough to require medical help. The hot flushes can be suppressed by the administration of oestrogen. This in turn may relieve the sleeplessness and help the depression. However, it will not resolve the patient's changed situation if that is troubling her, nor remove family problems. Hormone therapy is an adjunct to counselling in many cases. It may also be helpful if dyspareunia is a cause of marital disharmony.

For flushes ethinyloestradiol is given in small doses such as 10 micrograms daily, increasing or reducing the dose according to the effect. As an alternative, equine combined oestrogen (Premarin) 0.625 mg daily is often used, or oestradiol valerate (Progynova) 1 mg daily. For symptoms caused by atrophic changes in the genital tract, larger systemic doses are often required, but for this purpose oestrogens can also be administered locally as dienoestrol cream.

Most doctors would give endocrine treatment for several weeks to relieve symptoms, but would then gradually reduce the doses and discontinue the treatment. An entirely different policy is that of long-term replacement therapy. Those who advocate this regard the postmenopausal woman as suffering from a hormonal deficiency disease. They argue that many of the disorders traditionally regarded as concomitants of age, such as arteriosclerosis, obesity and osteoporosis, can be prevented by replacement therapy. For effective prevention of osteoporosis oestrogen treatment would have to be given for as long as 10 years. The case for continuous and prolonged hormone therapy is not yet proved, and most doctors will use hormone therapy with caution, and only for the relief of symptoms.

Those who give long-term therapy either prescribe oestrogens alone or in combination with progestogens. If unopposed oestrogen is used, it should be in the smallest effective dosage and given intermittently, three weeks out of four. Alternatively, it may be given in cyclical fashion with added progestogen; for example, ethinyloestradiol 10 micrograms might be given daily for 21 days, with norethisterone 0.1 mg daily for the last 7 days of this course. Withdrawal bleeding would follow, and the next course would be started on the 28th day. The advantage of this is that, by causing a predictable withdrawal bleed each month, any irregular bleeding can be recognized, but most women would not welcome the nuisance of the monthly bleeding. A patient with menopausal symptoms after hysterectomy is sometimes treated with a subcutaneous implant of ethinyl oestradiol 50 mg.

The amount of oestrogen required to suppress vasomotor symptoms is only about one-third of the smallest amount in the contraceptive pill, and most of the reservations about the use of the pill in older women for fear of thrombosis hardly apply. The major concern is related to the long-continued stimulation of the target epithelium in the breast and endometrium by oestrogens. Not only may oestrogens induce endometrial carcinoma, but they may enhance the growth of pre-existing carcinoma of the breast. It should be established as far as possible that no such tumour is present when oestrogen therapy is employed. The risk is small and it is claimed that addition of a progestogen prevents the danger of uterine cancer. If there is any irregular or excessive bleeding endometrial biopsy should be performed without delay.

# 6

# Examination of the gynaecological patient

Before making any examination it is essential that a careful history is taken, and the following outline is suggested.

Name, age, civil state and address.
A brief statement of the general nature and duration of the complaint.
*Obstetric history*
1. Number of children with ages and birthweights.
   Any abnormalities of pregnancy, labour or the puerperium.
2. Number of miscarriages, with stage of pregnancy when they occurred, and any complications.
3. Any termination of pregnancy, with method and reason.
*Usual menstrual cycle.* Age when periods began. Regularity of cycle. Usual duration of each period and length of cycle, counting from the first day of one period to the first day of next. First day of last period. This information is generally recorded thus: 'M.H. 13 5/28 regular', meaning the periods began at the age of 13, last for 5 days and occur every 28 days.
*Previous medical history.* Details of any serious illnesses or operations, with dates.
*Family history.* Occasionally of value.
*Detailed history of present complaint.*
1. Abnormal menstrual loss. The pattern of bleeding — regular or irregular. Amount of loss — greater or less than usual. Number of sanitary towels or tampons used. Passage of clots or flooding. Any pain with the loss.
2. Pelvic pain. Site, nature and relation to periods. Anything that aggravates or relieves it.
3. Vaginal discharge. Amount, colour, odour, presence of blood.
*Enquiry about other systems.*
1. Bowels. Regular or constipated. Any alteration of habit.
2. Micturition. Frequency, dysuria, urgency, incontinence (real or stress) or haematuria.
3. Intercourse. Any discomfort or pain. In cases of infertility, whether intercourse is normal; frequency and time in cycle.
4. Contraception. The use of the intrauterine device or oral contraceptives may be particularly relevant because of their possible effect on menstruation.
*Emotional problems.* Tactful enquiry. Relations with husband or sexual partner. Family problems. Bad housing or occupational stress.

## Examination of the patient
Much information about the general condition of the patient may be obtained by observing her while the history is being taken, and the student should train himself to do this in every case. Thus a note should be made as to whether the woman looks ill or well, whether she is abnormally fat or thin, or pale. Is the history given in a matter-of-fact manner, or is the patient unduly introspective? Is she trying to hide something, or making

light of symptoms which she thinks may lead to the diagnosis of some condition that she dreads? Is she depressed or anxious, or suffering from an emotional upset which is producing symptoms which are an unconscious expression of her need for help?

Before attention is directed to the abdomen or pelvis it is advisable to make a quick general examination, noting the appearance of the conjunctivae and the tongue, and examining the pulse. The urine should be examined to exclude the presence of protein or sugar. Physical examination should begin with the chest and breasts and only after this is the abdominal and pelvic examination made.

# Abdominal examination

The patient should lie flat, and if the abdomen is at all rigid she should draw up her knees to relax the muscles. The bladder should be empty.

### Inspection

The size and shape of the abdomen is noted. Fullness in the midline might indicate a tumour of uterine or ovarian origin; fullness in the flanks may occur with ascites. The condition of the skin, whether showing lineae albicantes, rashes, pigmentation or scars, is observed.

### Palpation

The abdomen should always be examined with a warm hand and with the flat of the hand rather than the tips of the fingers, as deep palpation can then be done without hurting the patient. Some patients who seem to be unable to relax their abdominal muscles when lying in the dorsal position, even with their knees drawn up, can relax when lying on the side. If abdominal rigidity is encountered, it must be determined whether this is due to nervous tension or is true rigidity of the muscles guarding some underlying tender spot. Tenseness may be overcome by asking the patient to breathe deeply with her mouth open, or by engaging her in conversation. If the rigidity is true guarding the abdominal muscles will neither relax nor move when the patient takes a deep breath.

If a tumour is discovered, its position, size, shape, mobility and consistency must be noted. As a general rule midline tumours are of uterine or ovarian origin, whilst those in either iliac fossa tend to arise from the ovary, tube or bowel. Malignant ovarian tumours, because of adherence, may give rise to swellings in the iliac fossa, and so may fibromyomata which are growing from the side of the uterus. Tumours arising from the pelvis, if not impacted or fixed by adhesions, are mobile from side to side but not up and down, and it is generally not possible to feel the lower border of the tumour. Tumours may be solid or cystic, and cystic tumours may be tense or flaccid. If sufficiently large, they may exhibit a fluid thrill, felt with a flat hand when the cyst is tapped with the other hand.

Ascites may also give a fluid thrill, but its presence is determined by shifting dullness on percussion. If there is free fluid in the peritoneal cavity, it is necessary to dip down by sudden but gentle movements of the fingers to feel whether there is any solid growth lying more deeply.

**Percussion**
This enables one to decide whether a swelling is in contact with the abdominal wall and therefore dull on percussion, or whether bowel intervenes between the tumour and the abdominal wall. If the abdomen is resonant in the centre and dull in the flanks, and the dullness shifts when the patient changes her position, free fluid can be diagnosed.

**Auscultation**
On listening with a stethoscope, bowel sounds are normally present, and apart from aortic pulsation are the only sounds that can be heard. The silent abdomen is an indication of intestinal paralysis, being found in cases of severe shock, generalized peritonitis and postoperative paralytic ileus.

On auscultation over a tumour two additional sounds may be heard. (1) The uterine souffle. If the tumour is the pregnant uterus or a large fibromyoma it will contain hypertrophied uterine vessels; should the stethoscope happen to be placed over one of these, a blowing sound will be heard which is synchronous with the patient's heart beat. (2) If the tumour is the pregnant uterus the fetal heart sounds can be heard after the 24th week, at a rate of 140–160 beats per minute.

## Vaginal examination

The procedure in making a vaginal examination is: (1) inspection of the vulva; (2) inspection of the vagina and vaginal cervix; (3) palpation of the vagina and vaginal cervix; and (4) bimanual palpation of the pelvic organs.

There are four positions which are commonly used for vaginal examination. Each position has its advantages and disadvantages.

*1. Lateral position*
After the abdominal examination is finished the patient simply turns onto her left side and draws up both knees. It is a comfortable position, is easily assumed, does not expose the patient unduly and permits of a reasonably thorough examination.

*2. Semi-prone or Sims' position*
This position, in which the patient lies on the left side with the left arm behind her and the right knee drawn up slightly more than the left, gives a good view of the external genitalia. It is especially useful for examining the cervix and anterior vaginal wall. On passage of a speculum, air enters the vagina and the anterior vaginal wall falls away. Sims used this position for the exposure of vesicovaginal fistulae.

*3. Dorsal position*
This position, with the patient lying on a couch on her back with the

knees flexed, does not afford such a good view of the vulva and does not permit the easy introduction of a speculum, but is a convenient position for bimanual palpation, and for that reason is most frequently used.

### 4. *Lithotomy position*

If the examination is made under anaesthesia, this is the best position. The patient lies on her back, with the buttocks drawn to the edge of the table and the thighs abducted and flexed on the abdomen, and kept in position by supports. Because of the extent of the exposure, unanaesthetized patients do not like this position; nevertheless it is routinely used in other countries and in departments of genito-urinary medicine.

For vaginal examination the bladder must be empty. The examination is made in a methodical manner. First the presence or absence of vaginal discharge is noted, then the labia and clitoris are examined for signs of infection, ulceration, new growths or swellings. The labia are separated and the urethral orifice is inspected; the urethra is compressed from behind forwards to see if there is any urethral discharge. The patient is asked to strain and cough; the presence of any stress incontinence is noted. The orifices of Bartholin's ducts are examined.

To make a visual examination of the vagina a speculum is employed. Care must be taken to avoid hurting the patient. A sterile lubricant is used. This should be presented from a tube, so that it cannot become contaminated and cause cross-infection of one patient by another. It should be transparent, so that discharge can be distinguished, and should not contain antiseptics which will interfere with bacteriological examination or the search for other organisms such as trichomonads.

Two forms of specula are in common use. (Fig. 6.1).

1. *Sims' speculum.* This was devised to display vesicovaginal fistulae. It consists of two concave blades of different sizes, with a handle connecting them.

2. *Cusco's or bivalve speculum.* This consists of two blades fixed together by a hinge at the vulval end of the instrument. It gives an excellent view of the cervix, and when screwed open remains steady in the vagina without being held.

### Examination of discharge.

The amount and nature of any discharge should be noted. Patients will occasionally complain of discharge when little or none exists, or alternatively deny all knowledge of an obviously copious discharge. A discharge may be mucoid; thick and white with infection with *Candida albicans;* purulent and offensive with infection with *Trichomonas vaginalis;* or blood-stained with a malignant ulcer or with a foreign body.

Although it is often possible to make a diagnosis of the probable cause of the discharge by clinical examination, diagnosis cannot be final without examining the discharge by the methods described in Chapter 13 (p. 108).

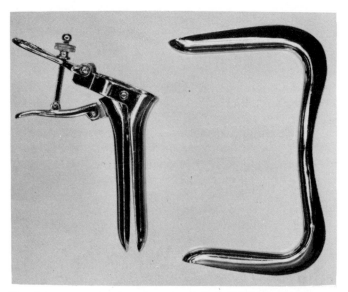

**Fig. 6.1** Cusco's bivalve speculum (left) and Sims' speculum.

When a discharge is associated with urethritis, gonococcal infection is a possibility, and swabs should be taken for examination, not only from the cervix but also from the urethra.

A cervical smear should be examined in all cases for the early detection of carcinomatous cells which are being exfoliated. This is best done before vaginal digital examination, and for that reason it is often preferable to pass the speculum before this. The technique of taking the smear is described later (p. 53).

**Digital examination**

Using the right index finger, guarded with a rubber glove and well lubricated, the vaginal walls are palpated. A growth or cyst, or a foreign body, may be discovered. The fornices are then examined, and it is noted whether they are obliterated or made to bulge by swellings inside the pelvis. Bands of scar tissue of traumatic origin may be found passing across the vault of the vagina.

The vaginal cervix is next examined, noting its direction, size and shape. Its surface may be smooth or irregular. The external os may be small, as is usual in nulliparae, or large and patulous, admitting the tip of the finger. The dilatation does not as a rule extend to the internal os, unless there is something inside the uterus which it is trying to extrude. The cervix may be torn on one or both sides, and the lips of the cervix may be everted. The cervix may be ulcerated and the site of a malignant growth, or there may be a polypus growing from it or coming through it. Occasionally the cervix can be reached only with difficulty, as when it is pushed upwards

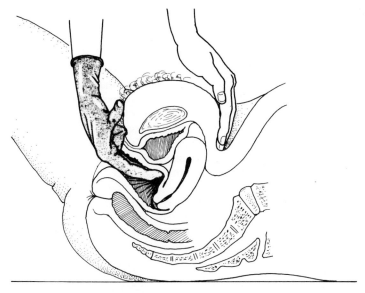

**Fig. 6.2** Bimanual palpation.

by a tumour in the rectovaginal pouch, or when the retroverted gravid uterus is incarcerated.

**Bimanual palpation**
For this examination the gloved index and middle fingers of the right hand are lubricated and introduced into the vagina, and the left hand is placed on the hypogastrium, so that the pelvic organs can be palpated between them. (If the vaginal orifice is small or tender only one finger is used.) Bimanual examination is carried out with the two hands palpating together. The direction of the cervix is first noted and then the fingers of the right hand are moved into the anterior fornix; by counterpressure of the left hand on the abdomen, the body of the uterus can be felt between the two hands if it is anteverted. It it is retroverted it will not be so felt, but felt if the fingers are transferred to the posterior fornix. The size, position and mobility of the uterus are determined, and then an attempt is made to examine the structures lying on either side of it by palpation between the fingers in the lateral fornix and counterpressure from the hand on the abdomen. A healthy Fallopian tube is not palpable, but if it is thickened it may be felt. The normal ovary is recognized as a small, oval movable structure, which is sensitive to pressure.

Should a tumour be felt in the pelvis, its size, consistency, mobility and attachments are noted. Especially must its attachment to or freedom from the uterus be determined. If the swelling is free from the uterus, it probably arises from the tube, ovary or bowel.

A loaded pelvic colon may be misdiagnosed as a pelvic tumour. Solid faeces indent on pressure.

# Rectal examination

It is sometimes impossible to do a vaginal examination on a virgin without an anaesthetic but, by rectal examination, the size, position and mobility of the uterus can be determined and any abnormal swelling felt. In certain patients it is essential to do a rectal as well as a vaginal examination. This is particularly important in cases of carcinoma of the cervix, for it is possible to examine the parametrial cellular tissue more easily by rectal than vaginal examination. The base of the broad ligaments and the uterosacral ligaments can only be palpated rectally. A finger in the rectum is situated further back in the pelvic cavity and may detect a small tumour in the rectovaginal pouch which is uncertainly felt by vaginal palpation. A combined examination with one finger in the vagina and one in the rectum may help to elucidate the physical signs in a difficult case.

# Examination of the urinary organs

### Urethra

The meatus should first be examined for redness, discharge or a growth. The finger is next passed into the vagina to squeeze the urethra from behind forwards, and any discharge is examined. It should be spread as a thin film on a microscope slide, stained and examined for organisms. Swabs are also taken for culture.

### Examination of the urine

Catheterization, which carries the risk of introducing infection, is seldom required for gynaecological diagnosis. In most cases, collection of a midstream specimen is adequate. The patient must be told exactly what to do. She should separate the labia with the fingers of her left hand and then pass a sterile swab moistened with sterile water over the meatus. (Antiseptics will interfere with the bacteriological examination.) The patient then passes urine and part of the stream is caught in a sterile container.

Many now believe that suprapubic bladder puncture is safer than catheterization, and the bacteriological results are more reliable. For this procedure the patient is told to hold her water until the bladder is uncomfortably full. A fine sterile needle is passed directly through the abdominal wall just above the symphysis pubis into the bladder. After 5 or 10 ml of urine have been withdrawn with a syringe, the patient immediately empties her bladder.

Whichever method is used for the collection of the specimen, it is essential that it is sent to the laboratory as soon as possible. Organisms multiply in urine if there is any delay, and a false estimate of the bacteriological population will be made.

# Vaginal and cervical smears for exfoliative cytology

Taking smears from the vagina and cervix for exfoliative cytology is an essential part of routine gynaecological examination.

The surface cells of any epithelium are constantly being shed and replaced by new ones, so that by sampling the fluid bathing the surface, or by scraping it, it is possible to examine cells from all parts of it. Since cells are shed from the surface of a carcinoma in even greater profusion than they are shed from normal epithalium, it is possible to find malignant cells during the earliest stages of a carcinoma, while it is still pre-invasive or before it can be seen on clinical examination.

A cervical smear should be taken from every woman who has a pelvic examination immediately after passage of the speculum and exposure of the cervix. Cervical smears are taken in family planning clinics, in antenatal clinics, and in many doctors' practices at regular intervals. Positive findings are more common after the age of 30 and after childbearing, but smears should be taken in younger women who are having regular intercourse.

The first two smears should not be more than one year apart in case a positive result is missed on the first occasion. Thereafter smears should be taken at intervals of not more than three years. However, if facilities are available, there is much to be said in favour of taking smears annually.

### Collection of material
In gynaecological work there are two methods in common use for the collection of material for cytological examination.

The most common method is to use Ayre's spatula. This is made of wood or plastic. It has one plain rounded end with which material can be collected from the posterior fornix. The other end is shaped so that it can be placed in the external os and rotated to obtain a very superficial scraping of the cervix, including the whole of the squamo-columnar junction. It is often better to use the rounded end to obtain material from a lacerated or patulous cervix. The spatula has the advantage that it collects cells directly from the cervix, but it may also be desirable to collect secretion from the posterior fornix with it, since endometrial cells tend to collect there.

A glass pipette may also be used, about 15 cm long and 0.5 cm in diameter, with a strong rubber bulb at one end and slightly curved at the other end. It is passed into the vagina and material is aspirated from the posterior fornix. This method has the advantage that it is not necessary to use a vaginal speculum, and patients can be taught to collect specimens (and make smears) from themselves. This method may also be useful in assessing the endocrine status or response of patients to treatment, as it is possible to make repeated examinations at frequent intervals with little inconvenience to the patient.

Supplementary methods that are occasionally used are the collection of material from the endocervical canal with an ordinary throat swab, and from the endometrium by aspiration through a cannula.

### Preparation, staining and examination of smears

The material must at once be spread on a microscope slide and immediately be put into fixative. It must not be allowed to dry, or the preparation will be spoilt. It is convenient to use a slide that is ground at one end so that the patient's name can be written on it in pencil.

Papanicolaou's staining method is the one most commonly used, and this employs as fixative a mixture of equal parts of absolute ethyl alcohol and diethyl ether. The nuclei are stained with haematoxylin. A mixture of stains is used for the cytoplasm which stains differentially according to the type of cell and the hormonal state of the patient.

Each slide must be examined completely so that every cell is looked at. With a normal smear being examined by a trained cytologist, this may take about 5–10 minutes, though it will take longer for an abnormal or difficult smear.

### Purposes

The principal use of the method is for the discovery of carcinoma-in-situ of the cervix and the early diagnosis of cervical and corporeal cancer. Much less often, malignant cells from carcinoma of the vagina, Fallopian tube or ovary, or from a metastasis in the genital tract, may be found. It may be used in the follow-up clinic to detect recurrence of a treated carcinoma.

It may also be of use in assessing the hormonal state of the patient, but endocrine assays are now available and are more reliable.

The frequency with which malignant cells are found in patients with invasive carcinoma of the cervix or body of the uterus, in whom the diagnosis was not suspected on clinical grounds, varies in reports from different centres, but is of the order of 1 per 1000. In addition about 5 cases of carcinoma-in-situ are found for every 1000 patients examined. Since this condition cannot be detected or even suspected by clinical examination, it is only by exfoliative cytology that one can search for it. (Also see p. 175).

The method is not restricted to gynaecological clinics, and it can also be employed on a large scale as a screening procedure in clinics for the detection of cancer in apparently healthy women. While programmes aimed at the examination at regular intervals of the entire female population at risk will allow of the eradication of many cases of in situ carcinoma, the hope that invasive carcinoma will be completely prevented is unlikely to be achieved. There are difficulties in persuading women to attend for examination, particularly poorer women with large families who are most at risk; it is not easy to find and train enough technicians to examine the smears; and it is by no means certain that all invasive carcinoma is preceded by in situ carcinoma. Nevertheless, invasive cancer is likely to be discovered at a much earlier stage if regular examinations are made.

**Normal cytological appearances**
In the normal cycle the majority of cells seen in the smears are squamous cells shed from the surface of the stratified squamous epithelium of the vagina and cervix. There are also varying numbers of polymorphs and histiocytes, endocervical columnar cells and, during menstruation, endometrial cells. The degree of cornification of the superficial cells of the squamous epithelium depends on the amount of circulating oestrogens. There is a great contrast between the histological appearance of the squamous epithelium seen at about the time of ovulation, when oestrogenic activity is at its maximum, and that seen in an elderly postmenopausal woman. This is reflected in the type of squamous cell predominating in the vaginal smear, and it is convenient to describe these cells as being of *superficial, intermediate or parabasal* type, according to which layer of cornified squamous epithelium they most resemble. However, these are merely descriptive terms. The cells seen can only come from the surface layer, unless there is ulceration with exposure of the deeper layers; hence, if parabasal cells predominate, it means that the squamous epithelium has failed to develop to the mature cornified state.

*Menstrual phase* (approximately days 1 to 5)
The squamous cells tend to have large nuclei, basophilic cytoplasm, irregular cell borders, and to be gathered into large groups. Mucus, red blood corpuscles and polymorphs are present. Endometrial cells occur singly and in groups. Histiocytes appear towards the end of menstruation.

*Follicular phase* (approximately days 5 to 14)
During this phase there is a decrease in the amount of mucus and the number of polymorphs. The squamous cells become larger, the nuclei decrease in size and there is an increase in the proportion of acidophilic cells. The cells tend to be discrete.

   At the end of this phase the cells are large, have brightly stained cytoplasm, pyknotic nuclei and sharply defined cell borders. There is little mucus, and few polymorphs and bacteria (Fig. 6.3).

*Luteal phase* (approximately days 14 to 28)
The cells become arranged in groups and show curling and folding of their edges, which are more irregular than in the previous phase. There is a decrease in the proportion of acidophilic cells. The nuclei are larger and less pyknotic. In the later part of this phase, as menstruation approaches, polymorphs and mucus reappear (Fig. 6.4).

*Postmenopausal appearances*
After the menopause the epithelium becomes less cornified and the appearances seen vary. Vaginal secretion is scanty and there may be few cells present. Parabasal cells may predominate to such an extent that very few superficial or intermediate type cells may be found (Fig. 6.5).

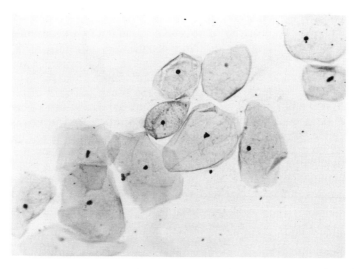

**Fig. 6.3** Vaginal smear: follicular phase × 300. Papanicolaou's stain. Large superficial squamous cells with pyknotic nuclei.

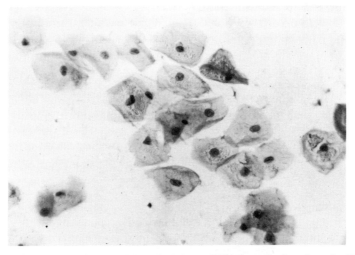

**Fig. 6.4** Vaginal smear: luteal phase × 300. Papanicolaou's stain. Nuclei not pyknotic. Cell borders folded over.

**Abnormal smears**

The characteristics of malignant cells found in smears are illustrated in Fig. 6.6. In brief, the nuclei of such cells are hyperchromatic, or irregular shape and with abnormal mitotic figures. The cell as a whole may be of bizarre shape, sometimes with multiple nuclei.

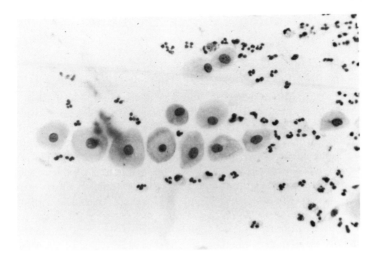

**Fig. 6.5** Vaginal smear: atrophic postmenopausal × 300. Papanicolaou's stain. Parabasal cells.

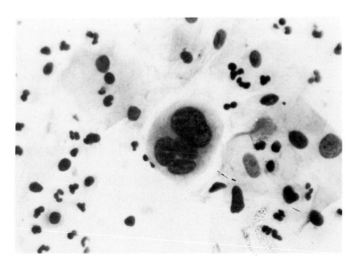

**Fig. 6.6** Vaginal smear. Squamous carcinoma of cervix × 600. Papanicolaou's stain. Multinucleated malignant cells showing altered nuclear/cytoplasmic ratio, nuclear hyperchromasia and variation in nuclear size.

# Further gynaecological investigations

## Colposcopy

A colposcope is a low-powered microscope used for examining the vaginal aspect of the cervix. It is attached to a stand which can be adjusted for height and angle, with a light for illuminating the field. The patient is placed in the lithotomy position and the cervix is exposed with a bivalve speculum. The colposcope is focused onto the cervix, which is painted with dilute acetic acid which temporarily stains abnormal epithelium white.

Normal squamous epithelium on the vaginal aspect of the cervix looks pale, smooth and opaque. Normal columnar epithelium of the cervical canal and of the surface of the cervix near to the external os shows many fine folds, which when magnified appear as small translucent villous processes.

Colposcopy is of great value in detecting areas of dysplasia, carcinoma-in-situ or early invasive carcinoma (see pp. 166–171).

## Endometrial biopsy

The most reliable method of examining the endometrium, whether for diagnosis of functional disorders of menstruation, of tuberculosis, or of carcinoma, is by curettage after dilatation of the cervix under general anaesthesia.

In cases of infertility, endometrial biopsy in the latter part of the cycle will demonstrate the presence or absence of the luteal phase, and thus show whether ovulation has taken place in that cycle.

It is possible to obtain tissue for endometrial biopsy by using a small suction aspirator (Vabra aspirator) without general anaesthesia, but many gynaecologists believe that, whenever there is the least suspicion of malignant disease, curettage should be performed under general anaesthesia.

In cases of suspected tuberculosis not only is premenstrual endometrium examined histologically, but also fragments are used to set up bacteriological cultures.

## Hysteroscopy

This procedure is under trial in some centres. Under general anaesthesia a small telescope is passed through the cervix. After distending the uterus with fluid or gas a limited view of the uterine cavity can be obtained.

## Laparoscopy

Inspection of the pelvic organs through an endoscope was formerly carried out through the posterior vaginal fornix with the patient in the knee-chest position (culdoscopy). This method has been superseded by the insertion of an endoscope with a fibre-optic light cable and a small telescope through the anterior abdominal wall (laparoscopy). An excellent view of the pelvic organs is obtained. For technique see p. 359.

**Tests for patency of the Fallopian tubes.** See p. 267.

**Ultrasonic examination**
In any case in which there is diagnostic uncertainty after abdominal and vaginal examination an ultrasonic examination is requested. The progressive enlargement of the Graafian follicle during a menstrual cycle can be observed. The examination may be useful in assessing the extent of malignant disease, including the follow-up of patients after treatment. A missing intrauterine contraceptive device may be located.

**Computerized tomography**
This can also be used to investigate abdominal or pelvic tumours and to establish their relationships.

# 7

# Determination of sex; intersex

The Oxford Dictionary defines a male as 'being of the sex that begets offspring', and a female as 'being of the offspring-bearing sex'. Although this simple distinction between a normal man and a normal woman seems obvious enough, in cases of incomplete or abnormal development the determination of sex is often far from easy. The description of a male as an individual with testes and a female as one with ovaries is only an extension of the dictionary definitions, and is not always adequate. Some individuals have the body form (phenotype) of one sex but the gonads of the other, while some have both ovarian and testicular tissues. In other cases, stimulation with an inappropriate sex hormone may cause virilization or feminization. The issue can be complicated further by psychological abnormalities which can produce inversion of sexual behaviour.

## Chromosomal or genetic sex

Chromosomal studies have improved our understanding of sexual differentiation. For this purpose cells are grown in tissue culture, active mitosis is arrested with colchicine, the cells are then squashed between slides to disrupt their nuclei, and after staining it is possible to count and classify the pairs of chromosomes in a particular nucleus. Every normal human somatic cell contains 46 chromosomes. These are classified according to their size, the position of the centromere, and the relative length of their arms. They may be arranged and numbered in order from the largest to the smallest, but so many of them are similar in appearance that it is easier arrange them in seven groups, labelled A to G. The pattern of chromosomes in any patient is described as the *karyotype*.

During mitotic division of any body cell, each chromosome divides along its length into two apparently similar parts. One part passes into each daughter cell, so that each new cell again contains 46 chromosomes. However, during the meiotic (reduction) division of the sex cells, the chromosomes group themselves in 23 pairs, and one member of each pair passes into the daughter cell, so that after the division each oöcyte or sperm contains half the ordinary complement. Forty-four of the 46 chromosomes, which are called *autosomes,* form apparently similar pairs, but the other two chromosomes, called *sex chromosomes,* may be dissimilar. In the normal male every body cell contains two sex chromosomes, a large X chromosome (resembling those in the C group) and a small Y chromosome (resembling those in the G group); after the reduction division half of the spermatozoa will carry an X chromosome and the other half will carry a Y chromosome. In normal female cells there are two X chromosomes, so that after the reduction division every oöcyte will carry an X chromosome. Conjugation of sperms and oöcytes give rise to XX and XY pairs again.

Every normal body cell has this male (XY) or female (XX) constitution, and in many body cells this difference in their nuclei can be recognized in ordinary stained preparations. In cells from a buccal smear, for example, or in polymorphonuclear leucocytes, a tiny nodule of chromatin (the Barr body, or 'nuclear drumstick') can be seen near the nuclear membrane of many cells in normal females, but not in normal males. This chromatin nodule is probably the second (inactive) X chromosome; hence its absence in males.

Normal women are therefore 'chromatin positive' and normal men are 'chromatin negative', but the presence or absence of this chromatin nodule is not complete proof of the chromosomal status of the individual; only study of cell cultures gives a completely reliable picture.

The Y chromosome can also be recognized because part of it has a selective affinity for the fluorescent stain quinacrine dihydrochloride.

The basic sexual differentiation is determined by genes, which are invisible parts of the chromosomes, and it is probable that the genes which determine the phenotype are not only located on the sex chromosomes, but also are scattered among the autosomes. Abnormal chromosomal patterns may arise by 'non-disjunction' during mitosis, when a pair of chromosomes do not separate properly so that an extra chromosome is carried to one cell while one chromosome is missing from the other cell; or else abnormal division of one or more chromosomes may occur. An abnormal chromosome may be wholly or partly attached to another chromosome (translocation).

In certain abnormal individuals with male phenotype (Klinefelter's syndrome, see p. 64) the chromosomal structure is XXY, and in them a chromatin nodule is seen. In other abnormal individuals with female phenotype (Turner's syndrome, see p. 64) there is only one X chromosome, and there is no visible nuclear nodule. In very rare instances mentally retarded, but otherwise apparently normal, females may have a XXX chromosomal structure, and such persons have two chromatin nodules.

Chromosomal studies have also proved to be of value and interest in the investigation of congenital abnormalities, and abnormal patterns have been found in up to 70 per cent of spontaneously aborted pregnancy sacs. Often the chromosomal defect is so gross that no embryo is formed.

## Differentiation of the gonad

As early as the 5th week of embryonic life the site of development of the gonad can be recognized as an area of thickening of the coelomic epithelium over the ventral surface of the mesonephros. Amoeboid cells which are *primordial germ cells* migrate into the developing gonad from the region of the yolk sac, where they can be recognized in the 3rd week. If the migration of these cells is prevented, partial development of the gonad will continue, but no germ cells appear in it.

Before the 6th week, the sex of the gonad cannot be determined, but thereafter the development of the testis and ovary differ. The testis can be distinguished by the formation of *sex cords* in the medulla, which later give rise to the seminiferous tubules, and these cords are joined by the rete testis to the mesonephric tubules, which will eventually form the epididymis.

In the female the cells of the cortex of the gonad proliferate to a much greater extent than in the testis, and by the 12th week the bulk of the ovary consists of a crowded mass of germ cells intermixed with cells derived from the epithelium which covers the ovary, but without the formation of distinct sex cords. By the 16th week the *primary oöcytes* can be distinguished, each surrounded by a single layer of flattened cells derived from the epithelium which covers the ovary; these cells later become the granulosa cells.

Although the migration of the primitive sex cells into the gonad is essential for the proper development of that organ, the early development of the female genital tract does not seem to be dependent on the ovary. The female genital pattern may be regarded as neutral, for early removal of the gonads in animals of either sex leads to prodominance of the Müllerian system and suppression of the Wolffian derivatives. In the female the Müllerian tract gives rise to the tubes, uterus and vagina, and the Wolffian duct is merely the excretory duct of the transitory mesonephros. In the male the development of the cortex of the gonad is suppressed and the medulla develops into a testis, while Müllerian development is inhibited and the Wolffian apparatus is modified to become the male genital tract. Although the male characteristics of the gonad itself are genetically determined, the development of the Wolffian system may depend on the local influence of the testis, for in hermaphrodites the Wolffian system is usually developed on the same side as the testis, whereas a tube and uterine horn may be found on the ovarian side. The Sertoli cells are believed to produce a Müllerian inhibition factor, a non-steroid protein substance.

## Later sexual differentiation

The ovary secretes mainly oestrogen and progesterone, while the testis secretes mainly androgens. These potent substances cause further sexual differentiation. In the female the final development of the genital tract, breasts and body form occurs only after full ovarian function is established at puberty, but androgens can modify the basic structure even while the fetus is still *in utero.* The male fetus is not affected by the large quantities of oestrogen to which it is subjected *in utero,* but small quantities of androgens, perhaps inadvertently given to the mother during early pregnancy, may virilize a female fetus. However, once the main pattern of development of the Müllerian or Wolffian system or of the mammary glands has been established, the sex hormones can produce only minor changes, such as enlargement of the clitoris by androgens in the female or activity of the breasts by oestrogens in the male.

In a normal female the hypothalamus at puberty secretes releasing hormone (GnRH) in a pulsatile manner, leading to the cyclical release of anterior pituitary hormones. Animal experiments suggest that in the male fetus the hypothalamus is imprinted by male sex hormones, with the result that in the male the hypothalamus eventually has a non-cyclical release pattern.

The psychological orientation of the individual and the pattern of behaviour is only partly determined by the balance of the sex hormones. Social custom and upbringing dictate many of the mental attitudes which predominate in men or women in any particular civilization or society; but this is not the place to pursue these speculations. It is enough to say here that abnormal sexual behaviour usually stems from psychological immaturity or disorder rather than from any anatomical, hormonal or genetic disorder.

## Intersex

Although it is usually easy to decide whether an individual is male or female, in a few cases this is very difficult and the ill-defined term *intersex* is applied to these. Many factors − chromosomal, gonadal, hormonal and psychological − combine to determine a person's social sex, and it may not be possible, to select a single factor as over-riding. In the human the basic pattern is female; male external characteristics (the male phenotype) are caused by androgens secreted by the testis. With failure of testicular activity the degree of masculinization will be determined by the stage of development reached when the failure occurred. There are, for instance, cases of early failure (testicular feminization, see p. 66) in which the external body form and psychological orientation are female although testes are present. In late failure of masculinization, hypospadias may be the only abnormality.

Virilism of a female fetus may be caused by androgens given to the mother during pregnancy, or by abnormal secretion of androgens by the suprarenal cortex in cases of the adrenogenital syndrome.

In rare instances, an individual may have both a testis and an ovary (true hermaphrodite), although these organs are seldom normal or capable of function. More frequently, owing to a developmental abnormality such as hypospadias, the anatomical sex is wrongly diagnosed in infancy, and the error is only discovered at puberty (pseudohermaphrodite).

Quite apart from any genetic, anatomical or hormonal abnormality, there may be abnormal homosexual behaviour, or there may be a psychological urge to adopt the clothing and physical characteristics of the opposite sex (tranvestism).

Outward genital structure and the general body form (the phenotype) will often affect the psychological orientation, partly because the pheno-type may dictate the way in which a child is brought up.

In the normal person the genetic pattern, the hormonal predominance, the anatomy of the genitalia and the psychological orientation are all in concord. Deviation of any of these may occur, but the 'sex' is still to be judged by the final balance of structure and function, and only relatively gross departures from the normal can be regarded as intersexual. For example, a boy with hypospadias and undescended testes could hardly be regarded as anything but male, and a girl with adrenogenital virilism is essentially still female.

In cases of intersex legal problems might arise in respect of inheritance or in relation to sexual offences. The true sex of some 'female' Olympic athletes has been questioned. There is no legal definition of sex, and decision is difficult if the chromosomal and gonadal sex conflict.

Some, at least, of the cases of intersex can be separated into categories, but only the better recognized groups can be mentioned here, and some of the groups may overlap.

## Klinefelter's syndrome

These cases only concern the gynaecologist indirectly, as they occur in patients whose appearance, although characteristic, is essentially male. They usually have scrotal testes, which are small and azoospermic, and they are therefore infertile. The penis may be small but potency is often normal. These patients usually have 47 chromosomes, with an additional sex chromosome, giving the structure XXY, and they are therefore 'chromatin positive'. In rare cases 48 XXXY, or mosaics of XX and XY are found.

## Gonadal dysgenesis

This term has been employed for patients with female habitus in whom the gonads are imperfectly formed, usually being represented by white streaks of connective tissue containing no germ cells or granulosa cells. The external body form is immaturely female, with an infantile vulva, vagina and uterus.

A variety of gonadal dysgenesis with short stature and other somatic abnormalities is known as *Turner's syndrome.* It may occur in more than one member of a family. There is often a web-like skin fold on each side of the neck. There is no breast development, nor feminine contour to the body, but the vulva appears to be that of a normal female. Although the uterus and vagina are present there is complete amenorrhoea and lack of secondary sexual characters because no hormones are produced by the gonads. Axillary and pubic hair is absent. The ovaries are thin streak-like structures without follicles and with a uniform fibrous stroma. Other abnormalities, including cubitus valgus and aortic coarctation, may be

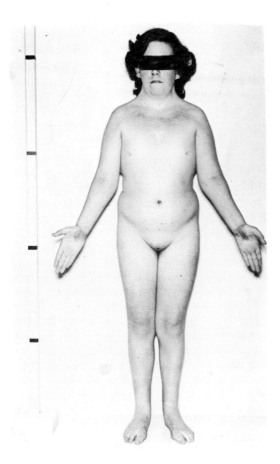

**Fig. 7.1** Turner's syndrome.

found. The urine contains no oestrogens, but gonadotrophic hormones are present. In most cases of Turner's syndrome there are 45 chromosomes; one X chromosome is missing, and the complement is written as 45 XO. Because there is only one X chromosome the nuclei will show no sex chromatin nodule.

Other patients with streak gonads do not have all of the somatic deformities of Turner's syndrome. Most of them have 46 chromosomes XX, or a mosaic of XO/XX or even XO/XY.

In *'simple' gonadal dysgenesis* the chromosomal structure is 46 XY, and the patient is a tall, apparent female, with primary amenorrhoea and no breast development, but with pubic and axillary hair. It is presumed that the Y chromosome is defective.

## True hermaphroditism

True hermaphrodites, with an ovary on one side and a testis on the other, are very rare indeed, and in such cases one or both of the gonads is almost invariably abnormal in structure and without function. Sometimes differentiation of the gonad is incomplete, and is described as an ovotestis. The chromosomal pattern may be 46 XY or a mosaic.

## Testicular feminization (androgen insensitivity syndrome)

Another recognized type of intersex is so-called testicular feminization. This may occur in more than one member of a family. The patient has an attractive female appearance, and usually presents with amenorrhoea. The skin is smooth and hairless, and the voice is female. Although scalp hair is luxuriant there is often a lack of pubic and axillary hair. The breasts are well formed. The vulva appears to be normal and, although the uterus is usually absent, there is a vaginal pit and sexual activity may be normal. If the gonads, which may be situated in the abdomen or in the groin, are examined they are found to be testes, with an excessive development of the interstitial cells. The chromosomal structure is XY.

In this disorder the gonads produce testosterone, usually in normal amounts. However, one of two deficiencies may be responsible for failure of the testosterone to bring about the normal changes seen in a male fetus. The nuclear receptor which binds testosterone and thus initiates activity in the target cell may be missing. Alternatively, the enzyme which converts testosterone into the active dihydrotestosterone may be deficient. In the latter case some virilization does take place after birth, but in the absence of the specific nuclear receptor testosterone is totally ineffective.

Malignant disease (disgerminoma, see p. 205) may develop in the abnormal testes, and it is therefore usual to remove these and to give hormone replacement therapy.

## Adrenogenital syndrome

Abnormal production of androgens by the cortex of the suprarenal gland will cause virilism in the female, and if the disorder arises in fetal life it will cause one form of pseudohermaphroditism. In these cases there is a functional disorder of the suprarenal cortex, which may be familial, in which the normal conversion of 17α-hydroxyprogesterone to cortisol is blocked, most commonly because of a deficiency of the enzyme 21-hydroxylase. Cortisol normally inhibits the production of adrenocortico-trophin, which stimulates the suprarenal cortex. The abnormal cortex cannot produce cortisol, and responds instead by producing an excess of androgens, which appear in the urine as oxosteroids. There is no detectable chromosomal abnormality, and the abnormal androgens will only produce structural changes in the female genital tract if they operate early in fetal life, at about the 11th to the 16th week.

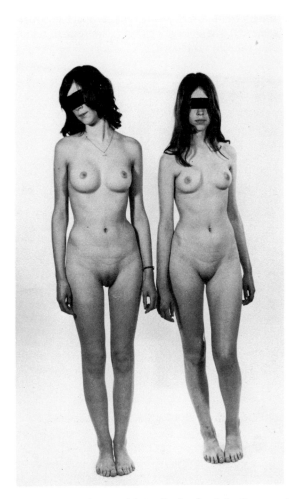

**Fig. 7.2** Two sisters with testicular feminization syndrome.

When the child is born, enlargement of the clitoris and fusion of the labia minora may be noticed, raising some doubt about the sex. Further examination will show that there is a vagina and uterus, and if (unnecessarily) a laparotomy is performed, normal ovaries will be found. A diagnostic point is that the excretion of 17-oxosteroids and of pregnanetriol are raised. It is important that a correct diagnosis is made because treatment with cortisone or related substances, which inhibit the output of adreno-corticotrophin, will prevent the further results of the disorder.

If no treatment is given, the growth of the child is slower than normal, there is excessive muscular development and precocious growth of pubic hair followed by general hirsutes. With treatment with cortisone, controlled by estimations of the urinary excretion of oxosteroids, normal menstruation and fertility will be achieved. The enlarged clitoris may require removal, and the membrane closing the vulva is incised.

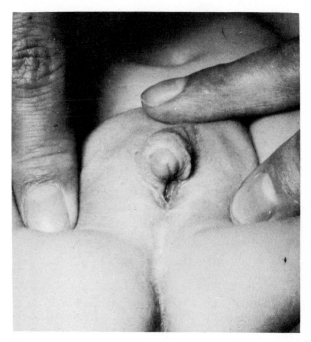

**Fig. 7.3** Enlargement of clitoris in a case of adrenogenital pseudo-hermaphroditism.

## Management of cases of intersex

It is important to make a correct assessment of the case as early in childhood as possible, and any newborn infant with abnormalities of the external genitalia should be very carefully examined. If an incorrect diagnosis of sex is made in infancy subsequent social adjustment may be most difficult.

Some patients will not present until defective growth is noticed (Turner's syndrome) or until secondary sexual characteristics or menstruation fail to appear. In a few cases an adult will seek advice because of amenorrhoea, infertility or difficulties with sexual intercourse.

After obtaining a history of the case, including the family history, a general examination is made, noting the height and general body build. Hernia should be looked for, with a possible inguinal gonad. A careful examination of the genital tract is made, under anaesthesia if necessary. An examination of a buccal smear or of leucocytes for nuclear drumsticks is helpful, although it has already been explained that this is *not* a test for 'sex' in itself. More elaborate chromosomal studies are available in special centres. An estimation of the urinary excretion of oxosteroids will lead to the diagnosis of adrenogenital pseudohermaphroditism. Laparotomy (or laparoscopy) is only occasionally justified.

If the general configuration of the body and genitalia is female, and the nuclear chromosomal mass is absent, the patient may have:
1. Turner's syndrome (45 XO).
2. Gonadal agenesis (46 XY).
3. Testicular feminization (46 XY).
4. Hypospadias and undescended testes (46 XY).

If the configuration is male, and the nuclei show chromosomal masses, the patient may have:
1. Congenital adrenogenital syndrome (46 XX).
2. Masculization by androgens given to her mother during pregnancy (46 XX).
3. Klinefelter's syndrome (47 XXY).

Patients with no breast development are likely to be true males, or else to have gonadal dysgenesis.

Management of cases of intersex is often difficult. Except in cases of the adrenogenital syndrome, it will hardly ever be possible to secure full function and fertility, and the aim of treatment must be to help the individual to fit into society in whichever sex is most appropriate. Sexual intercourse is sometimes possible and desired, and may be facilitated by surgical treatment.

In a child the first decision is the best sex for upbringing. Most cases of intersex are 'neuter' and therefore nearer to the female phenotype, and such simple procedures as removal of the phallus may assist them. In cases of testicular feminization the gonads should be removed after pubertal development because they are often subject to malignant change. Hormone replacement therapy will usually be needed.

In gonadal agenesis the secondary sexual characteristics may be developed and pseudomenstruation produced by giving sex steroids, sometimes with psychological benefit.

In older patients nothing should be done to alter the sex of a patient who has made a good social adjustment, whatever the result of scientific investigation, and some discretion should be exercised in revealing these results. If, however, the patient is ill suited to the situation in which he finds 'himself' and is willing to accept the social inconvenience of a change of sex, then surgical measures such as removal of the phallus or even more extensive surgical procedures may be considered.

Psychological difficulties are often very great, and treatment of these unfortunate individuals demands team work, with close cooperation of gynaecologist, psychiatrist and other appropriate specialists.

# 8

# Other malformations of the female genital organs

In addition to the malformations described in the preceding chapter, other abnormalities occur in most of which there is no evident chromosomal abnormality or defect of the ovaries or hormonal secretion.

## Deformities of the vulva

The hymenal opening may be very small or cribriform, but complete imperforation is rare. In most cases in which there is a membrane obstructing the entrance to the vagina it is situated above the hymen.

Enlargement of the labia minora may be congenital. In some primitive tribes considerable enlargement is produced by manipulation, the so-called 'Hottentot apron'.

Hyptertrophy of the clitoris occurs in virilism caused by androgens secreted by the adrenal cortex (p. 66) or ovarian tumours (p. 207).

## Deformities of the vagina

### Vaginal atresia

There may be a membrane obstructing the entrance to the vagina, situated above the hymen, as a result of failure of fusion of the part of the vagina derived from the Müllerian ducts with the part derived from the urogenital sinus. Less commonly, a considerable length of the vagina may be un-canalized, and sometimes the vagina is completely absent.

In cases with an obstructing membrane or partial atresia, the uterus is often normal, so that after puberty there is retention of the menstrual secretion, a condition known as *cryptomenorrhoea*. The menstrual fluid accumulates in the vagina and gradually distends it to form a *haematocolpos*. The accumulation of fluid is slow, for although the menstrual secretion each month may be 30 ml or more, some absorption of fluid occurs during the intermenstrual intervals, and the vaginal contents are concentrated to form a thick chocolate-brown fluid. If the fluid leaks back through the uterus and Fallopian tubes, the fimbriated ends of the tubes may become blocked by adhesions, and occasionally peritoneal endometriosis ensues.

Most girls with a haematocolpos present between the ages of 14 and 16. The vagina is easily distensible and at first there is little discomfort, but the accumulation of fluid gradually forms a tumour of considerable size

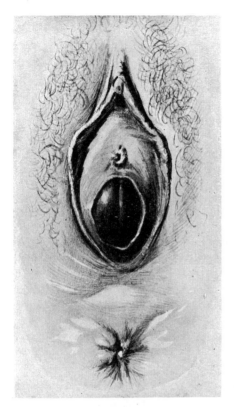

**Fig. 8.1** Vaginal atresia. The septum is seen bulging with the hymen spread out on its lower surface.

which may be felt above the symphysis pubis. If the uterus is not distended, it may be felt as a hard structure perched on top of the cystic swelling. Retention of urine may occur owing to the bladder being pushed upwards with the uterus, thus elongating the urethra. Enquiry will often show that the patient has had abdominal discomfort each month, although no external loss has occurred. Later, if the uterus or tubes are becoming distended, or if there is peritonitis, pain may be severe. The diagnosis is obvious on inspection of the vulva, when the bulging occluding membrane is seen, with a purple colour if it is thin. Rectal examination reveals a large, tense, cylindrical swelling filling the pelvis.

In newborn infants similar distension of the vagina, and sometimes of the uterus and tubes, occurs with mucoid fluid secreted by the cervix (*hydrocolpos*). A large abdominal mass is found, with a bulging membrane and urinary retention. Careful examination of the anal canal and urinary tract is most important, as there may be other congenital abnormalities.

In the rarer cases in which the atresia is at a higher level, the diagnosis is not so obvious. There is less distension of the vagina, and attacks of abdominal pain may be the most prominent feature.

Obstruction may affect one-half of a double uterus and vagina and give rise to a tumour which may cause considerable difficulty in diagnosis, since the patient menstruates regularly from the other half of the genital tract. Laparotomy may be needed to reveal the complete picture.

*Treatment*
The treatment of haematocolpos or hydrocolpos is simple. All that is necessary is to establish drainage. This is best done by excising the membrane; although simple incision will suffice immediately, stenosis may occur later and dyspareunia result. The risk of infection is considerable, and surgical technique must be meticulous. A vaginal examination should not be made when the membrane is excised. The contents may be aspirated with a vacuum extractor but should not be 'mopped out' with swabs, which could easily introduce infection. Antibiotic treatment should be started 24 hours before the operation and continued for 5 days afterwards.

If the stenosis is at the level of the cervix, it may be possible to open up the canal by dissection from below. If the vagina is absent, an artificial vagina may be constructed (see below).

The remote prognosis in cases of haematocolpos is satisfactory if the distension is confined to the vagina. If the uterus and tubes are distended, some patients become sterile as a result of sealing of the fimbrial ends of the tubes.

**Absent vagina**
In cases with complete absence of the vagina it is unusual to find a functioning uterus. There is often a shallow depression at the site of the normal vaginal orifice. If the patient wishes to marry, or if the abnormality is only discovered after attempts at intercourse, then an operation to form a cavity in the position of the vagina may be performed.

Williams' operation is a simple procedure in which the edges of the posterior parts of the labia majora are sutured together in the midline to form a perineal pouch. The artificial pouch runs in a more horizontal direction than the normal vagina, but results of the operation are often good.

A more extensive operation is that of McIndoe, in which a space is dissected in the fascial space between the rectum behind and the bladder and urethra in front. This cavity must be lined with skin or it will soon contract down. A split skin graft (Thiersch graft) is cut from the thigh and wrapped round a mould of compressed plastic foam. The graft is applied to the mould so that the basal active surface of the skin graft is directed outwards to come into close contact with the walls of the cavity. The mould is held in place with a few stitches at the introitus, and must be worn until the whole surface of the cavity is covered with living skin. The foam expands to give gentle pressure until the graft has taken.

Yet another operation that is occasionally performed is that of Baldwin, in which a section of ileum is isolated, and after intestinal continuity has been restored the isolated section is drawn down with its mesenteric blood supply to form a new vagina.

If a functioning uterus is present, it will usually be found that there is a patent cervix and an area of normal vaginal epithelium above the atresia, and that this epithelium can be freed by dissection and drawn down to the introitus.

In cases of congenital malformation of the vagina there are often also abnormalities of the ureters or kidneys, which should always be investigated by pyelography or ultrasound. In infants the anal canal must be carefully examined.

### Septate vagina
Sometimes the fusion of the two Müllerian ducts is incomplete, so that there is partial or complete duplication of the vagina, with an anteroposterior septum between the two passages. The uterus may also be duplicated. One vaginal passage may be larger than the other, and used for intercourse, or both may be equally developed. A vaginal septum may be completely missed on vaginal examination if the thin septum is displaced to one side and the other passage is not noticed. Sometimes a septum may obstruct delivery, but if it does not give way it can easily be divided.

## Deformities of the uterus

### Absent or rudimentary uterus
Complete absence of the uterus is very rare, but it may be rudimentary, when it is simply represented by a small thickening at the upper limit of the vagina. The endometrium is absent and there is amenorrhoea.

### Failure of fusion of the Müllerian ducts
Failure of fusion of the two Müllerian tracts will give rise to varying degrees of duplication of the uterus and vagina, as shown in Fig. 8.2. There may be associated abnormalities of the ureters and kidneys.

#### *Uterus didelphys*
In this condition there is a complete lack of fusion of the Müllerian ducts, with a double uterus and double vagina.

#### *Uterus bicornis bicollis*
The two horns of the uterus remain completely separate as far as their cavities are concerned, although there is some fusion of the muscular walls, and the cervix is double. There may or may not be a vaginal septum.

#### *Uterus bicornis unicollis*
The body of the uterus is bifid but the cervix is normally developed. The uterine horns may be unequal in size.

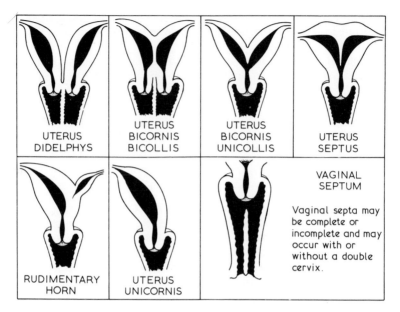

**Fig. 8.2** Diagram to show various uterine malformations.

### Uterus unicornis
Only one of the Müllerian ducts has developed to produce one Fallopian tube, the uterus and vagina. The second duct may be present in rudimentary form, with a canal which may not be patent. If the canal is not patent and the rudimentary horn contains functioning endometrium, a hemi-haematometra may form in it.

### Uterus septus
Although the ducts have fused externally the uterine cavity is partly or completely divided by a median septum. In addition, the vagina may be septate.

With all these deformities of the uterus, the vulva and hymen are usually normal, as these structures are not developed from the Müllerian cords.

In most cases of partial or total duplication of the uterus there are no gynaecological symptoms and there is normal menstruation. Pregnancy may occur in either or both sides. During pregnancy there is an increased risk of abortion, and difficulty may arise during labour because mal-presentations are more common, or because the empty horn of a double uterus comes to lie in the rectovaginal pouch below the presenting part and causes obstruction to delivery.

Pregnancy sometimes occurs in a rudimentary horn. Although such a horn may have a normal tube leading to it, there is sometimes no evident connection with the lower genital tract, and it must be assumed that the sperm which effected fertilization passed up through the opposite tube and across the peritoneal cavity. Such a pregnant horn will enlarge to accommodate the embryo for a time, but will eventually rupture, giving the same symptoms as those of tubal pregnancy, except that the accident occurs later, often at the 16th week. A rudimentary horn is easily excised.

### Congenital elongation of the cervix
This condition is mentioned here for convenience, although it is doubtful whether it is really congenital. The abnormality is nearly always discovered in adults, often in negresses. For reasons that are not understood, the vaginal portion of the cervix becomes greatly elongated, and the external os may appear at the vulva although there is no descent of the vaginal vault. If the elongation of the cervix causes any discomfort, the redundant tissue is excised.

## Abnormalities of the Fallopian tubes

The Fallopian tubes may be malformed or absent if the uterus is malformed. Congenital diverticula or accessory ostia may occur, but have no clinical significance.

## Abnormalities of the ovaries

Gonadal dysgenesis (see p. 64).

## Tumours and cysts of the broad ligament

Cysts may arise from developmental remnants in the broad ligament. Some cysts become pedunculated, but many grow between the layers of the broad ligament. They may be difficult to distinguish clinically from ovarian cysts. Small cysts are of no clinical importance, but large cysts may open up the layers of the broad ligament, push the uterus over to the opposite side, and displace the ureter upwards. With large cysts the ovary may be found flattened on the surface of the cyst.

### Fimbrial cysts
Although many broad ligament cysts arise from Wolffian remnants, some appear to arise from small remnants of ovarian tissue in relation to the fimbria ovarica. These so-called fimbrial cysts are the only broad ligament cysts to attain a large size.

The cyst originates between the abdominal ostium of the tube and the ovary. The fimbria ovarica is stretched over the cyst (Fig. 8.3). The cyst is unilocular and has a thin and translucent, but comparatively strong, wall loosely attached to the investing peritoneum. The inner surface is usually smooth, but may show a few papillary processes. The cyst contains almost colourless watery fluid of low specific gravity. On histological examination

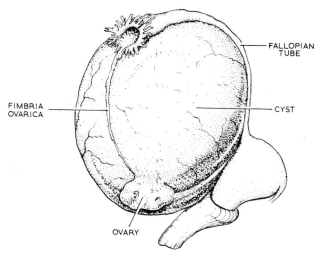

**Fig. 8.3** Fimbrial cyst showing the fimbria ovarica stretched over the cyst.

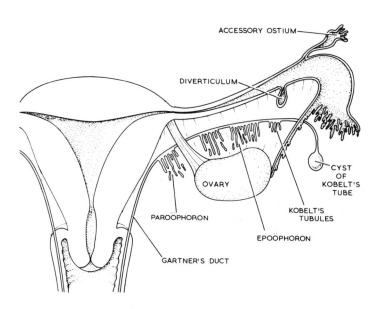

**Fig. 8.4** Diagram to show ultimate fate of the Wolffian duct and its tubules, and also tubal malformations.

the wall consists of connective tissue, lined by a single layer of low columnar epithelium.

### Cysts of Wolffian origin

If the broad ligament is held up to the light, the duct of Gartner (the Wolffian duct) may sometimes be seen lying between its layers below the Fallopian tube. It can be traced medially towards the body of the uterus, and it then turns downwards to run beside the wall of the vagina. The outer end of the duct may form a small translucent cyst about the size of a pea, which is often pedunculated (hydatid of Morgagni) and attached near the outer end of the tube.

Three sets of tubules pass from Gartner's duct towards the ovary. Kobelt's tubules form the outer set and are said to be of pronephric origin. The other tubules are mesonephric, the middle set being called the epoöphoron and the proximal set the paroöphoron. Small cysts may form in any of these, and Gartner's duct may give rise to lateral vaginal cysts.

# 9

# Genital injuries and fistulae

## Injuries to the vulva

Direct injury to the vulva can cause a large labial haematoma which may require surgical treatment; an incision is made to turn out the blood clot and any bleeding points are ligated before closing the incision.

## Injuries to the vagina

Penetrating injuries of the wall of the vagina can result from the accidental insertion of any pointed object or as a result of rape. Tearing of the hymen occurs with the first intercourse, and bleeding from a hymenal laceration can occasionally be profuse. Before any injury is sutured, careful inspection of the area, undertaken in the operating theatre with the patient anaesthetized, is essential to determine the extent of any injury.

Chemical injuries to the vagina result from caustic substances such as unduly strong antiseptic solutions used as a vaginal douche. In some primitive societies women introduce rock salt or alum into the vagina after childbirth; superficial ulceration so produced may heal well, but deeper ulceration causes dense scarring and fibrosis.

Foreign bodies left in the vagina may cause infection or ulceration. A vast range of objects have been found; the commonest are forgotten tampons, pessaries, or swabs left after vaginal operations. More bizarre objects are sometimes introduced by children or during some sexual activity.

Most vaginal injuries, however, are incurred during labour, either through prolonged pressure on the vaginal wall, by overstretching, or during obstetric operations. If the laceration of the posterior vaginal wall and perineum is extensive, the anal sphincter and the anterior wall of the anal canal may be torn. Unless the sphincter is repaired there will be incontinence of flatus and of faeces when the stool is fluid.

The most serious injuries are those which result in a fistula between the bladder or rectum and the vagina.

## Injuries to the uterus

The cervix may be torn during normal labour, or more often when forceps are used to deliver the fetal head before full dilatation has been achieved. Forcible dilatation of the cervix during gynaecological procedures, particulary prior to termination of pregnancy, may tear the circular fibres of the cervix, especially those of the internal os, with the result that the cervix becomes incompetent so that in a subsequent pregnancy mid-trimester abortion or premature labour may occur. When a patient who has had a termination becomes pregnant the cervix should always be examined regularly during the antenatal period to check that it is remaining closed.

The body of the uterus may be perforated during the operation of dilatation and curettage; this often goes unrecognized. If the operator realizes that he has perforated the uterus with a small instrument, such as a uterine sound, the patient's pulse and blood pressure should be observed half-hourly for a few hours after the operation. Usually nothing untoward follows, but occasionally, and especially if the perforation is caused by a larger instrument such as a cannula used for aspiration-termination of pregnancy, bleeding occurs into the peritoneal cavity, necessitating laparotomy and repair of the perforation. If injury to the bowel is suspected, laparotomy is immediately performed; if carcinoma of the body of the uterus is diagnosed, hysterectomy and bilateral salpingo-oöphorectomy is carried out.

The uterus may also be perforated during the insertion of an intrauterine contraceptive device.

## Fistulae

### Vesicovaginal fistula
This is a most distressing complaint. Urine constantly escapes from the vagina, making the underclothes wet and with a persistent smell of urine.

*Causes*
1. *Direct trauma.* Penetrating injuries of the anterior vaginal wall may involve the bladder, and if they are unrecognized will lead to fistula formation. The bladder may be opened during the course of obstetric and gynaecological operations, especially Caesarean section and abdominal or vaginal hysterectomy. If the injury is recognized and immediately repaired at the time of the operation, healing nearly always occurs, but failure to appreciate that damage has been done leads to a stormy postoperative course and fistula formation.

2. *Obstetric injury.* Prolonged labour in the presence of disproportion may cause compression of the bladder base between the fetal head and the pubic bone, leading to avascular necrosis of the bladder. Some days after the delivery the bladder base sloughs and a fistula develops. Although this type of vesicovaginal fistula has almost entirely disappeared in developed countries as a result of the free use of Caesarean section to prevent prolonged labour, sadly it still occurs in countries where obstetric services, particularly in rural areas, are absent or poorly staffed.

3. *Neoplastic fistulae.* Carcinoma of the cervix may invade the bladder and eventually cause a fistula. Bladder cancer rarely does this.

4. *Radiation.* Fistulae may be caused by vaginal application of caesium or other radioactive elements. They are most likely to occur during the treatment of advanced growths, and if the dose is excessive.

*Symptoms and diagnosis*
The diagnosis is generally obvious both from the history of a constant leak of urine from the vagina and from direct inspection of the anterior vaginal wall, using the speculum designed by Sims for the purpose. The position and size of the fistula vary considerably. Those caused by prolonged labour usually involve the bladder base and are situated in the midline half-way up the anterior vaginal wall; postoperative fistulae are generally higher up. Small fistulae hardly admit a probe, whereas large fistulae admit one or two fingers. With very large fistulae the whole of the urethra may have disappeared, leaving a gaping opening through which the bladder mucosa is seen, and sometimes the ureteric orifices. A pyelogram should always be done to detect possible ureteric involvement in the lesion.

Very small fistulae may not be immediately obvious, but they may be seen on cystoscopy, and injection of a solution of methylene blue into the bladder is sometimes helpful.

*Treatment*
Prevention is the best treatment, and in most cases fistula formation can be avoided. Better obstetric care is an essential preventive measure, but it may be difficult to secure when communities are poor, small and widely scattered. Village health teams which include midwives who can recognize obstructed labour early, or medical assistants who can perform an emergency Caesarean section, are increasingly being used, and should help to reduce the incidence of fistulae.

During pelvic operations the bladder must be treated with care to avoid operative injury. If damage to the bladder is suspected, every effort should be made to settle the question. Immediate repair of a hole in the bladder at this stage is easy and almost invariably successful, and will spare the patient the misery of the waiting period before secondary repair can be attempted.

Most vesicovaginal fistulae can be closed by an operation by the vaginal route. As already stated, fresh injuries are repaired at once, but in cases seen some days after the injury the timing of the operation is important. Two or three months should elapse between the time when the fistula developed and that when repair is attempted. This allows local tissue damage and infection to settle down and urinary infection to be eradicated.

The principle of the operation is to separate bladder mucosa from the vaginal skin, and then to close the mucosa carefully without tension, using fine catgut sutures in one or two layers. The vaginal skin is then closed with nylon sutures, care being taken to free the tissues laterally sufficiently to avoid tension on the suture line. When the opening is large and the tissues are deficient a flap can be fashioned from the fat in the adjacent labium majus or from the gracilis muscle and swung across between the vesical and vaginal suture lines. If the urethra has been destroyed, a new epithelial tube has to be fashioned from adjacent skin.

Postoperative care is very important; great care is taken to secure constant drainage of the bladder by catheter for three weeks to enable the repair to heal. An indwelling Bonnanno suprapubic catheter has many advantages.

Fistulae due to radiation damage may be difficult to close because the tissues are so avascular. Implantation of the ureters into an isolated loop of ileum may then be considered. Colpocleisis is occasionally employed; this consists of closing the vagina below the fistula so that leakage by that route is stopped.

Patients with vesicovaginal fistulae become very depressed as a result of the constant leak of urine and the accompanying odour, and they need a great deal of encouragement to enable them to face the discomfort of the condition and the surgical treatment. The problem is particularly difficult when successive operations are needed to close the fistula. The best results are obtained by surgeons who have had special experience of this work, and to whom difficult cases may well be referred.

Although the principles of treatment are the same in patients in under-developed countries, the problems are even greater because of malnutrition, local sepsis and very extensive scarring. In some primitive communities young girls who sustain vesicovaginal fistulae caused by pelvic disproportion during labour soon after puberty are cast out of the village when their condition makes them socially unacceptable. Unless they are able to reach a centre where treatment is available they are liable to starve and require many weeks of feeding-up and nursing before they are fit for operation. Sometimes several operations are needed to close the fistula. Expert obstetric supervision is most important for future labours, many of which are treated by Caesarean section.

### Rectovaginal fistula

Most rectovaginal fistulae are the result of third degree lacerations of the perineum and posterior vaginal wall which have not been repaired, or have broken down after repair so that an opening is left from the rectum into the vagina. Advanced carcinoma of the rectum or vagina is a cause. Burns caused by radiotherapy usually result in a stricture rather than a fistula.

If the fistula is very small there may only be a leak of mucus from the rectum, but with most fistulae flatus escapes and also faeces whenever the stool is loose. Any patient who complains of a faeculent discharge must be examined carefully for a fistula. Inspection of the posterior vaginal wall and the use of a probe will demonstrate the smaller fistulae.

The fistula is repaired after a course of phthalylsulphathiazole 2 g orally every 6 hours for 3 days. The edges of the fistula are excised and it is repaired in two layers. To repair fistulae low down near the sphincter it is often easiest to divide the perineum deliberately up to the fistula, and after dealing with the fistula the perineal body and sphincter are repaired. Whenever the sphincter is concerned in the damage, its torn ends must be exposed and sutured together if continence is to be restored. Exceptionally a temporary colostomy is needed.

### Colovaginal fistula

This is rare, but may result from rupture of a pericolic abscess into the posterior vaginal fornix; the abscess is usually secondary to acute diverticulitis. The subsequent fistula is usually small, but there is an intermittent faeculent discharge. The diagnosis is usually obvious if a barium enema is given. Closure of the fistula involves laparotomy and resection of the affected part of the colon.

### Ureterovaginal fistula

The close anatomical relationship of the ureter and the uterus occasionally leads to damage to the ureter during pelvic operations. The ureter may be damaged at the pelvic brim when the infundibulopelvic ligaments is being cut and tied during oöphorectomy. More commonly it is damaged lower down in its course during abdominal or vaginal hysterectomy when the uterine artery and transverse cervical ligament are being clamped or divided. Fibromyomata which extend into the base of the broad ligament may displace the ureter from its normal position and make it especially vulnerable. Apart from direct operative injury the ureter may develop a fistula as a result of interference with its blood supply when it is dissected out during a Wertheim's hysterectomy, especially if the patient has received previous radiotherapy.

Early diagnosis is essential, and the possibility of damage to the ureter should always be considered when a patient's postoperative course after hysterectomy is complicated by renal pain and pyrexia. When the ureter has been tied, acute pain and tenderness of the kidney is immediately obvious. When the ureter has been cut, the escape of urine into the extraperioneal tissues of the pelvis causes the patient to develop a high temperature, and she looks obviously ill. Once the diagnosis is suspected, an intravenous pyelogram will demonstrate which ureter is involved. That on the affected side is usually dilated down to the site of injury, or there may be failure of secretion on that side.

Sometimes the patient's immediate postoperative course is uneventful and the presence of a fistula becomes obvious only when she begins to leak urine constantly from the vagina, while she passes about half the normal output from the bladder. Although an intravenous pyelogram may show which ureter is damaged, and sometimes the fistulous track is seen, retrograde ureteric catheterization may be needed to demonstrate the exact site of the injury.

If the diagnosis is made within 72 hours of the operation an immediate laparotomy is performed; otherwise the operation is done electively later. If the ureteric damage is close to the bladder, the cut or tied end is freshened and then reimplanted into the bladder. Damage to the ureter at the level of the pelvic brim may call for the use of a bladder flap (Boari technique) to bridge the distance between the cut end of the ureter and the bladder.

When implantation of the cut end of the ureter into the bladder is not possible, ureteric anastomosis may be attempted, the two cut ends being sewn together with fine catgut sutures. A ureter repaired in this way will usually heal, but there is a risk of a stricture forming later at the site of anastomosis.

# 10

# Genital prolapse

In uterovaginal prolapse there is damage to, or weakness of, the structures which support the pelvic organs, so that some of these descend from their normal positions and finally herniate through the vaginal opening. Certain terms may first be defined (Fig. 10.1).

*Cystocele*
Prolapse of the bladder and anterior vaginal wall is known as a cystocele. Descent of the urethra and bladder neck may occur separately or accompany a cystocele; when sagging of the urethra occurs alone it is sometimes known as a *urethrocele.*

*Rectocele*
Prolapse of the rectum and posterior vaginal wall is known as a rectocele. It is usually accompanied by some deficiency of the perineal body.

*Uterine prolapse*
Prolapse of the uterus is accompanied by descent and inversion of the vaginal vault. Three degrees of uterine prolapse are described: (1) the uterus becomes retroverted and descends in the axis of the vagina though the cervix does not reach the introitus; (2) the cervix appears at or protrudes from the vaginal orifice; (3) the vaginal walls are everted to such a degree that the uterus lies outside the vulva; this complete form of uterine prolapse is known as procidentia.

Cystocele or rectocele or both may occur without uterine descent, but uterine prolapse is accompanied by descent of the bladder because of the close attachment of the bladder to the anterior aspect of the supravaginal cervix. Descent of the rectum does not necessarily accompany uterine prolapse because the prolapsing vaginal wall easily becomes separated from the rectum.

*Enterocele*
A hernia of the rectovaginal peritoneal pouch through the posterior vaginal fornix is known as an enterocele. Elongation of the rectovaginal pouch inevitably accompanies uterine prolapse, and small intestine may be found in the peritoneal sac behind the uterus in cases of procidentia. Enterocele may also occur without uterine prolapse, and cause a bulge of the upper part of the posterior vaginal wall which must be distinguished from a

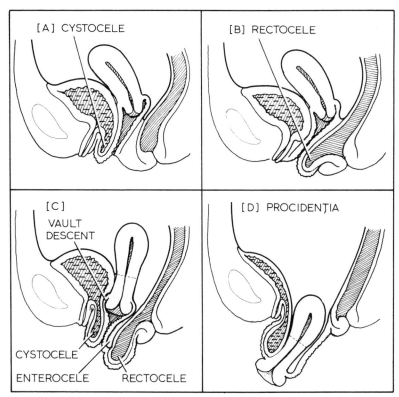

**Fig. 10.1** Diagrams to show varieties of prolapse. Note elongation of supravaginal cervix in C and D.

rectocele. Enterocele may occasionally occur after the uterus has been removed by abdominal or vaginal hysterectomy, and is usually combined with some degree of prolapse of the vaginal vault.

## Supporting structures

*Pelvic floor*
The floor of the pelvic cavity consists of a muscular diaphragm formed by the levatores ani muscles. The medial edges of the levator muscles (pubococcygeal portion) form the lateral boundaries of the urogenital aperture, through which pass the vagina and urethra; these muscles have a sphincteric action on the vaginal introitus. A few fibres from the medial edge of the pubococcygeus are inserted into the urethral and vaginal walls. These muscles may be regarded as slings which pass round the urethra, vagina and rectum; by their contraction they pull these structures upwards and forwards. The superficial group of perineal muscles and the deep trans-

verse perineal muscles also contribute fibres to the perineal body, but the levators are the most important supporting muscles.

Although the pelvic floor may be said to support the pelvic organs, it does so indirectly. The posterior vaginal wall is supported by the perineal body. Since the vagina has an oblique course upwards and backwards, when the patient is standing the anterior vaginal wall (above which is the bladder) rests on the posterior wall. Thus the perineal body and levator sling serve as an indirect support for all these structures.

The uterus does not rest on the levator muscles but is held in place at a higher level by the ligaments and connective tissues of the pelvic fascia. Deficiency of the perineal body, into which fibres of the pubococcygeal part of the levator ani are inserted, causes widening or laxity of the pelvic floor aperture, but this does not necessarily lead to uterine prolapse; indeed, a complete perineal tear may be present for many years without any uterine descent.

*Pelvic fascia*
Descent of the uterus is only possible if the fascial structures which support it are injured or atrophic. The most important ligaments supporting the uterus are the transverse cervical or cardinal ligaments, which attach the cervix and vaginal vault to the side walls of the pelvis. The uterus is also supported by the uterosacral ligaments, which pass upwards and backwards from the cervix and vaginal vault to blend with the fascia covering the front of the second and third sacral segments. Anteriorly the uterosacral ligaments cannot be separated from the cardinal ligaments, and both structures lie in the same oblique plane (Fig. 10.2). The rectum and the rectovaginal pouch lie between the uterosacral ligaments. Both the cardinal and the uterosacral ligaments contain smooth muscle and elastic fibres.

The bladder rests upon and is supported by the pubocervical fascia, which passes downwards and forwards from the cervix to the posterior surface of the bodies of the pubic bones. Although this fascia is sometimes described as a ligament, it is not so definite a structure as the cardinal or uterosacral ligaments.

The upper surface of the levator ani muscle is covered by a sheet of dense fascia. This fascia closes the genital hiatus between the medial edges of the levator muscles, except where the vagina and urethra emerge. Both the urethra and vagina have tubular sheaths of fascia, continuous below with the levator fascia. The periurethral fascia is continuous above with the fascia which invests the bladder, and at the bladder base lateral extensions of the fascia extend outwards towards the pelvic walls and form the major supports of the bladder.

The rectum also has a tubular investment of fascia, which can easily be separated from the vaginal fascia. The rectovaginal peritoneal pouch is not strongly supported between the uterosacral ligaments, and it is at this point that the pouch sometimes herniates downwards as an enterocele.

The broad ligaments and the round ligaments have little or no supporting function, and easily become elongated if the uterus descends.

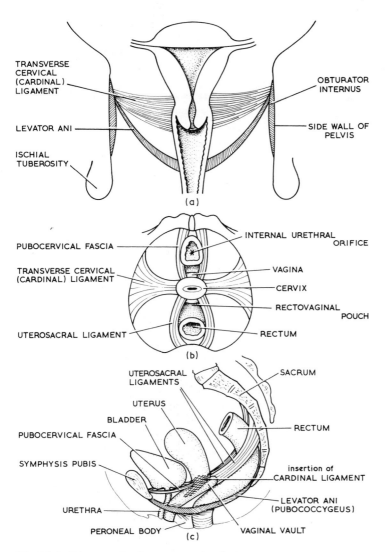

**Fig. 10.2** Diagrams to show supports of uterus.

### Causes of prolapse

Nearly all patients suffering from prolapse have borne children, and in some cases the prolapse becomes evident soon after a particular confinement. Prolapse is almost invariably the result of damage to the supporting structures during childbirth, yet in many cases the prolapse does not become evident until after the menopause, when some degree of atrophy of these structures occurs.

*Obstetric factors*

During delivery the fetal head stretches the supporting structures of the pelvic organs as it passes through the cervix and down the vagina. The perivaginal fascial sheath may be overstretched and the urogenital hiatus widened by separation of the levatores ani muscles.

If the patient is instructed to bear down before full dilatation of the cervix, or if the doctor applies forceps traction in the first stage of labour, the cervix will be dragged downwards in front of the fetal head and the transverse cervical ligaments may be overstretched.

A common obstetrical injury is tearing or overstretching of the perineal body, which removes the support of the posterior vaginal wall and, therefore, indirectly that of the anterior wall and bladder.

Prolonged labour, especially a long second stage, or delivery of a large fetus, increases the likelihood of damage, as does an occipito-posterior position of the head. Forceps delivery, by shortening the second stage of labour diminishes the risk of overstretching the perineum, although difficult forceps delivery may damage the other supporting structures.

Episiotomy is helpful in preventing perineal damage; a clean incision is preferable to an irregular tear, and episiotomy will prevent overstretching of the structures. Careful repair of the episiotomy or of any laceration diminishes the risk of subsequent prolapse.

Although considerable laxity of the vaginal walls may be evident immediately after delivery, this will as a rule diminish considerably within a few weeks as muscular tone recovers.

*Postmenopausal atrophy*

Prolapse often becomes more marked, or may appear for the first time, after the menopause, and most cases of procidentia are seen in elderly women in whom the uterus and its supports are atrophic. Atrophy of the ligaments and fascial structures is associated with diminished oestrogen secretion, and there is lowered muscle tone with increasing age. Rare cases of prolapse in nulliparous women are explained by atrophy of the pelvic supports with age. In these cases descent of the uterus and vaginal vault occurs, with little cystocele or rectocele.

*Intra-abdominal pressure*

Violent coughing, unaccustomed heavy work or a large intra-abdominal tumour may be contributory factors in cases of prolapse.

*Postoperative prolapse*

Abdominal hysterectomy involves division of the supporting ligaments of the uterus, but fortunately in most cases sufficient attachment of the cardinal and uterosacral ligaments to the vault remains, so that prolapse is an uncommon sequel of this operation; however, in cases with pre-existing prolapse, hysterectomy will do nothing to deal with the elongated ligaments, and will make matters worse rather than better unless it is combined with repair of these ligaments and the pelvic floor.

Prolapse of the rectovaginal pouch or enterocele sometimes follows vaginal hysterectomy or the Manchester operation for prolapse and may occur either because the operator has failed to recognize and remove a pre-existing pouch or because he has failed to close the gap between the uterosacral ligaments.

## Morbid anatomy

Most of the anatomical changes in prolapse have already been described, but other secondary changes may now be mentioned.

The vaginal epithelium becomes stretched and increased in area, and if it is exposed it soon becomes thickened, and sometimes dry and ulcerated. Ulceration may also arise from a neglected ring pessary.

In cases with gross prolapse of the vaginal walls, the drag of these structures on the cervix leads to elongation of the supravaginal cervix and to oedema and enlargement of the vaginal portion. If the cervix is exposed, it may become ulcerated, and secondary infection gives rise to mucopurulent or blood-stained discharge.

If there is a large cystocele, the bladder often empties incompletely and cystitis from bacterial infection is a common sequel. In cases with uterine descent the ureters are carried downwards with the cardinal ligaments, but are not usually obstructed.

## Symptoms

*Local discomfort* results from the prolapsed part bulging into the vagina and eventually protruding through the vaginal opening, with drag on the supporting structures. The sensation of prolapse is increased on coughing, standing or exertion. It is relieved when the patient lies down.

*Backache* sometimes accompanies the local discomfort, and similarly is worse on standing and relieved when the patient lies down. However, in the majority of patients with prolapse any backache will be found to have some other cause, and it is important to consider this possibility before promising patients that treatment of the prolapse will cure the backache.

*Urinary symptoms.* Frequency of micturition is almost invariable in patients who have a cystocele. Incomplete emptying of the bladder predisposes to urinary infection, causing dysuria. In procidentia the patient sometimes has to push up the prolapse before she can empty the bladder.

Stress incontinence is often associated with prolapse. In this condition the patient involuntarily passes a small quantity of urine whenever she coughs or strains. Strictly speaking, this is a separate lesion, for it can occur in the absence of any prolapse – and severe prolapse can occur without stress incontinence. Stress incontinence needs to be differentiated from urge incontinence caused by excessive detrusor tone (see p. 334).

*Bowel symptoms.* With a rectocele there may be difficulty in emptying the bowel. As the patient strains, the rectocele bulges into the vagina, preventing normal evacuation of the faeces through the anus unless she pushes the rectocele back with her fingers.

*Ulceration and bleeding.* In procidentia, exposed cervical and vaginal

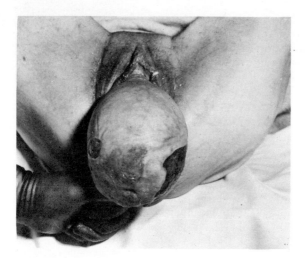

**Fig. 10.3**  Procidentia showing ulceration of the everted vaginal wall. The external cervical os is just above the surgeon's hand.

skin becomes keratinized and dry. Rubbing against clothing may lead to the formation of superficial ulcers, and a blood-stained discharge.

### Diagnosis
The diagnosis of genital prolapse may be obvious on inspecting the vulva with the patient lying on her back and straining down. With lesser degrees of prolapse the patient is best examined in the left lateral position. A Sims speculum passed in this position enables an assessment of anterior wall prolapse to be made. The degree of uterine prolapse is not easy to assess without pulling down the uterus with a volsellum attached to the cervix. As this may be uncomfortable for the patient, it is best performed prior to operation when the patient is already anaesthetized. Rectocele and enterocele are obvious on inspection of the posterior vaginal wall while the patient is straining, but a rectal examination may have to be made to distinguish between them. Stress incontinence can usually be demonstrated by asking the patient to cough when the bladder is full, when a small jet of urine may be seen to escape from the urinary meatus.

### Treatment

*Prevention*
The importance of preventing and limiting injury to the pelvic floor and supporting structures during delivery has already been mentioned. While the value of postnatal pelvic floor exercises as a means of preventing prolapse has not been strictly proven, they are probably beneficial.

Frequent pregnancies at unduly short intervals may increase the risk of prolapse.

*Surgical treatment*

Many women with slight prolapse have no discomfort and do not require treatment. A few may find pelvic floor exercises helpful.

Prolapse which is causing discomfort should be treated surgically unless (1) the woman intends to have another baby in the near future or (2) she is too old or ill for an operation. In fact, most elderly women tolerate vaginal surgery well, and the benefits of successful repair are so great that the majority of patients can and should be operated upon.

The details of the operations for the repair of prolapse are given on p. 350. In principle, anterior vaginal wall prolapse requires anterior colporrhaphy, particular attention being paid to supporting the urethra and urethrovesical junction. Posterior vaginal wall prolapse is treated by posterior colporrhaphy, which includes excision of the sac of any enterocele and repair of the perineal body (perineorrhaphy).

Uterine prolapse is best treated by vaginal hysterectomy combined with careful suturing together of the divided uterine supports, and such repair of the vaginal walls as may be necessary. If there is only first degree descent, an alternative procedure is the Manchester (Fothergill) operation. After partial amputation of the elongated cervix, the cut transverse cervical ligaments are joined to the front of the cervical stump, thereby shortening them and elevating the uterus, and the operation is completed by such repair of the vaginal walls as is needed. Amputation of the cervix reduces cervical mucus, which is probably necessary for successful sperm penetration and conception. The cervix should be left intact if the patient wishes to have another child.

*Pregnancy after operations for prolapse*

If a patient becomes pregnant after a Manchester operation there is a slightly increased risk of cervical incompetence and mid-trimester abortion because of damage to the internal os. Occasionally amputation of the cervix is followed by fibrosis, so that it fails to dilate during labour. But in the majority of cases both pregnancy and labour are normal.

There is a risk of recurrence of the prolapse after vaginal delivery, and Caesarean section must be considered. It is certainly wise for cases in which stress incontinence has been successfully treated, as this can be a difficult symptom to cure, but in other cases vaginal delivery may be allowed after episiotomy.

*Palliative treatment*

Treatment of prolapse with a pessary may be considered as a temporary measure in the early months of pregnancy, or in patients who hope to have another child or to postpone operative treatment. Occasionally a pessary may be advised when a patient is unfit for an anaesthetic, or when the operation is refused by the patient.

A ring pessary is used, made of polyethylene or 'flexible vinyl'. The diameters are given in millimetres; the correct size for the patient is the largest size of which she is unaware. If the ring is too small it may be

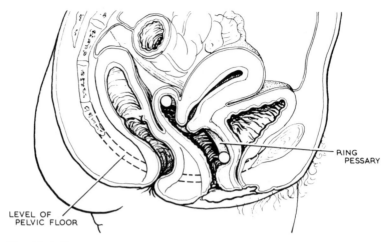

LEVEL OF
PELVIC FLOOR

RING
PESSARY

**Fig. 10.4**  Ring pessary in place.

expelled from the vagina on straining, and if it is too large it will cause discomfort and may cause pressure necrosis and ulceration of the vaginal walls.

Before a pessary is inserted a vaginal examination is made to exclude any other abnormality, to replace the uterus if it is retroverted and to assess the probable size of ring required. The pessary is compressed into an ellipse for passage through the vaginal introitus. As the ring passes into the vagina and above the pelvic floor, it returns to its circular form. The forefinger guides the upper part of the ring into the posterior fornix so that the cervix lies within the ring. The patient is re-examined to make sure that the vaginal walls are not unduly stretched, and she is then asked to strain down to see that the ring is large enough not to be expelled.

Rubber ring pessaries should not be used because they cause vaginitis. The polyethylene pessary causes little irritation and douching is not required. The ring need only be changed after 12 months. However, if any purulent discharge or bleeding occurs the patient should report at once, and the ring is removed before full investigation.

# 11

# Retroversion and inversion of the uterus

## Retroversion of the uterus

The uterus normally lies at an angle to the vagina so that the fundus is directed forwards and the cervix points backwards into the posterior fornix — the position of anteversion. If the fundus is directed backwards with the cervix pointing into the anterior fornix, the uterus is said to be retroverted. If the anteverted uterus is bent forwards on itself, it is said to be anteflexed; similarly the retroverted uterus may be retroflexed.

Retroversion is recognized on bimanual pelvic examination when the cervix is found to be directed forwards and, with the examining fingers in the posterior vaginal fornix, the body of the uterus can be felt. It is important to ascertain the precise position of the uterus before inserting an intrauterine contraceptive device or taking an endometrial biopsy, and if there is doubt a uterine sound can be passed.

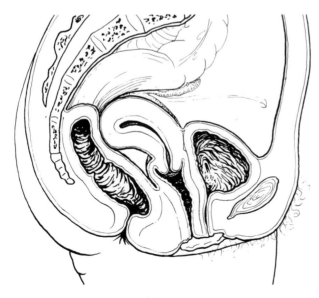

Fig. 11.1 Retroversion of the uterus.

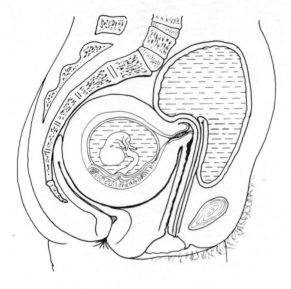

**Fig. 11.2**   Retroversion of the pregnant uterus.

## Retroversion uncomplicated by pelvic disease

In 20 per cent of normal women the uterus is retroverted. Although such cases of retroversion are described as 'congenital' the retroversion in fact occurs at the time of puberty. In the infant the uterus is straight and upright, with the cervix and body of equal length. As the body of the uterus enlarges at puberty it usually becomes anteverted and anteflexed, but it sometimes adopts the opposite position.

This form of retroversion is of little clinical significance. The uterus is mobile and can be pushed forwards into the position of anteversion by pressure in the posterior fornix. If pregnancy occurs, as the uterus enlarges it nearly always rises up into the abdomen in the normal way at about the 12th week, and after delivery it resumes its retroverted position. If the uterus is observed to be retroverted in early pregnancy, no attempt should be made to correct the position.

In rare instances the fundus of the retroverted gravid uterus becomes impacted under the sacral promontory, and the uterus is then said to be incarcerated in the pelvic cavity. The cervix is directed forwards and slightly *upwards,* as shown in Fig. 11.1. Because the bladder base is attached to the supravaginal cervix the urethra becomes stretched and elongated, and retention of urine may occur at about the 14th week. The distended bladder should not be mistaken for the pregnant uterus if the direction of the cervix is noted. A catheter must be passed to relieve the retention; spontaneous anteversion almost invariably occurs as the bladder is emptied, especially if the patient lies prone.

Uncomplicated retroversion does not cause infertility, and in the absence of incarceration it will not cause miscarriage.

The uterus is sometimes discovered to be retroverted in the puerperium or at a postnatal examination. Most of these cases are merely instances of pre-existing retroversion in which the uterus has returned to its usual position. Symptoms such as backache and dyspareunia are sometimes attributed to retroversion discovered after delivery. Some women do have backache in the first few months after delivery, but this is more often the result of fatigue and poor muscle tone than of the position of the uterus. If these patients are left untreated, the backache usually resolves spontaneously.

Deep dyspareunia has been attributed to prolapse of the ovaries into the rectovaginal pouch in cases of retroversion, but unless the ovaries are fixed in the pouch by endometriosis or inflammatory adhesions it is most unlikely that they would be pressed upon during intercourse.

If the uterus is tender and movement of it reproduces the discomfort that the patient experiences during intercourse, then it is justifiable to correct the retroversion by the operation of ventrosuspension. One method (Gilliam's operation) is to open the abdomen through a small transverse incision, and then to shorten the round ligaments on each side so as to pull the uterus forwards and hold it in anteversion. Alternatively, this can be done by a laparascopic technique.

## Retroversion incidental to other pelvic diseases

(a) *Prolapse*
In cases of prolapse the uterus becomes retroverted as it descends through the vagina. Any symptoms are those of prolapse, not of retroversion, and the treatment is that for prolapse.

(b) *Fixation by pelvic adhesions*
In chronic salpingo-oöphoritis or endometriosis adhesions may form behind the uterus (Fig. 11.3) and hold it in retroversion. If the uterus is found to be fixed in the retroverted position, especially if this is comfirmed by examination under anaesthesia, the presence of such adhesions should be suspected. The history of the case, or the discovery of tubo-ovarian swellings behind the uterus, will often suggest the cause. Such symptoms as menorrhagia, dysmenorrhoea or dyspareunia may be present, but are due to the underlying disease, not the retroversion. This type of retroversion is sometimes corrected by ventrosuspension at the conclusion of operation for the underlying disease.

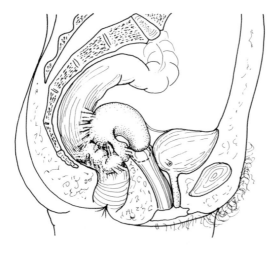

**Fig. 11.3** Fixed retroversion caused by adhesions following salpingo-oöphoritis.

## Inversion of the uterus

Inversion of the uterus, in which it is turned inside out so that the fundus passes through the cervix into the vagina, is a rare but dangerous complication of the third stage of labour, sometimes caused by attempts to deliver the fundally inserted placenta by traction on the cord before placental separation has occurred, and while the uterus is not contracting. (See 'Obstetrics by Ten Teachers'.)

In a non-pregnant woman inversion may occur from the slow but progressive extrusion through the cervix of a submucous fibromyomatous polyp arising from the uterine fundus. The cervix dilates to allow the passage of the fibromyoma and ultimately the fundus itself. On bimanual examination a depression may be felt in place of the fundus. Removal of the polyp by vaginal myomectomy may allow the inversion to be corrected, but in most cases the best treatment is hysterectomy.

# 12

## Infection and inflammation of the vulva

### Vulvitis

The skin covering the vulva may be involved in any generalized dermatological disorder but its special anatomical situation makes it liable to a number of inflammatory conditions which are confined to the genital area. Although micro-organisms abound in the vulval and perineal regions, normal skin is resistant to invasion by most of these. However, if the skin is continually moist because of vaginal discharge or urinary incontinence irritation may occur, which leads to scratching and damage to the macerated skin. Resistance of the skin to infection is also reduced if there are atrophic or degenerative changes as a result of disease or reduced oestrogen levels after the climacteric.

Specific organisms may also cause infection; for example, staphylococci may infect sebaceous glands or hair follicles, *Candida albicans* may grow freely if there is glycosuria, and treponemata or other organisms may be transmitted at coitus.

In addition, non-infective dermatitis may be caused by sensitivity reactions to chemical agents such as medicinal applications or toilet preparations.

Because there are so many causes of vulvitis, careful investigation is always necessary. A full gynaecological history and examination are required. Special attention must be paid to any skin disorders elsewhere. The urine must be tested for sugar and examined bacteriologically. Any vaginal discharge must be investigated. On occasion rectal swabs should be examined and proctoscopy may be required. The skin may be examined bacteriologically and by histological examination of scrapings or a biopsy.

Vulvitis may be acute or chronic, but such a classification helps little, and an aetiological one is more satisfactory:

1. Vulvitis due to specific infections.
2. Vulvitis due to sensitivity reactions.
3. Vulvitis secondary to vaginal discharge or urinary disorders.
4. Vulval dystrophies.

## Vulvitis due to specific infections

### (1) Virus infections

(a) *Condylomata acuminata (viral warts).* These soft pink or whitish papillomata may occur on any part of the vulva. They consist of numerous fine frond-like processes. The warts vary in size from 1 mm to about 2 cm, and rarely the whole vulva may be obscured by them. They may extend up into the vagina. Sometimes there is severe irritation.

Although infection with *Trichomonas vaginalis* is often found, this is coincidental and the possibility of other sexually transmitted infections must also be considered. The condylomata are caused by a human papilloma-virus (HVP 6) which is usually transmitted by sexual contact, with an incubation period of several weeks. The male partner may have or may develop penile warts. Condylomata may enlarge and spread during pregnancy. The virus cannot be cultured by the techniques which are ordinarily available.

The warts have the structure of papillomata; a central core of connective tissue with blood vessels is covered with a thick epidermal layer consisting of an overgrowth of the prickle cells. Electron microscopy shows that these cells are filled with virus particles.

The best treatment is to remove the warts with cutting diathermy under general anaesthesia. The resulting small burns are uncomfortable and require frequent bathing and simple antiseptic dressings to prevent infection. When there are very few warts the excision can be done under local anaesthesia. They can also be treated by cryosurgery or with a laser. Any coincidental vaginal discharge must be investigated and treated. There is a tendency for the warts to recur, and more than one session of treatment may be needed. Any male contacts should be followed up.

Warts can also be treated by application of 20 per cent podophyllin in benzoin tincture. This is a painful and not very effective treatment.

(b) *Herpes genitalis.* This viral infection is transmitted venereally. It is described on p. 140.

(c) *Molluscum contagiosum* is caused by a pox virus which is transmitted by body contact or towels or clothing. Pearly-white umbilicated nodules can occur anywhere on the skin. They are treated by application of phenol to the centre of each papule. Diathermy or cryosurgery can also be used.

### (2) Bacterial infections

(a) *Chancroid (soft sore).* This is caused by Ducrey's bacillus, which is transmitted sexually. Multiple painful shallow ulcers occur on the vulva. There is inguinal adenitis and secondary infection generally occurs with the formation of a bubo (abscess) in the groin (see p. 141).

(b) *Gonorrhoea.* Gonococci do not invade the vulval skin, but may cause infection of Skene's tubules at the lower end of the urethra. They may also cause a Bartholin's abscess, although this lesion is more commonly due to other organisms.

(c) *Syphilis.* The vulva may be affected by a primary chancre. In the secondary stage condylomata lata appear as raised plaques with a slightly indented top which is covered by a greyish exudate.

(d) *Lymphogranuloma venereum.* This chronic sexually transmitted disease is caused by a strain of *Chlamydia trachomatis* (see p. 142). It is rare in Britain, but may be encountered in ports where it is introduced by seamen.

(e) *Granuloma inguinale.* This is another sexually transmitted disease, of tropical origin. The organism causing it is uncertain (p. 142).

(f) *Tuberculosis.* Vulval tuberculosis is very rare. Infection is secondary to other lesions higher in the genital tract. An ulcer is formed with bluish undermined edges.

(g) *Furunculosis.* Staphylococci may infect the hair follicles on the outer aspect of the labia majora. Bacteriological examination of the pus will decide the choice of an antibiotic.

### (3) Fungal infections

(a) *Candidiasis.* In diabetic patients with glycosuria, vulvitis due to infection with *Candida albicans* may occur. The whole vulva is inflamed with an appearance described as that of raw beef. The urine should be tested for sugar in all cases of vulvitis. However, infection with *Candida* is not confined to diabetics, and is common during pregnancy especially if the renal threshold for sugar is lowered. It may also occur in patients who are using oral contraceptives or who have recently been given antibiotics. The modern use of tight-fitting nylon underwear prevents normal skin aeration and encourages recurrent infection. The vagina is often the primary site of infection and the fungus is usually easily found there, but it can also be demonstrated by staining scrapings of the vulval skin.

Treatment of diabetes, if that is present, will often clear up the infection. Vulval infection will usually resolve if the vaginal infection is treated with fungicidal pessaries or creams (see p. 110). In resistant cases, an alternative treatment is to paint the vagina and vulva with an aqueous solution of gentian violet (0.5 per cent). The dye will stain clothing, and the patient should be warned of this.

(b) *Tinea cruris (ringworm).* Bright red circumscribed lesions may occur in association with ringworm of the feet. Scrapings of the skin are examined microscopically to show the fungus. Treatment is with benzoic acid compound ointment or zinc undecenoate ointment. Some fungi (*Trichophyton rubrum*) will respond to griseofulvin 500 mg twice daily by mouth for 4 weeks.

### (4) Parasitic infections

(a) *Phthirus pubis.* Lice may inhabit the pubic hair. Because of scratching and lack of hygiene there may be vulvitis. The crab louse and its eggs are found on the hairs. Treatment is by application of gamma-benzene hexachloride. After rubbing the preparation into the hair the area should not be washed for 24 hours. Repeated applications may be required.

(b) *Scabies.* Infestation with *Sarcoptes scabiei* can affect the vulva as well as other parts of the body. The parasite burrows through the skin, laying ova in its tunnel. Vesicles and pustules result and, because of the intense irritation, scratching causes excoriation. Benzyl benzoate application is used.

(c) *Enterobius vermicularis.* Threadworms from the anus may cause vulval irritation in children. The worms are easily seen in the stools, and the irritation is relieved when they are eradicated from the bowel.

### Vulvitis due to sensitivity reactions

The vulval skin may become sensitized to many agents, with resulting dermatitis. These agents include ointments prescribed by doctors or bought by the patient from chemists for the relief of pruritis, and detergents, deodorants and dusting powders. Sensitivity may occur to contraceptive creams, to the rubber of contraceptive caps or condoms, or to powder used with them.

In any case of vulvitis careful enquiry must be made about any local applications to the vulval area and any recent changes in the use of toilet preparations or contraceptives. Patch tests can sometimes identify the offending agent. Any substance under suspicion must be withdrawn and zinc or calamine cream applied. Betamethasone valerate ointment (Betnovate) or hydrocortisone ointment may be used; but ointments containing benzocaine or antihistamines should be avoided, as sensitivity to these is not uncommon. Many successes will be obtained merely by withdrawing all local applications and by stopping the patient scratching. To do this it is often necessary to give a sedative at night to ensure that the patient sleeps soundly without scratching.

### Vulvitis secondary to vaginal discharge or urinary disorders

Vulvitis may be secondary to vaginitis; for example, in cases of profuse discharge due to infection with *Trichomonas vaginalis.* Irritation will occur if there is sufficient vaginal discharge from any cause to keep the vulval skin continually moist, and scratching will add to the damage to the skin. If there is urinary incontinence, especially if the urine is also infected, vulvitis may ensue. The association with glycosuria has already been mentioned. In vulval dermatitis of long standing there may be some thickening and pigmentation of the skin, but the skin soon recovers when the cause is removed.

### Vulval dystrophies

These conditions have previously been classified under the three headings leukoplakia, lichen sclerosus et atrophicus, and kraurosis. The term leukoplakia (Greek, white plate) has been criticized because it has no clinical or pathological precision, and the term kraurosis (Greek, dry) became unsuitable because it was used to imply contraction of the vulva, which could be the end result of more than one condition. Indeed those who believe that these vulval disorders are all stages or varients of a single process have placed them under one heading — *vulval dystrophy* — but we believe that some subdivision should be made. The following classification is used here:

Primary atrophy, often formerly described as kraurosis.

Lichen sclerosus et atrophicus.

Hypertrophic dystrophy, often formerly described as leukoplakia.

**Primary atrophy**

For unknown reasons the skin of the vulva may undergo atrophy. This tends to occur at the time of the climacteric, and it is natural to assume that withdrawal of oestrogens is the cause. However, atrophy may take place before the climacteric, and atrophy does not always occur after the menopause, so some other factor may be involved.

Histological examination of normal skin shows a well defined wavy line between the epidermis and the dermis. There is progressive maturation in the epidermis from the basal cells through the prickle cells to the keratinized cells on the surface. As the superficial cells are rubbed off, they are replaced from the deeper layers. The dermis consists of collagen fibrils with associated fibroblasts.

In primary atrophy the whole epidermis becomes thin and the wavy line between it and the dermis becomes flattened. There are very few prickle cells and almost no keratin. Immediately below the epidermis, the dermis shows hyalinization and the fibrillary structure is lost. There is also infiltration with lymphocytes and plasma cells.

The clinical appearances mirror the histological changes, for the skin looks red and shiny because of its thinness. The labia minora are shrunken, and the introitus may contract so that dyspareunia occurs. The complaint is of soreness rather than pruritus. The skin involved is that of the genital area; the adjacent skin of the thighs and perineum is not involved.

An initial trial of treatment with oestrogens is worth while, although many cases of true primary atrophy show no response. Dienoestrol cream is applied locally, or ethinyloestradiol 10 micrograms daily is given by mouth. Otherwise bland ointments such as calamine cream, or zinc and ichthyol cream are used to reduce soreness. If there is superadded inflammation, betamethasone cream or hydrocortisone cream may be helpful.

These patients must be followed up for many years, as hypertrophic changes (see below) may appear later. If there is any doubt about this, biopsy should be performed.

**Lichen sclerosus et atrophicus**

This disorder is of unknown cause. Similar lesions are sometimes found on other parts of the body. There are areas of slightly thickened ivory-coloured skin, which are often symmetrical and may extend onto adjacent parts of the thighs or perineal region. (Primary atrophy and hypertrophic dystrophy

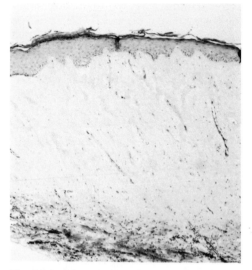

**Fig. 12.1**  Primary atrophy of vulva. The epidermis is thin and the rete pegs are small. There is a hyalinized zone beneath the epidermis.

do not extend onto these regions.) There is hyperkeratosis, and it is this increase in the keratin layer which helps to distinguish this condition from primary atrophy; otherwise the histological picture is similar in the two conditions. There is intense pruritus rather than soreness.

There is no specific treatment. Treatment with bland applications, as described in the previous section, is given. Although excision of affected skin by simple vulvectomy is sometimes performed to relieve pruritus, the disease may recur at the margins of the area of excision. Hypertrophic changes may follow, for which biopsy may often be wise.

**Hypertrophic dystrophy or leukoplakia**
This change in the vulval skin often occurs on a basis of previous atrophy, therefore the histological picture is a compound of the two processes. The rete pegs of the epidermis dip deeply into the dermis. The cells of the basal layer show active mitosis, the prickle cell layer is increased in thickness and there is a heavy accumulation of keratin on the surface. In the dermis there is infiltration with inflammatory cells, and the fibrillary structure is lost. In advanced cases the basal cells break through the basement membrane and frank squamous-celled carcinoma is established. These hypertrophic changes are patchy, but are confined to the inner aspects of the labia majora, the labia minora, the introitus and the prepuce of the clitoris. These are the sites at which carcinoma of the vulva occurs; malignant change is very rare in perianal or perineal skin.

On examination, irregular patches of hypertrophied skin may be seen. White patches are due to thickening of the keratin layer. However, it must

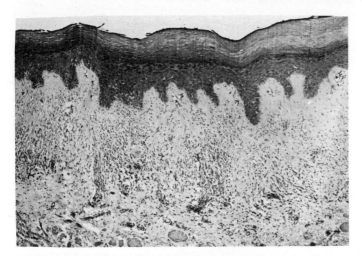

Fig. 12.2 Hypertrophic leukoplakia of vulva. The epidermis is thick with enlarged rete pegs. There is a thick keratin layer, which would appear as a white plaque on the surface. There is infiltration with inflammatory cells in the dermis.

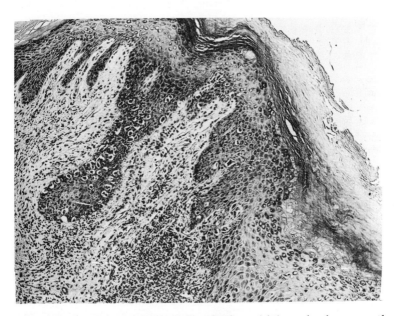

Fig. 12.3 Hypertrophic leukoplakia of vulva, with irregular downgrowth of papillae and abnormal basal cells. Superficial keratinization.

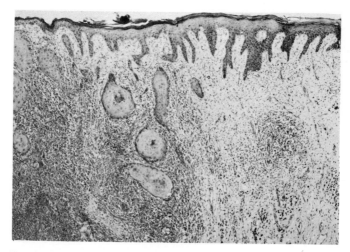

**Fig. 12.4** Leukoplakia of vulva progressing to epithelioma. On the right of the section typical leukoplakia is seen. On the left there are cell nests of epithelioma invading the dermis and surrounded by inflammatory cells.

be realized that histological hypertrophic changes may be present without the clinical appearance of white patches. The diagnosis must be established by biopsy, and for this specimens may have to be taken from several sites.

The initial treatment is the same as that already described in previous sections, but if there is no response or if hypertrophic changes are severe, local vulvectomy should be considered. This is partly to relieve pruritus, but also to remove skin which could become the site of an epithelioma. Any chronic dystrophy must be followed up for many years because of the possibility of malignant change.

### Behçet's syndrome

This is a rare condition of unknown causation in which painful shallow ulcers appear on the vulva and in the mouth, sometimes with associated conjunctivitis. The ulcers heal slowly and spontaneously, but may recur from time to time. Treatment is unsatisfactory, but oral prednisolone may be tried.

## Bartholinitis

The vestibular gland of Bartholin on each side lies beneath the posterior third of the labium minus and its duct opens into the posterior part of the vestibule. The gland may be infected by gonococci, staphylococci or streptococci, or with mixed organisms including *Escherichia coli*. The result is an abscess which forms a red and painful swelling and expands the

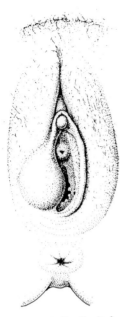

Fig. 12.5  Bartholin's cyst.

posterior part of the labium minus. It causes severe discomfort in walking or sitting.

In the very early stages it may be possible to abort the infection with an antibiotic such as ampicillin but the patients almost always come too late for this. The treatment is then to drain the abscess, and this is best done by excision of an elliptical piece of skin and the abscess wall including the site of the duct. The pus is cultured so that the appropriate antibiotic can be chosen.

### Bartholin's cyst
The duct of the gland may become blocked. It then becomes distended by the mucoid secretion of the gland, forming a cyst which lies beneath and expands the posterior part of the labium minus. Such a cyst may become infected, but otherwise is painless. If treatment is demanded, the cyst is marsupialized by excision of an elliptical piece of skin with the underlying cyst wall, and then sewing the lining of the cyst to the skin. In a few days the wide opening contracts down. This simple procedure is much easier and more effective than excising the cyst and gland from the vascular field in which they lie.

## Pruritus vulvae

Pruritus is the term used to describe a sensation of irritation from which the patient attempts to gain relief by scratching. It is a symptom, not a disease in itself. The irritation often increases when the patient is warm in bed, and she may scratch the area during sleep and wake to find that she has made herself bleed.

## Physical causes

There is always some underlying cause for the onset of pruritus, but scratching soon damages the skin and causes secondary changes which may obscure the primary cause. In addition, the skin may become sensitized to some local application prescribed by the doctor or obtained by the patient herself. In cases of long standing, the diagnosis of both the initial cause and also of the reason for the maintenance of the irritation may become extremely difficult, particularly when more than one factor is involved. Successful treatment depends on two cardinal principles: (1) to remove any underlying cause, and (2) to stop further damage to the skin by scratching or by unsuitable applications.

The causes of pruritus have been described in preceding pages, and may be summarized as follows:

1. Vaginal discharge.
2. Urinary conditions, including glycosuria and incontinence.
3. Disease or sensitization of the vulval skin.
4. General diseases. Pruritus is a manifestation of liver disease and Hodgkin's disease, but is seldom confined to the vulva.

*Pruritus ani* can usually be distinguished from pruritus vulvae, but in some cases both areas are involved, and irritation may spread from one area to the other. Pruritus ani may be caused by threadworms, especially in children, or by irritating discharge from the anus, such as sometimes occurs with the constant intake of liquid paraffin, with haemorrhoids, or if the patient neglects to keep this area clean.

## Psychogenic causes

While any physical cause must be sought and treated appropriately, many patients who complain of pruritus have no identifiable lesion of the vulva. Even when there is a simple local initial cause for the irritation, the symptom may be increased and maintained almost indefinitely by scratching.

Psychological problems may present as pruritus, and when relief is not obtained by local treatment a deeper history is required. Sexual anxieties including ideas of menopausal inadequacy and fears of venereal or malignant disease are not unusual, but a wide spectrum of anxiety may be involved.

The first task is to find the cause of the disorder and, whenever possible, to remove it. This may not be easy or immediately possible, and while investigation is in progress it is essential to avoid further damage to the skin by scratching. Sometimes admission to hospital is well worth while, but in all cases an adequate sedative must be given at night to secure sleep and stop scratching. Great care should be used in prescribing any of the antipruritics that are advertised so lavishly. Many of these relieve the irritation temporarily, but themselves produce more irritation later on.

Corticosteroid applications such as hydrocortisone cream or beta-methasone valerate cream (Betnovate) are useful means of stopping local inflammatory and allergic reactions, and can be safely used as long as any underlying cause for the pruritus is not overlooked. While pruritus of psychological origin requires to be recognized, local disease must also be excluded.

# 13

# Vaginitis and vaginal discharge

Changes in the activity of the vaginal epithelium and in the vaginal secretion at different ages have a profound influence on the defence against vaginal infection. In the adult the normal vaginal moisture or secretion consists of vaginal transudate containing desquamated vaginal epithelial cells which may give it a creamy colour, mucus secreted by the cervical glands and, to a small extent, secretion from the endometrial glands. Its viscosity depends mainly on the cervical component. Apart from menstruation, there is a cyclic variation in the amount of secretion; it is heavier premenstrually and there is an increased secretion of clear cervical mucus at the time of ovulation. There are no glands in the vagina; the transudate passes through the stratified epithelium. Under oestrogenic influence the epithelium contains glycogen, which is converted to lactic acid by Döderlein's bacilli, which are normally present in the vagina. As a result, the vaginal fluid is acid (pH 4) and this prevents multiplication of most pathogenic organisms. In the presence of infection large numbers of leucocytes reach the vaginal cavity, presumably by diapedesis through the vaginal wall.

The vaginal transudate lubricates the vaginal surfaces, and with sexual arousal the amount of transudate increases, as does the mucoid secretion of Bartholin's glands and the cervical glands.

In children and postmenopausal women oestrogen levels are low, and although at these ages the vagina may be less exposed to infection, vaginitis may still occur because of the loss of the acid barrier.

## Vaginal discharge

Vaginal discharge is a very common gynaecological symptom. Its significance is sometimes difficult to assess, and the complaint is occasionally the patient's way of expressing anxiety about matters about which she feels less free to talk – sexual problems or fear of cancer, for example. Discharge may be of varying significance in different cases; an increase which causes complaint in one woman may be less than that which others call normal; the change in amount is the significant point. Vaginal discharge seldom has an odour noticeable at a distance and a complaint that 'everyone can smell it' is sometimes evidence of a psychological overlay in her story.

Assessment of the amount of discharge can be difficult. Persistent moistness, a stain on the underclothes, or the need to wear a pad give a rough guide when related to an estimate of the patient's normal standard of hygiene.

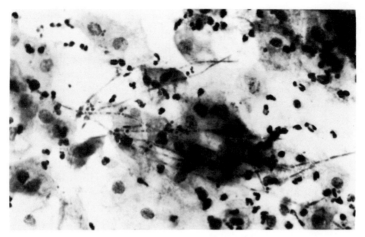

**Fig. 13.1** *Candida albicans.* Filaments seen in a vaginal smear.

There is a natural increase in the vaginal moisture or 'secretion' at the time of ovulation, premenstrually and during pregnancy. The contraceptive pill may cause an increase in cervical secretion and a cervical erosion. The term leucorrhoea, which is now infrequently used, should be confined to an increase in the physiological secretion. When infection supervenes, the clear or white secretion becomes purulent and yellow. Vulval irritation often accompanies infection.

Common organisms causing infective vaginal discharge in adult women are *Candida albicans, Trichomonas vaginalis, Neisseria gonorrhoeae* (see p. 138) and *Gardnerella vaginalis.* Infection with *Chlamydia trachomatis* (see p. 139) may also occur, although this does not produce much evident discharge. There may be simultaneous infection with more than one of these organisms, and in departments of genito-urinary medicine all these possibilities are routinely investigated, together with a serological test for syphilis. In every case tactful but thorough enquiry about sexual contacts must be made; one sexual partner cannot be infected by venereal disease unless one of the two partners has had a third contact.

**Vaginal thrush (mycotic vaginitis)**
Infection with *Candida albicans* is especially likely to occur in patients who have glycosuria; the urine must be examined for sugar in every case in which this infection is found. Apart from cases of diabetes, infection may occur during pregnancy when the renal threshold for glucose may be low. Infection may also occur in patients who are using oral contraceptives or are being treated with antibiotics for some other condition. The infection is not usually transmitted sexually.

There is intense vulval irritation and accompanying vaginal discharge. There is sometimes redness and inflammation of the vulval skin, which may spread to the thighs. Examination may be difficult because of tenderness. With heavy infection the discharge is thick and white, when it is removed the vaginal wall is seen to be red and inflamed. Not every case shows the typical white discharge, and diagnosis must not depend on naked-eye appearances alone.

The fungus can be demonstrated in the clinic in wet preparations. Mycelial threads are seen (Fig. 13.1). The organism grows easily in laboratory cultures in which gram-positive mycelia and spores are seen.

### Treatment
A fungicide is inserted into the vagina. Nystatin pessaries (100 000 units) are often used, being inserted for 14 successive nights. This will be more effective if nystatin cream is also applied to the vulva and nystatin tablets (500 000 units) are taken twice daily by mouth to combat possible re-infection from the bowel. Other drugs which can be used are clotrimazole vaginal tablets (Canesten), amphotericin pessaries (Fungilin) and miconazole nitrate pessaries (Gyno-Daktarin).

### Infection with Trichomonas vaginalis
The infection is usually transmitted by a male carrier during sexual intercourse, but it may also be carried on toilet articles from one woman to another. Cross-infection in antenatal and gynaecological clinics may occur, and disposable gloves should be used for examination.

There is usually a profuse and offensive discharge which produces irritation and soreness but in a few cases the discharge is less, and it is not sufficient to rely on naked eye appearances for diagnosis. The onset is

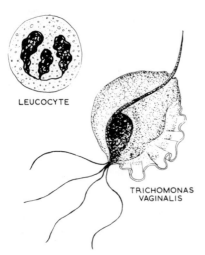

LEUCOCYTE

TRICHOMONAS
VAGINALIS

**Fig. 13.2** *Trichomonas vaginalis,* showing flagella and undulating membrane, with a polymorphonuclear leucocyte drawn to the same scale.

sudden, and there may be a history of previous similar attacks. This infection can occur in women of any age, and is often seen during pregnancy.

There may be inflammation of the vulva, and vaginal examination may be difficult because of soreness. There is a profuse thin greenish-yellow discharge with a characteristic odour which contains minute bubbles of gas. The vaginal wall is intensely red and inflamed, and numerous minute punctate ulcers ('strawberry spots') may be seen.

The diagnosis is easily established in the clinic by examination of the discharge. A little of it is taken with a wire loop or pipette and placed in a drop of normal saline on a glass slide and, after application of a coverslip, examined at once with a microscope, using a 4 mm objective. If the specimen is examined without delay there is no need to warm the saline or the slide. The *Trichomonas* will be recognized by its motility. Numerous leucocytes, will also be seen. The trichomonads are a little larger then leucocytes, and if stained can be shown to have flagella at one end and a spear-like protrusion at the other, with an undulating membrane at the side.

*Treatment*

Metronidazole (Flagyl) is given orally, 200 mg three times daily for a week. Since patients are often reinfected by their sexual partners, the male should be given the same treatment. Alternatively, 2 doses of 2 g may be given in one day, followed by 1 g daily for 7 days. If patients on metronidazole take alcohol they may suffer headaches and flushing. Subsequent recurrence of the infection calls for a further course of treatment and examination of the consort; the *Trichomonas* may be found in the urethra or under the prepuce.

**Infection with Gardnerella vaginalis**

Doubts have been expressed about the role of this organism in vaginal infections. It is a small gram-negative rod. The diagnosis is possible when a patient complains of a smelly non-irritating greyish-white discharge, which may contain small bubbles like those of trichomonal infection. If a drop of discharge is mixed with a drop of 10 per cent solution of potassium hydroxide there is an ammoniacal odour (Amies test), but the same occurs if trichomonads or spermatozoa are present. A smear preparation may show clue cells — epithelial cells which appear stippled because of adherent bacteria. For laboratory culture some discharge should be sent in Stuart's transport medium.

The treatment is the same as that for trichomoniasis (see above).

**Gonorrhoea (see p. 138)**

**Other causes of vaginitis and vaginal discharge**

Vaginitis may result from sensitivity to spermicides used for barrier contraception, or from the accidental use of some unsuitable fluid for a douche (e.g. lysol). A retained pessary or a forgotten tampon or swab will produce a most offensive purulent discharge. With cervical erosions or polypi there is increased secretion of mucus from the cervix, sometimes with a little bleeding. Early cervical cancer may cause postcoital bleeding, but advanced cancer will give rise to offensive, purulent and blood-stained discharge.

## The menopausal patient

After the cessation of menstruation slow atrophy occurs in the vulva and vagina. There is thinning of the vulval and vaginal epithelium, loss of glycogen in the vaginal epithelial cells and a fall in acidity. Local resistance to infection is further diminished by the reduced blood supply.

### Atrophic vaginitis

Vaginitis in postmenopausal women was formerly termed senile vaginitis, but the term atrophic vaginitis is preferable. It is not due to any specific organism. The patient complains of a profuse purulent and sometimes blood-stained discharge, which produces discomfort and soreness at the vulva. The vaginal walls are inflamed. There may also be atrophic endo-metritis and if this occurs discharge will be seen coming from the cervix. If vaginitis has been present for some time, desquamation of the epithelium of the vagina may lead to the formation of bands and adhesions.

It is important to remember that this condition can be accompanied by malignant disease of the uterus. If the slightest doubt exists — for instance, if there is bleeding or improvement does not rapidly follow treatment — diagnostic curettage must be performed.

*Treatment*

When malignant disease has been excluded as a cause of the discharge, the vaginitis is treated with oestrogens such as ethinyloestradiol 10 micro-grams by mouth twice a day for 14 days. Rapid regeneration of the epithelium of the vagina and an increase in blood supply are to be expected, but unfortunately endometrial bleeding may also occur. Unless this is of short duration and not recurrent, diagnostic curettage must be performed. The possibility of bleeding may be reduced, but not entirely eliminated, by administering the oestrogen in the form of pessaries or creams which act locally on the vaginal epithelium.

## Vulvovaginitis in childhood

Because vaginitis in children is usually accompanied by secondary vulvitis, the term vulvovaginitis is often used. Protection of the non-oestrogenized vagina by the hymen is usually effective, but infection may occur as a result of poor hygiene, of insertion of a foreign body by the child, or of sexual interference. A few instances of streptococcal infection appear to be associated with infections of the throat or scarlatina. Candidiasis and trichomoniasis are uncommon, but infection may be carried from an adult if the family standard of hygiene is poor. Gonococcal infection may occur.

The child usually complains of soreness and discomfort on micturition. The vulval skin is reddened, and discharge may be evident; but sometimes the 'discharge' is only a slight stain on clothing noticed by an anxious mother — she, rather than the child, may require reassurance. A copious purulent discharge suggests the presence of a foreign body. Anal thread-worms may cause pruritus and scratching.

Advice on hygiene may be necessary. The vulval region should be bathed daily, but irritant antiseptics should not be added to the water, and care must be taken to rinse out detergents from clothing. It is seldom necessary to give an anaesthetic for examination; a small wire loop or pipette may be passed into the vagina to obtain discharge for bacteriological examination. A foreign body may be felt by rectal examination, or possibly seen with the aid of a small nasal speculum. Oestrogens may be tried (ethinyloestradiol 5 micrograms daily by mouth for a small child) or dienoestrol cream locally before any more thorough investigation. Trichomoniasis is treated with oral metronidazole but with half the adult dose. Candidiasis is treated with oral nystatin suspension (400 000 units three times daily).

# 14

# Cervicitis and cervical erosion

## Acute cervicitis

The endocervical columnar epithelium may be infected by the gonococcus or *Chlamydia trachomatis* (see p. 139). Cervical infection may also follow childbirth or operative dilatation of the cervix, and spread into the base of the broad ligament (parametrium).

## Cervical erosion, chronic cervicitis and cervical ectropion

Terms must first be defined. The term *cervical erosion* is applied when, in an adult, the stratified epithelium which normally covers the vaginal portion of the cervix is replaced by columnar epithelium which is continuous with that of the cervical canal. An erosion is *not an ulcer* – as the word would imply. Although chronic cervicitis is sometimes found in association with an erosion, most erosions are *not infected*, nor are they inflammatory lesions.

In newborn infants, columnar epithelium is commonly found on the ectocervix; such a 'congenital erosion' is not abnormal, and it may persist into childhood.

The term *chronic cervicitis* is often used loosely, but it should be strictly confined to cases with true inflammation of the cervix. This may occur as a sequel of acute cervicitis.

The term *cervical ectropion* is used when the cervix is so badly lacerated and everted (usually at delivery but sometimes by surgical injury) that the normal endocervical columnar epithelium is exposed  in the patulous os.

### Cervical erosion

This is one of the commonest findings in the genital tract. An erosion often starts during pregnancy, but may not be discovered until the patient is seen in the postnatal clinic or afterwards. Many erosions resolve after delivery when the stratified epithelium returns to replace the ectopic columnar epithelium, but a few persist. Erosions are seldom seen after the climacteric. These facts suggest that the erosion is dependent on the hormonal status of the patient, and this is supported by the fact that many women who are taking oral contraceptives containing oestrogens develop erosions, which resolve when the pills are discontinued.

*Pathology*

It is surprising how much uncertainty there is about the pathogenesis of such a common and accessible lesion.

During pregnancy, under the influence of the high concentration of hormones, the glandular tissue of the endocervix proliferates extensively, and there is increased vascularity. The cervix is softened and enlarged, and the cervical lips roll outwards to expose some of the endocervical mucosa. This may well explain the appearance of some of the erosions so frequently seen during pregnancy; and some hold that all erosions are of this nature.

However, it is difficult to believe that this process explains the extensive erosions which are often seen on the firm non-pregnant cervix with a tightly closed os. Microscopical examination shows that the squamo-columnar junction is an irregular and unstable transformation zone, with 'ebb and flow' of the two types of epithelium (Figs. 14.1 and 2). With the hormonal stimulus of the contraceptive pill or pregnancy the columnar epithelium may proliferate and extend outwards to replace the stratified epithelium. On the other hand, in many places the stratified epithelium will be seen actively growing to displace the columnar epithelium, and it may even grow down into the cervical glands. This process has been called *epidermidization*, and it must not be mistaken for carcinoma. In a section cut obliquely there may seem to be deep islands of stratified epithelium, but this epithelium shows normal architecture with regular and well

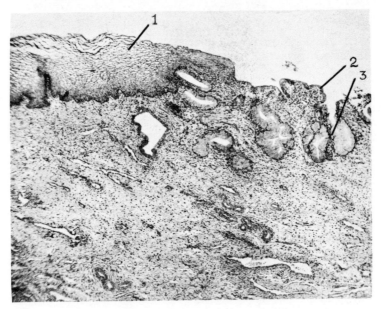

**Fig. 14.1** Section of normal cervix at the level of the external os. 1, Squamous epithelium; 2, columnar epithelium of canal; 3, cervical gland.

differentiated cells, and there is no invasion of the basement membrane.

The proliferation of stratified epithelium in the process of epidermidization sometimes obstructs the orifices of cervical glands, which then become distended with secretion and desquamated cells to form small cysts called *Nabothian follicles*. They have no clinical significance.

However the change from stratified to columnar epithelium (or the reverse) comes about in a cervical erosion, the process is unrelated to dysplasia, which is a premalignant condition, described on p. 167.

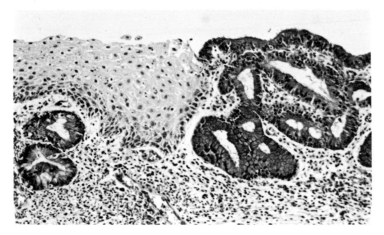

**Fig. 14.2** Cervix: squamocolumnar junction. There is some underlying infiltration with inflammatory cells; this is almost invariably seen.

*Symptoms and signs*

Many patients with erosions have no complaint. The only symptom caused by an erosion is a mucoid discharge. This comes from the columnar epithelium of both the glands in the cervical canal and from the erosion itself. Discharge from an erosion can often be dated to the birth of a child or to the start of oral contraception.

A brown intermenstrual discharge or slight postcoital bleeding may be noticed, but should not be attributed to the erosion without smears and possibly colposcopy and biopsy to exclude carcinoma. During pregnancy slight bleeding from an erosion may lead to suspicion of placenta praevia. If the bleeding is more than slight, it must never be attributed to the erosion.

Pain is never caused by an erosion, nor is it a cause of backache or dyspareunia.

Only in a few cases can an erosion be detected by palpation. They are said to feel 'velvety', but the sign is unreliable. The diagnosis is made by inspecting the cervix with a speculum. A red granular area is seen around the external os, where the pink stratified epithelium has been replaced by red columnar epithelium. The lesion may be flat or thrown up into small papillary folds.

*Treatment*
See below.

### Chronic cervicitis
True cervical infection may persist after bacterial invasion at the time of delivery or abortion. In such cases mucopus is seen coming from the external os. Bacteriological examination is seldom helpful because so many cases show a very mixed flora by the time the patient is seen.

The symptoms hardly differ from those of cervical erosion, except that the discharge is more purulent; the same treatment is applied. Small vascular tags of proliferating cervical epithelium may project from the cervical canal in some of these cases. These tags are not of the same nature as cervical adenomatous polypi (see p. 162).

The cervix may also be infected with *Chlamydia trachomatis* during intercourse with a male with chlamydial urethritis. No local symptoms may be noticed but the organism can spread upward to cause chronic salpingitis. *Chlamydia* is difficult to culture by ordinary bacteriological techniques, but an immuno-fluorescent antibody test is available. If a male is found to have non-gonococcal urethritis the possibility of chlamydial infection of any sexual contact must be considered, and she should be treated with tetracycline 500 mg orally 6-hourly for 2 weeks.

### Cervical ectropion
Often the cervix is partly split during childbirth. The split may be on both sides of the cervix or on one side only. Such lacerations may be very small or so large that they extend right up to the vaginal fornix. When the tear is bilateral, eversion of the two lips of the cervix exposes the columnar epithelium of the cervical canal, and such a lesion is often wrongly diagnosed as an erosion.

A small ectropion does not cause symptoms, but there may be mucoid discharge from a large one. In a few cases, especially if abortion has occurred and cervical incompetence is thought to be the cause, trachelorrhaphy is performed. The edges of the tears are excised, and the resulting raw surfaces are sutured together to reconstitute the cervical canal.

### Treatment of cervical erosion or chronic cervicitis
Erosions found on routine examination should not be treated unless they are causing troublesome discharge. A cervical smear must be taken in all cases, and if there is any doubt about the smear colposcopy and cervical biopsy should be undertaken.

If patients taking an oral contraceptive complain of discharge and are found to have an erosion, another contraceptive method may be advised. However, some patients will wish to continue with the pill. Sometimes it is worth treating the erosion (see below) but it may recur while the hormonal stimulation continues. Otherwise, the patient will have to accept the discharge as a side-effect of the pill and put up with it.

Erosions are not treated during pregnancy; most of them resolve after delivery.

When a patient has troublesome discharge, the erosion is treated. Three methods are commonly employed: (1) thermal cauterization with diathermy or an electrically heated wire cautery, (2) freezing to produce tissue necrosis (cryosurgery), or (3) a laser.

*Thermal cauterization.* It is usual to perform diagnostic curettage before cauterization, and in many cases cervical biopsy is performed. The cervix is insensitive, and superficial cauterization without anaesthesia is possible, but anaesthesia permits more thorough diagnostic examination. After dilating the cervix the lower part of the cervical canal and the whole area of the erosion are cauterized to a depth of about 2 mm. The patient should be warned that discharge will increase for 2 or 3 weeks until the cauterized tissue, which inevitably becomes mildly infected, separates and the burn heals.

In a few cases the infection is followed by secondary haemorrhage about 10–14 days after the operation. Daily postoperative instillation of sulphonamide cream into the vagina may reduce the risk of this complication. If secondary haemorrhage does occur, the patient, who has usually left hospital soon after the operation, is readmitted. A speculum is passed and the blood cleared away from the vagina so that the cervix can be inspected. A single bleeding point can seldom be seen, and attempts to suture the area are unsatisfactory. It is usually best to pack the vagina firmly with gauze so that pressure is applied to the cervix. The pack is removed about 48 hours later. If treatment is not delayed, blood transfusion can be avoided.

*Cryosurgery.* This gives equally good results. It is claimed that there is less risk of postoperative infection and secondary haemorrhage with this method, and it can be used without anaesthesia. The appliance consists of a 'probe', the head of which is cooled to temperatures below freezing point by the rapid expansion of gas which is passed through it. Nitrous oxide from a cylinder is very convenient. Application to the cervix for about 2 minutes freezes the tissues to a depth of about 2 mm. The probe adheres to the tissue until the temperature rises again, and should not be pulled away before this. Separation of the necrotic tissue causes discharge for 2 or 3 weeks.

A *laser* may be used to destroy the superficial epithelium.

# 15

# Endometritis, pyometra and haematometra

During reproductive life endometritis is uncommon except after delivery or abortion. The cavity of the uterus is protected against bacterial invasion by the acid barrier of the vagina and the cervical mucus, and in addition the shedding of the endometrium at each menstrual period prevents organisms from obtaining a foothold for long. However, after delivery or abortion lochial discharge forms an excellent culture medium and organisms may enter the tissues at the site from which the placenta has separated.

Endometritis may follow operations such as curettage, or the insertion of an intrauterine device. When an intrauterine device is in place the subjacent endometrium shows infiltration with polymorphonuclear leucocytes. This may only be a response to the foreign body, but in a few cases actinomyces-like organisms have been noticed in smears or cultured from the uterus.

Gonococcal infection may spread upwards from the cervix to the endometrium and tubes, while tuberculous endometritis often follows tuberculous salpingitis.

With advanced carcinoma of the endometrium or of the cervix, especially if the cervical canal is obstructed, infection occurs.

After the menopause there may be ascending infection which causes what was formerly called senile endometritis, but for which we prefer the happier term atrophic endometritis.

## Atrophic endometritis

After the menopause, with the loss of vaginal acidity, atrophy of the vaginal epithelium and of the endometrium, and diminution of blood supply, ascending infection may occur with organisms of low virulence.

There is extensive infiltration of the endometrium with polymorphonuclear leucocytes and plasma cells, and ulceration of the surface of the atrophic endometrium may ensue. The purulent discharge either drains into the vagina or may accumulate in the uterus to form a pyometra.

### Symptoms and signs
The patient complains of vaginal discharge which may be blood stained. Pelvic examination shows atrophic vaginitis and purulent discharge may be seen coming from the cervix. If a pyometra is present, the uterus will be enlarged, soft and tender.

### Diagnosis

The symptoms and signs of carcinoma of the endometrium are similar to those of atrophic endometritis, and in both a pyometra may be present. The diagnosis can only be determined by curettage. The material obtained in atrophic endometritis will be granulation tissue with scanty endometrium. In carcinoma of the endometrium or cervix a large amount of necrotic material may be removed.

### Treatment

Efficient drainage is provided by the cervical dilatation necessary for diagnosis. Healing occurs rapidly after administration of oestrogens. Ethinyloestradiol 0.01 mg daily for about 4 weeks should be sufficient. Recurrence is uncommon, but should it occur hysterectomy may be necessary.

## Pyometra

The uterus may become distended with pus as a result of obstruction of the cervical canal by carcinoma of the cervix, especially an endocervical growth, or by carcinoma in the lower part of the body of the uterus. It may occur after treatment of cervical cancer with radium or caesium.

Pyometra can also occur after the menopause in patients with atrophic endometritis, in the absence of malignant disease.

The organisms responsible for a pyometra may be coliforms, streptococci or staphylococci, but not infrequently no organisms are grown on culture. A tuberculous pyometra is now very rare.

The patient may complain of an intermittent blood-stained purulent discharge. Abdominal pain and fever are seldom present. The body of the uterus may be enlarged to a diameter of about 10 cm, and may feel cystic. It may be tender.

The diagnosis is made by dilatation of the cervix, when pus escapes. It is not sufficient merely to diagnose a pyometra; in every case a most careful examination must be made to exclude a carcinoma. Much care must be taken because there is a risk of perforating the thin wall of a pyometra during dilatation of the cervix and curettage.

### Treatment

In the absence of any evidence of carcinoma the pyometra is drained by dilatation of the cervix and stitching a drainage tube into the uterus for a few days. If carcinoma is present, the usual treatment is given after initial drainage of the pus. Pyometra not associated with carcinoma sometimes recurs, when hysterectomy is performed.

## Haematometra

This is described here for convenience, although it may not be accompanied by infection. It is a collection of blood in the uterine cavity, caused by

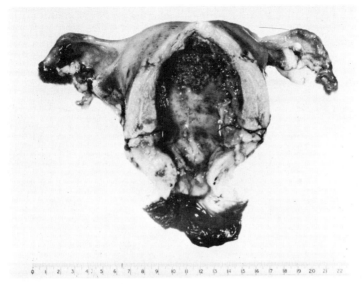

**Fig. 15.1** Uterus showing distension by pyometra which was caused by carcinoma of the cervix.

obstruction in the genital tract at or below the level of the cervix.

A haematometra may, rarely, occur together with a haematocolpos due to vaginal atresia or absence of the vagina. A functioning rudimentary horn or one half of a double uterus may become distended with menstrual blood because it does not communicate with the vagina.

Haematometra may result from stenosis of the cervix caused by operations such as amputation of the cervix, cone biopsy or cervical cauterization.

Carcinoma of the cervix or of the lower part of the body of the uterus may obstruct the cervical canal to cause a haematometra. This may occur after the menopause, when the bleeding comes from the growth rather than the endometrium.

When there is obstruction to the outflow of menstrual discharge there will be apparent amenorrhoea with discomfort at monthly intervals. If a haematometra accompanies a haematocolpos, the enlarged uterus may be felt, but only after evacuation of the haematocolpos. A haematometra in an accessory horn, or in one half of a double uterus, is difficult to recognize because the patient menstruates normally, and the cystic swelling may be mistakenly diagnosed as an ovarian cyst or pyosalpinx.

**Treatment**
When a haematometra is associated with a haematocolpos the latter is evacuated by incision of the obstructing membrane, and the haematometra will be evacuated spontaneously in the course of time. It is entirely wrong to perform hysterectomy.

When a functioning uterus occurs with absence of the vagina it may be possible to construct a new vagina by insertion of a Thiersch graft and then to connect the uterus to it (see p. 72). If a rudimentary horn or one half of a double uterus has become distended with blood it may be excised.

If stenosis of the cervix has caused a haematometra with dysmenorrhoea, simple dilatation of the cervix is usually all that is needed.

# 16

# Salpingo-oöphoritis

Salpingitis is an inflammatory condition of the Fallopian tubes caused by bacterial infection. In most cases both tubes are involved. Since the ovary is also infected in many cases, the term salpingo-oöphoritis is usually more correct.

## Aetiology

Organisms can reach the tube by various routes.
1. Ascending infection through the vagina and uterus.
   (a) Infection may occur after abortion or delivery. The common organisms are streptococci and staphylococci.
   (b) Gonococcal infection.
   (c) Recent studies indicate that *Chlamydia trachomatis* is a common cause of salpingitis. It is likely that the organism is derived from a sexual partner with chlamydial urethritis. The organisms are thought to colonize the cervix, without producing noticeable symptoms, but may subsequently ascend to infect the Fallopian tubes. Direct culture of the organism is difficult and requires techniques which are not in general use, but an immuno-fluorescent antibody test is available.
   (d) Tubal infection may rarely follow therapeutic abortion, salpingography or the insertion of an intrauterine contraceptive device. It is possible that many of these cases are caused by reactivation of pre-existing infection. In rare instances actinomycosis has been found in association with the use of an intrauterine contraceptive device (see p. 308).
2. Infection from the intestinal tract. Infection of the right tube and ovary can occur in appendicitis, or both tubes may be involved in pelvic peritonitis or abscess. The organisms are usually *Escherichia coli* or *Streptococcus faecalis*. Bacteria from the intestinal tract may also infect a tube previously damaged by gonorrhoea.
3. Infection through the blood stream. Tuberculosis is the only example (see p. 130).

In practice it is usually difficult to demonstrate the organisms causing tubal inflammation because most cases of acute salpingitis are not treated by operation, and in chronic cases the organisms tend to die, so on examination the pus in the tube may be sterile, or a secondary infection from the bowel may have occurred.

## Pathology

The various pathological appearances of the tubes that may be found can be tabulated as follows.
1. Acute salpingitis.
2. Chronic salpingitis:
    (a) hydrosalpinx.
    (b) pyosalpinx.
    (c) chronic interstitial salpingitis.

In acute salpingitis both tubes are red and oedematous and there is usually a purulent exudate. The plicae of the tubal mucosa are swollen, and the epithelium covering them is shed in places. It is possible for this type of inflammation to subside without leaving any gross changes, but in most cases damage is done to the ciliated epithelium of the tube, causing infertility or possibly delay in the transport of the fertilized ovum and an ectopic pregnancy.

Frequently the tube becomes occluded. The lumen of the interstitial part is so fine that the slightest inflammatory reaction blocks it. At the other end of the tube the fimbriae adhere together and are drawn in, and the abdominal ostium is sealed. Once the ends are closed, inflammatory exudate collects and distends the tube. When the collection of fluid is more or less clear it is called a *hydrosalpinx,* or if it is purulent a *pyosalpinx.* Because the ampullary end of the tube distends more easily than the isthmus the tube becomes retort shaped (see Fig. 16.1).

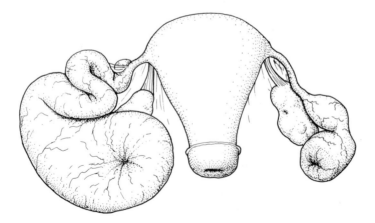

**Fig. 16.1** Hydrosalpinx of left tube showing typical retort shape. There is a smaller hydrosalpinx on the right side.

A hydrosalpinx may become 7 cm in diameter or even larger, but because the infection has not been very active the wall of the tube remains thin and dense peritubal adhesions are not usually found. Should the infecting organisms be more virulent they pass deeply into the wall of the tube, which becomes thickened, and as the covering peritoneum becomes involved in the inflammation peritoneal adhesions occur.

In most cases of suppurative salpingitis the ends of the tube are blocked and therefore the pus collects in the tube to form a pyosalpinx. However, if the pus is rapidly poured out it will pass through the abdominal ostium and infect the peritoneum and surrounding structures before there has been time for this to be closed by adhesion of the fimbriae. A peritubal abscess may result, the pus being localized by the formation of adhesions between the surrounding structures, including the ovary. Peritoneal fluid is poured out between the coils of intestine and other organs adjacent to the abscess, and this in turn becomes localized by the formation of adhesions. In this way a mass may be formed consisting of peritoneal exudate and adherent intestine and omentum which is many times bigger than the peritubal abscess and is palpable abdominally. In a few cases the pus reaches the rectovaginal pouch to form a pelvic abscess. It is extremely rare for limiting adhesions not to confine the infection to the pelvis, and general peritonitis is not to be feared.

The ovaries soon participate in the inflammation. They become enlarged by oedema and adhere to the tubes by filmy adhesions. If the infection is severe the ovary develops small abscesses within its substance or may, with the tube and adjacent structures, form part of the wall of an abscess cavity. A distended tube may communicate with a cyst of the ovary, forming a *tubo-ovarian cyst* or abscess.

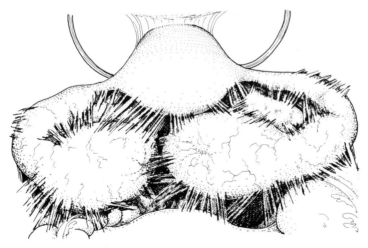

**Fig. 16.2** Bilateral pyosalpinges seen from above with adhesions to uterus and rectum.

Adhesions, which may be filmy or very dense, develop between the tubes and ovaries, the uterus, the rectum and intestines, and the omentum. The uterus is often drawn backwards into a position of retroversion.

In some cases the inflammation does not result in the collection of pus within the lumen of the tube. Inflammatory changes within the muscle wall produce areas of variable thickening and fibrosis, often with kinking. This condition is called *interstitial salpingitis,* and is often found as a residual lesion in patients whose symptoms have resolved.

## Symptoms and signs

### Acute salpingitis

The patient feels ill and complains of lower abdominal pain. The pain is worse on movement and the patient usually takes to her bed. Vomiting may occur at the onset and the bowels are constipated. The pulse rate is increased and the temperature is raised, often above 39.5°C. The tongue is dry but not usually furred. Because there is pelvic hyperaemia there may be a mucous discharge from the uterus, and if there is cervicitis this may be purulent. Often there is a profuse purulent discharge because of co-incidental infection with trichomonads. Because there is oöphoritis the menstrual cycle is often upset, and periods may be heavy from pelvic hyperaemia. In many cases in which the infection is of low virulence all symptoms disappear in a few days, and the true nature of the illness is never proven.

Examination shows diffuse tenderness and rigidity on palpation over the lower abdomen. Slight abdominal distension may be present. Pelvic examination causes pain, especially on movement of the uterus. In many cases the tenderness in the fornices is such that no other physical signs can be made out. In less acute cases a sense of fullness is noticed on bimanual examination in the lateral fornices. The converse is perhaps more useful; if bimanual pressure to the side of the uterus is not painful, the patient is certainly not suffering from acute salpingitis.

If there is a peritubal abscess, the encysted serous peritonitis around it forms a mass, which may become palpable above the symphysis pubis. It is irregular in outline, and partly resonant on percussion because of coils of intestine adherent to it. In order to relax the abdominal muscles over this tender mass the patient often lies in bed with both knees flexed.

Abscess formation, within or without the tube, is shown by deterioration of the patient's condition. She looks and feels ill, and complains of increasing pain. Her appetite deteriorates and she sleeps badly. Temperature and pulse rate increase and rigors may occur. There is increasing leucocytosis. The pelvic mass increases in size, and if left alone the abscess usually points and drains into the rectum; this event is often preceded by mucous diarrhoea.

With modern antibiotic treatment the formation of a large pelvic mass is seen less often, and in any case it tends to absorb after one or two weeks.

The tender Fallopian tubes may then be felt as oblong tender and fixed masses behind the uterus. The patient may be left with blocked tubes and more or less dense pelvic adhesions.

### Chronic salpingitis

A patient with chronic salpingitis may be ambulant and even follow her regular employment. She does not, however, feel well and many ordinary daily tasks become a burden. The menstrual loss is often heavy and preceded by dysmenorrhoea of congestive type, with pain preceding and throughout each period. The inflammation of the ovaries may upset the menstrual cycle and produce irregular bleeding. In addition to menstrual pain there is often continuing dull pain or aching in the lower abdomen or back. There is dyspareunia, and there may be an excessive cervical discharge.

It is not to be expected that the above formidable list of symptoms will be present in every case; as a rule, one symptom is predominant while the others are slight or absent. Patients with chronic pelvic inflammation are liable, at intervals of a few weeks or months, to recurrent acute exacerbations of the disease, each resembling an attack of acute pelvic peritonitis. These attacks may be due to secondary coliform infection, or to an exacerbation of the inflammation caused by the organisms originally present.

Chronic salpingitis can be a crippling disease, particularly in a young woman. She may be too unwell to work, with menorrhagia, dysmenorrhoea and dyspareunia, and sometimes with a complaint of infertility for which treatment is unlikely to be successful.

## Diagnosis

At its onset acute salpingitis must be distinguished from acute appendicitis. If the appendix is pelvic, the signs may be much alike. The history will often be helpful, for in salpingitis there will generally be a history and signs of recent abortion or delivery or of gonococcal infection. In appendicitis the pain usually starts near the umbilicus and later becomes localized to the right iliac fossa, whereas in salpingitis the pain starts in the lower abdomen and is bilateral. The temperature with salpingitis is usually higher, often reaching 39.5°C, whereas in appendicitis it seldom exceeds 38.5°C; the pulse rate, however, is not so much raised in salpingitis as in appendicitis. Vomiting may occur with either condition but is more constant with appendicitis. A furred tongue suggests appendicitis. In cases of salpingitis, vaginal examination shows tenderness in both lateral fornices; in appendicitis the signs will be more marked on the right side.

Occasionally acute infection of the urinary tract may resemble salpingitis. Urinary tract infection often starts with a rigor and may produce a high temperature. Even if frequency of micturition is not present there will be pain and tenderness in the loin, and there will be no pelvic signs. Examination of the urine will settle the diagnosis.

Later, when there is more exudate around the Fallopian tubes and in the rectovaginal pouch, the physical signs may resemble those of a pelvic haematocele resulting from an ectopic gestation. If the salpingitis follows an abortion there may be a period of amenorrhoea preceding the abdominal pain, but with an ectopic gestation the amenorrhoea is seldom longer than 6 weeks, whereas with uterine abortion it is more often 8 or 12 weeks. The onset of the pain in a ruptured ectopic gestation is generally more sudden and more severe than in salpingitis. If a pyosalpinx has formed, the history will usually make the nature of the swelling obvious, but if the patient is first seen at this stage the swelling will have to be differentiated from an ectopic gestation with a tubal mole or from a small ovarian cyst.

Ovarian endometriomatous cysts may cause pelvic pain and menorrhagia, and the physical signs closely resemble those of chronic salpingitis with bilateral tubal swellings. The absence of a history of infection after abortion or delivery, of gonorrhoea, or of any suggestion of tuberculosis, and the absence of pyrexia, help in reaching the correct diagnosis.

All experienced gynaecologists have had difficulty in the differential diagnosis. If doubt remains, laparoscopy should be performed — both for the immediate safety of the patient in making the correct diagnosis and for planning treatment.

## Treatment

### Acute salpingitis
The patient should be kept in bed and may need admission to hospital. Heat applied to the lower abdomen is comforting. Pain is treated symptomatically, and may require pethidine. Should an intrauterine contraceptive device be in place it is removed.

Bacterial swabs are taken from the cervix and urethra, but treatment with ampicillin 500 mg 4 times daily is begun without waiting for the bacteriological report. It is hoped that immediate treatment will prevent permanent damage to the tubes. If the bacteriological investigations suggest that the infection is gonococcal ampicillin is continued, with probenecid 1 g daily for 14 days. In severe cases ampicillin or benzyl penicillin may be given intramuscularly or intravenously.

If gonococci are not found treatment may be changed to tetracycline 500 mg 4 times daily with metronidazole 400 mg twice daily for 14 days.

If there is no clinical response or if there are allergic reactions other drugs which may be used are spectinomycin or cefuroxime.

Surgical treatment of acute salpingitis is seldom called for; the indications may be listed as follows:

1. When, in the early stages, the diagnosis is doubtful and appendicitis is a possibility. If at laparotomy it is found that the tubes are acutely inflamed they should not be removed if there is any hope of restoration of function. Bacterial swabs should be taken from any pus and from the lumen of the tubes before closing the abdomen.

2. In the very rare cases of deterioration in spite of active medical forms of treatment.

3. When there is definite evidence of a pelvic abscess, this must be drained.

4. When the patient suffers from repeated recurrent attacks of acute salpingitis, operation is advised in a quiescent phase.

### Chronic salpingitis

Frequently after an attack of acute salpingitis an abscess does not form yet the disease obviously fails to resolve completely. The patient complains of variable low abdominal discomfort or pain, low backache, heavy menstrual loss, discharge and dyspareunia. On pelvic examination there is tenderness and residual thickening of one or both tubes. Only prolonged antibiotic treatment and convalescence have any prospect of resolving this condition. It may be necessary to continue treatment for 3—6 months, changing between the various broad-spectrum antibiotics, such as ampicillin, co-trimoxazole, tetracycline and the cephalosporins, and metronizadole. Chlamydial infections, which may be difficult to diagnose by laboratory investigations, respond to tetracyclines or erythromycin. A sensible life, with light work and adequate rest, is essential if further exacerbations are to be avoided.

Sometimes these measures fail, and surgical treatment is indicated. While tissue which is healthy should be conserved, it is no kindness to the patient to leave her with infected tissues which will call for further subsequent surgical treatment. Both tubes may have to be removed, and in that case, especially if there is menorrhagia and discharge, total hysterectomy is often wise. An effort is made to find and conserve any healthy ovarian tissue.

### Prognosis

Even in the worst cases the prognosis as regards life is good, as the infection is almost always confined to the pelvis. In the past restoration of function of the Fallopian tubes was exceptional, but now if the diagnosis is made early and the patient is treated with appropriate antibiotics the prospects are improved. If there is delay and suppuration occurs in the tubes, the progress of the disease can usually be stopped and the formation of a pyosalpinx or pelvic abscess avoided, but the hope of restoration of fertility is poor.

For the investigation and treatment of tubal blockage caused by salpingitis see pp.267 and 272.

# 17

# Tuberculosis of the genital tract

Tuberculous infection of the genital tract is becoming uncommon in Britain; it is seen more often in developing countries. The infection is almost invariably secondary to a tuberculous infection in the lung, although by the time the genital infection becomes manifest the primary lesion may be quiescent or healed. Although it is theoretically possible for a patient to be infected directly from a male with tuberculous epididymitis, this event is almost unknown.

The Fallopian tube is the most common site of initial infection in the pelvic organs. The problem is to discover how the bacilli reach the tubes. At one time it was thought that the route was transperitoneal, the tubes being secondarily infected from a tuberculous peritonitis or adenitis. However, nearly all tubal infections are caused by the human type of bacillus, whereas many peritoneal infections are caused by bovine bacilli. It is now generally agreed that the lung is the primary site, and that the organisms are carried in the blood to the pelvis. The initial pelvic infection may occur soon after puberty, and cases are most often diagnosed in young women.

Genital tuberculosis has become less common as the incidence of pulmonary tuberculosis has diminished, and early treatment with anti-tuberculous drugs has also reduced the risk of dissemination.

## Pathology

In early cases small tuberculous nodules can be seen at the ampullary end of the Fallopian tube. These spread along the lining of the tube and may reach the endometrium. Unlike infection with the gonococcus or strepto-coccus, with tuberculous infection the tube tends to remain patent for some time, although its walls may be much thickened. It is only when the nodules become caseous and break down that infected material is discharged into the lumen of the tube; when this occurs the ampullary end of the tube becomes sealed and a pyosalpinx forms. Secondary pyogenic infection may play a part in causing this.

If the infection involves the peritoneal cavity, small tubercles may be seen on the serosal surface of the tube. Spread of infection to the ovary is often late, unless the peritoneum is involved or unless there is a pyosalpinx, when the ampullary end of the tube is often adherent to the ovary.

If the infection spreads to the endometrium, typical foci with giant

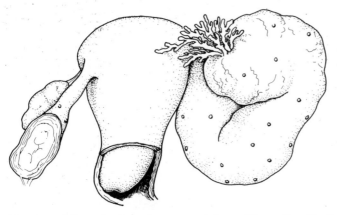

**Fig. 17.1** Bilateral tuberculous pyosalpinges. The walls of both tubes are thickened and they contain caseous material. Tubercles are seen on the peritoneal surface.

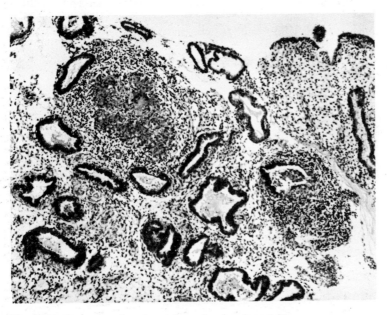

**Fig. 17.2** Curetting showing tuberculous endometritis.

cell systems surrounded by round-celled infiltration may be found when curettings are examined; but they do not have time to develop into mature tubercles before they are shed at menstruation, and they are easily missed unless the endometrial sample is taken immediately before a period. Although most of the infected endometrium is shed at each menstruation, reinfection occurs from persisting lesions in the deeper layers, or from the tubes. Rarely, the infection spreads to the myometrium, and if caseation occurs a pyometra results.

Tuberculous infection of the cervix is rare. It forms a raised red nodule on the vaginal portion, which resembles carcinoma and bleeds easily on examination. Later the granulomatous material may break down to form a shallow ulcer. Tuberculous ulcers of the vagina or vulva are extremely rare. All these lesions are secondary to disease of the upper genital tract.

## Symptoms and signs

The symptoms and signs vary greatly. When the lesions in the tubes are only small tubercles, with little fibrosis or caseation, there may be no symptoms unless the patient complains of infertility. The tubes are only slightly thickened, and on bimanual palpation this may not be detected.

When the disease is more active, with caseation in the tubes, the symptoms are those of chronic salpingitis. There is pelvic discomfort or pain, often worse at the time of the periods, and if the ovaries are involved there may be more frequent periods with increased loss. There may be slight evening pyrexia, with lymphocytosis and a raised erythrocyte sedimentation rate.

Occasionally, if the disease follows a very active course, the picture is that of acute salpingitis with severe pain and high fever.

In both these more severe varieties the enlargement of the Fallopian tubes and the inflammation and oedema of surrounding structures will produce swellings in the lateral fornices which can be felt on bimanual palpation. There will be tenderness and fixation of the pelvic organs.

Finally, if there is widespread infection of the peritoneum there may be ascites and general abdominal distension, pyrexia and ill-health. If the patient acquires the disease at about the time of puberty the onset of menstruation may be delayed, and amenorrhoea is sometimes seen in cases in which the patient's general health is much impaired. It is therefore seen that any type of menstrual irregularity can occur in the various stages of the disease, but tuberculosis is the only pelvic infection to be associated with amenorrhoea.

## Diagnosis

The diagnosis of a condition with such a wide variation in symptoms and signs may be difficult, although a previous history of other tuberculous lesions or of close contact with another member of the family with active disease will raise the index of suspicion.

In the absence of major symptoms or signs the diagnosis is only likely to be made in the course of investigation of a complaint of infertility, when the tubes may be found to be occluded. Since in nearly every case of active tuberculous salpingitis the endometrium is involved, histological examination of curettings will show the presence of tubercles. For this purpose a small endometrial biopsy is not sufficient because the lesions are often few and scattered, so a thorough curettage should be carried out just before a period is due, and several sections should be examined. Part of the material is sent for bacterial culture or guinea-pig inoculation.

If the patient presents with signs of pelvic inflammation it may be difficult to arrive at a certain diagnosis. The history may be helpful; the onset of tuberculosis is often insidious, whereas the more common coccal infections can be traced to a puerperal or gonococcal infection. If the patient is a virgin, a tuberculous infection is much more likely than an ascending one.

In every case a radiological examination of the chest must be made, although by the time the genital infection is manifest any primary pulmonary lesion may have healed. Other organs may be secondarily involved, and any patient with pus cells in the urine must have a full investigation of the urinary tract.

## Treatment

The treatment of tuberculous infection of the genital tract is primarily medical. In the common type of case in which the infection is discovered during investigation for infertility a prolonged course of medical treatment is given. This now usually consists of rifampicin 450—600 mg with isoniazid 300 mg by mouth daily. Rifinah 150 is a convenient preparation containing 150 mg of rifampicin and 100 mg of isoniazid in a single tablet. During the acute stage of the disease ethambutol hydrochloride, 15 mg per kg body weight orally daily, is often added, but is discontinued as soon as investigations give negative results. This drug may cause loss of visual acuity and should be stopped at once if the patient notices any change. The rifampicin and isoniazid are continued for at least a year.

After about a year of treatment the endometrium is re-examined. If tubercles are present treatment must be continued, but even if they are not found the endometrium should be re-examined at intervals of about six months. At least two negative reports, including both histological and bacteriological examination, are required before the patient can be considered cured.

With this regimen of treatment any tubo-ovarian swellings may gradually diminish in size until they can no longer be felt. If this occurs and repeated endometrial biopsies remain negative it is best to do nothing further except follow-up the patient.

If, however, tubo-ovarian swellings persist, and particularly if endometrial examination shows that the disease is still active, surgical treatment may be necessary, especially if there are also symptoms. This will entail removal of both tubes and ovaries and total hysterectomy. The operation is often difficult because of dense adhesions, and there is a risk of injury to the bowel and the production of fistulae. Fortunately, with modern medical treatment these difficult operations are now seldom necessary.

## Prognosis

With early diagnosis and modern treatment there is now little risk to life from tuberculosis of the genital tract, and symptoms are usually relieved, but fertility is seldom restored. After the infection has been cured the tubes are patent in nearly half the cases. In spite of this, few patients become pregnant, probably because of fibrosis of the walls of the Fallopian tubes and damage to their ciliated epithelium. If pregnancy occurs there is a high incidence of ectopic pregnancy and of abortion.

# 18

# Sexually transmitted diseases

The list of sexually transmitted diseases is long, and the number of cases is increasing in Britain and in many parts of the world. These diseases include, in rough order of frequency of occurrence, chlamydial infections, gonorrhoea, trichomoniasis, herpes, syphilis, chancroid, lymphogranuloma venereum and granuloma inguinale. Other diseases which are sometimes transmitted by sexual contact include candidiasis, genital warts, hepatitis, acquired immune deficiency syndrome, pediculosis, scabies and molluscum contagiosum.

In public health these diseases are very important. It will often be best to refer a patient with suspicion of sexually transmitted disease to a special department of genito-urinary medicine which has a full range of facilities for laboratory investigation, and social workers to help in the follow-up of contacts.

In treating a woman with venereal disease psychosexual problems are frequently encountered. There may be anger or resentment against the person who donated the infection, or there may be feelings of guilt or depression. Marital discord will be exacerbated if there is dyspareunia from pelvic inflammatory disease or herpes genitalis, or an offensive discharge such as that caused by trichomoniasis. Exaggerated fear of the consequences of 'VD' may lead to a variety of psychosexual symptoms.

These diseases may be of medico-legal importance. They may affect proceedings for divorce, and for a doctor to assert to a third party that anyone is suffering from venereal disease might be slanderous. None the less the doctor has a duty to protect others, and may have to give advice with this purpose.

## Syphilis

Syphilis is now far less common than non-specific infection, gonorrhoea and herpes genitalis, but it may accompany any of them. It has a double importance; first because if it is untreated it can cause serious lesions of the heart and blood vessels, the nervous system, the eyes and the bones; secondly because during pregnancy it may cause fetal death or the birth of an infected child. It is caused by a spirochaete, *Treponema pallidum*.

The disease may be described in three stages:

*Primary stage*
An abrasion of the skin, which may be minute, allows the organisms to

reach the subcutaneous tissues in which they multiply. After an incubation period of 9—90 days the multiplication of the spirochaetes gives rise to a lesion which usually ulcerates, and is termed a *chancre*. This ulcer is typical of the first stage of syphilis.

A chancre is rarely observed in women. Being almost painless, unless it is in a situation where it may be palpated, it may not be noticed by the patient and will heal spontaneously in 3 to 10 weeks, leaving a very slight scar. The chancre is most common on the cervix, but it may occur on the labia. Extragenital chancres may occur anywhere, but are most often seen on the lip, anus, nipple or finger. It is rare for there to be more than one present.

In an exposed situation the chancre first takes the form of a raised papule with an indurated base, but usually the patient is not seen until this has broken down to form a shallow punched-out ulcer with well defined edges and a smooth shiny floor. It exudes a serous discharge unless secondarily infected, when the discharge is more purulent. When it is on the labium the whole area becomes oedematous and tense. About a week after the appearance of the chancre the related lymphatic glands enlarge; they become rubbery, but remain painless, discrete and mobile. They do not suppurate unless secondary septic infection occurs.

To demonstrate spirochaetes the edge of the lesion is gently wiped with a swab dipped in normal saline until serum, but not blood, exudes. The serum is transferred to a glass slide and examined under dark ground illumination. Under an oil-immersion lens the treponemata appear as motile white corkscrew-shaped organisms against the dark background. The examination is repeated on 3 successive days. Confirmation by serological reactions on the patient's serum (see below) is obtained 6 weeks after the appearance of the chancre.

A cervical chancre differs from a carcinoma in the lesser degree of friability and lesser tendency to bleed on examination, and the sharp outline of the ulcer.

*Secondary stage*
Usually about 2 months after the appearance of the chancre the first evidence of dissemination of the spirochaetes occurs in the form of a rash, usually symmetrical. This may be a coppery coloured maculopapular rash on the trunk and limbs. It can also appear on the face and forehead (corona veneris). The rash does not irritate and can often be seen more clearly if the skin is cooled by stripping the patient and waiting a few minutes. In addition, there may be anaemia, slight pyrexia and headache. Alopecia can occur. There may be a sore throat, and 'mucous patches' within the mouth, which are whitish areas seen on the inner aspects of the lips, cheek and palate.

Another manifestation of syphilis which occurs soon after the appearance of the rash is the formation of *condylomata lata* in moist areas, especially around the vulva and anus. They appear as raised plaques which may be bilaterally symmetrical. They tend to become macerated, and so appear as raised discs with a slightly indented top which is covered by greyish exudate.

A slight generalized enlargement of all the lymphatic glands may be present at this stage; those in the posterior triangle of the neck and just above the elbows are sometimes especially noticeable.

In this stage the disease is contagious and spirochaetes can be found very easily, especially in the moist lesions. The serological reactions are always positive.

*Tertiary stage*
In the later stages of the disease, perhaps years after the chancre has healed, lesions occur which are due to endarteritis. These gummata may occur in skin, mucosae, bones and viscera, although they are very rare in the female genital organs.

Neurosyphilis includes meningovascular disease with focal lesions, tabes dorsalis and general paralysis of the insane. Cardiovascular lesions include aneurysms of the aorta and large arteries.

Many patients are found to be suffering from syphilis who have never experienced any symptoms. Sometimes the disease is discovered as the result of a routine serological test during an antenatal visit. If the patient becomes pregnant soon after acquiring the disease the fetus may die, usually in the last half of pregnancy, and spirochaetes may be found in its liver or in the intima of the umbilical cord. If untreated, subsequent pregnancies may proceed nearer to term until a child is born alive with signs of congenital syphilis.

Blood serological reactions are strongly suggestive of syphilis, but this diagnosis should never be made on the basis of only one type of test. While the tests are almost completely reliable in the secondary stage, they do not become positive for 4 to 10 weeks after the infection. All the tests are positive with other treponemal infections, such as yaws.

The *VDRL test* (venereal disease reference laboratory test) is a non-specific flocculation test for antibody (reagin). Transient false reactions may occur after some viral infections, after immunization against typhoid and yellow fever, and in some autoimmune diseases.

Specific tests for treponemata include the *absorbed fluorescent treponemal antibody test* and the *Treponema pallidum haemagglutination test*. These tests may remain positive for many years, even after the disease has been effectively treated. The best combination of screening tests is the VDRL test and the haemagglutination test.

## Treatment
Treatment should be begun at once with daily intramuscular injections of procaine penicillin 600 000 units in aqueous solution. If the patient is sensitive to penicillin, tetracycline 500 mg 6-hourly for 21 days, or erythromycin 500 mg 4 times daily for 10 days may be given. Careful follow-up is essential, and clinical or serological relapse will call for further treatment.

Patients treated in early pregnancy may expect a healthy child, but mother and child must be treated until they become seronegative and then observed for at least 2 years. During this period the serological reactions must remain seronegative, and a final cerebrospinal fluid examination must also be negative before a cure is certain. The mother is advised to have further treatment during each subsequent pregnancy.

## Gonorrhoea

This is caused by infection with the gonococcus. The gram-negative organisms are kidney shaped, and are seen under the microscope in pairs with their long axes parallel; they are often intracellular. Culture is not easy, and the inoculum must be incubated immediately. The gonococcus is grown on blood-agar or hydrocele-agar media in an atmosphere of 10 per cent carbon dioxide. After 6 weeks the gonococcal complement fixation test on the patient's serum may become positive.

Chronic cases may be difficult to diagnose, and repeated specimens for microscopy and culture should be examined, especially soon after menstruation.

Squamous epithelium such as that of the adult vagina is resistant to infection by the gonococcus. In children the vaginal epithelium is thinner and less resistant. Glandular epithelium, such as that of the cervix, urethra or Bartholin's gland, is easily invaded. The deeper layers of the connective tissue are little affected, but the infection spreads along a mucous membrane; thus after infection of the cervix it may ascend to the endometrium and Fallopian tubes, causing acute salpingitis. The initial symptoms are usually noticed within 2—7 days after exposure.

In rare cases the organisms enter the blood stream, causing endocarditis, arthritis and iritis.

### Symptoms and signs

These may be slight in women. The patient may notice a little discomfort on micturition, with slight urethral and cervical discharge. Acute infection of Bartholin's glands can occur and severe symptoms will arise if the infection spreads upwards to the Fallopian tubes. A patient may harbour gonococci, and transmit the infection, without having any symptoms.

Infection in small children will cause both vaginitis and vulvitis, with evident discharge.

### Diagnosis

If there is profuse discharge, this is most likely to be due to infection with *Trichomonas;* both infections may be acquired together. The most likely places to obtain pus containing the gonococcus are the urethra and cervical canal. After wiping away gross discharge, specimens of urethral and cervical discharge are taken with a wire loop. An immediate diagnosis can sometimes be made by examination of a stained smear but this alone should not be relied on. Warm culture plates, as described above, are innoculated directly in the clinic; otherwise, swabs may be sent to the laboratory in Stuart's transport medium.

## Treatment

Gonorrhoea in adult women is treated with a single dose of ampicillin 2 g with oral probenecid 1 g. If the patient is allergic to the penicillin group of drugs a single dose of spectinomycin 2 g is given by intramuscular injection.

After 7 days bacteriological tests are repeated. The woman should not have intercourse until these tests are clear. All sexual contacts should be traced and examined.

Complications will need additional or alternative treatment. Gonococcal salpingitis is treated in hospital with large doses of ampicillin together with oral probenecid, and a Bartholin's abscess will require drainage or marsupialization.

Gonorrhoea and syphilis can be contracted at the same time. Serological tests for syphilis should be carried out monthly while the patient is under observation.

*Treatment of the infant and child.* The treatment of gonococcal conjunctivitis in the newborn child is described in *Obstetrics by Ten Teachers.*

Gonococcal vulvo-vaginitis in an older child is treated with a single injection of cephotaxime in a dose related to age. If the child is allergic to cephotaxime spectinomycin 40 mg per kg is used.

## Chlamydial infection

Cases formerly described as non-specific genital infection in women or non-gonococcal urethritis in men are now recognized to be sexually transmitted and often caused by *Chlamydia trachomatis.* This organism is a gram-negative obligate intracellular bacterium, which reproduces inside host cells by binary fission. There are a number of strains.

*Chlamydia* cannot be isolated from patients by routine bacteriological techniques. It must be cultured by inoculation into suitable cells, in which occlusion bodies develop and can be stained and recognized. Material for examination must be conveyed to the laboratory without delay in a special buffered transport medium containing calf serum and antibiotics.

Serological tests are available. The complement fixation test is of limited value, but immunofluorescent tests can be used to detect specific antibodies for particular strains.

In men *chlamydia* is the cause of many cases of non-gonococcal urethritis, and may cause epididymitis. Some men harbour the organism without evident urethral discharge.

In women *chlamydia* may be found in the cervix, where it causes chronic cervicitis, often without symptoms. However, the infection may spread upward to the tubes, causing chronic salpingitis with the usual symptoms, and consequent infertility.

Ophthalmia neonatorum may be caused by *chlamydia* derived from the mother's cervix during delivery, and chlamydial neonatal pneumonia has also been reported.

Lymphogranuloma venereum (see p. 142) is caused by particular strains of *chlamydia*.

Fortunately these infections respond to tetracyclines and to erythromycin. Oral tetracycline, 500 mg 6-hourly for 2 weeks, is adequate for genital infection, and the same treatment may justifiably be given to the sexual contact of any male with non-gonococcal urethritis, even if she has no symptoms. In pregnant women erythromycin stearate, 500 mg 12-hourly for 2 weeks, is the best alternative to tetracycline.

As in all cases of sexually transmitted disease, serological tests for syphilis should be carried out.

## Herpes genitalis

It is estimated that in Britain there are now more than 10 000 new cases of genital herpes every year, and the number seems to be increasing. This is an unpleasant disease, with at present no cure, and which recurs from time to time.

There are two types of herpes simplex virus. HSV I causes herpes labialis. HSV II is the usual cause of herpes genitalis, although HSV I causes occasional cases through oro-genital contact. The virus invades cells, which it disrupts and in which it reproduces.

Symptoms of the first attack usually appear less than 7 days after sexual contact. The man concerned may have evident genital herpes, but in both sexes a few infected individuals may have such slight symptoms that the lesions are not noticed. Usually small extremely painful vesicles appear, which break down to form small ulcers and then scabs. Virus is shed from the lesions until healing is complete in about a fortnight.

In women the vesicles appear most commonly on the clitoris, labia and vestibule, but they may also occur on the vaginal wall and cervix, and sometimes on the perianal skin or thighs. Micturition may be very painful, and retention of urine may occur. In the initial attack there is often fever and malaise, and the inguinal lymph glands may be enlarged. The diagnosis is usually made on clinical examination, but viral cultures can be employed. For culture, serum is obtained from a vesicle or by rubbing a sterile swab over an ulcer, and sent to the laboratory in viral transport medium kept at 4°C.

In some patients the virus remains dormant, but in others recurrent attacks occur at irregular intervals. Although recurrent attacks may be milder and shorter than the first attack they cause much discomfort and misery to both partners, not infrequently leading to the breakdown of relationships and depressive symptoms.

Serious problems arise in relation to pregnancy. A primary attack of genital herpes during early pregnancy may cause abortion. If a primary or recurrent attack occurs during late pregnancy the fetus can be infected during delivery, and suffer damage to the central nervous system. Among infants with neonatal herpes the mortality is high, and those that survive may have neurological damage. If a mother has active herpes when she is in labour, delivery by Caesarean section before the membranes rupture is recommended.

Herpes virus has been linked with cervical dysplasia and cancer. There is certainly an association between herpes and cervical cancer, but the evidence that HSV II causes cancer is not convincing. Cervical dysplasia and cancer occur more frequently in women who have had several sexual partners and in those who began intercourse at an early age; such women might be more likely to be infected with herpes.

**Treatment**

Saline baths may relieve the local pain. Application of idoxuridine, 40 per cent solution in dimethyl sulphoxide, is expensive and probably useless. Recently acyclovir, which inhibits the intracellular synthesis of DNA by the virus, has been found to reduce the severity of the attack and the time during which virus is shed, but unfortunately it does not prevent recurrence. It may be used locally, but is better given orally in doses of 200 mg 5 times daily for 7 days. It can also be given intravenously, and might be so used for neonatal infection. A vaccine to confer immunity is now under trial.

Patients of both sexes should be warned that they are infectious whenever any lesions are evident. Women should have annual cervical smears.

## Chancroid (soft sore)

This is caused by infection with *Haemophilus ducreyii*. Small shallow ulcers occur on the vulva and vagina. The ulcers are multiple and painful, and may be surrounded by a zone of hyperaemia. They are irregular in outline with undermined edges. Their bases are covered with a greenish slough.

The glands in the groin become enlarged. They are tender and soft, thus differing from the adenitis associated with syphilis, in which the glands are discrete, firm and painless. As secondary infection with pyogenic organisms is common, these glands frequently suppurate.

The sores tend to heal spontaneously if kept clean, but if secondary pyogenic infection occurs there may be considerable destruction of tissue and consequent scarring.

The disease has to be differentiated in the early stage from simple pyogenic infection of hair follicles. Such furuncles have the ordinary appearance of boils elsewhere, and there is a hair follicle in the centre of each. It is distinguished from primary syphilis by the short incubation period, the multiplicity of lesions, and the inguinal glands which are soft, painful and tend to suppurate. Ducrey's bacillus can only be found with difficulty and diagnosis cannot rest on a search for it.

Chancroid may be treated with co-trimoxazole 960 mg twice daily by mouth. Persistent cases respond to tetracycline. If the glands suppurate, they are aspirated through healthy tissue, not incised.

## Lymphogranuloma venereum

This is caused by a strain of *Chlamydia trachomatis* which is transmitted sexually. It most commonly occurs in seaports of the Far East, Africa and South America.

In women the earliest genital lesion is an almost painless shallow ulcer, which gradually deepens and extends. The inguinal glands may be enlarged, and may break down to form multiple sinuses. The ulcers eventually heal, leaving irregular scars, and characteristic 'windows' in the labia minora where the tissue has been destroyed. The urethra may also be destroyed; and involvement of the rectum causes stenosis, sometimes with a recto-vaginal fistula. After some years epithelioma may develop in the involved skin. The diagnosis is made with a complement fixation test. The disease responds to tetracycline. Surgical treatment may be required if the urethra is destroyed or there is a rectal stricture.

## Granuloma inguinale

This disease occurs in the Caribbean, Southern United States and Africa. It is transmitted venereally. Mononuclear cells whose cytoplasm contains Donovan bodies are found in the lesions. The nature of these is uncertain; they have been described as bacilli or aggregations of virus. Discrete papules break down to form painful ulcers which extend over the vulva, perineum and groins, and the vaginal epithelium or rectal mucosa may be involved. Healing is followed by dense fibrosis, and there may be extensive swelling of the vulva (pseudo-elephantiasis). Epithelioma may occur in the damaged skin. The diagnosis is made by discovery of Donovan bodies in a biopsy. The ulcers heal with streptomycin or tetracycline, but residual fibrosis may require surgical treatment.

## Acquired immune deficiency syndrome (AIDS)

This is caused by human T-cell lymphotrophic virus (HTLV III), which is found in blood, semen and brain cells of infected individuals. It is diagnosed by antibody tests. The virus invades T-4 lymphocytes and causes immune deficiency, so that a variety of bacterial infections occur.

While it commonly occurs in male homosexuals after anal intercourse, it is uncommon in women after normal intercourse. It may be transmitted by blood transfusion, to haemophiliacs in blood products, and with infected needles during intravenous drug abuse. There is at present no treatment.

# 19

# Cysts and new growths of the vulva, urethra and vagina

## Vulval cysts

**Sebaceous cysts** arise from blockage of the ducts of sebaceous glands and most frequently lie in the area between the labia majora and minora. They contain a characteristic cheesy material, and may become infected.

**Bartholin's cyst.** A cyst may result from blockage of Bartholin's duct by inflammation or by inspissated secretion. It appears as a swelling situated to the inner side of the posterior end of the labium majus. As it grows it bulges across the vaginal introitus, and the posterior end of the labium minus is stretched over it. Small cysts may not give rise to symptoms, but large cysts cause discomfort and may become infected, to form an abscess with surrounding cellulitis.

A Bartholin's cyst is treated by marsupialization; an incision is made into the cyst and the lining epithelium is stitched to the skin. The opening contracts down to form a small sinus, and the gland may continue to function.

Recurrent cysts are best excised. Careful dissection is required and there is always free bleeding from the deep bed left after its removal. It is important not only to tie every bleeding vessel but also to drain the cavity; otherwise a very large haematoma may result.

**Cyst of the canal of Nuck.** Part of the processus vaginalis (p. 1) may persist to form a cyst beneath the anterior part of the labium majus.

## Benign tumours of the vulva

**Infective papilloma (condyloma acuminatum)** is caused by a virus. It is described on p. 98.

**Fibroma** and **lipoma** may occur, often becoming pedunculated.

**Hidradenoma** arises in the apocrine glands. It forms a sharply circumscribed, partly cystic swelling, rarely larger than 1 cm in diameter. Histological examination shows cystic spaces enclosing a papillary adenomatous mass, with cubical epithelium. Simple excision is adequate treatment.

**Pigmented moles or naevi.** These are relatively common on the vulva. They vary in colour from pale to black and may be smooth or hairy. Hairy naevi rarely become malignant, but other pigmented moles may become extravagantly malignant (see p. 146).

**Endometriosis** may appear as a vulval tumour, usually near the point of insertion of the round ligament into the labium majus. It may be a solitary lesion or part of widespread endometriosis. The tumour grows during reproductive life, and becomes tender during menstruation.

**Elephantiasis.** See Filiariasis, p. 341.

## Malignant tumours of the vulva

**Carcinoma of the vulva.** Carcinoma of the vulva accounts for about 5 per cent of the cases of genital cancer in the female. In Britain it is most often seen in elderly women, with a median age of 60. In about two-thirds of the cases leukoplakia or other dystrophic changes are found in the vulval skin. If patients with the histological changes of hypertrophic leukoplakia are followed up over a long time, about one-third will develop a vulval epithelioma.

In other countries where schistosomiasis, lymphogranuloma inguinale and granuloma venereum occur, these lesions may be followed by epithelioma, which then occurs in much younger women.

Most vulval cancers appear as ulcers, often with raised everted irregular margins, but sometimes the edge is abrupt and indurated. Hypertrophic growths may be quite large and even partly pedunculated; sooner or later they too break down and ulcerate. The histological appearance is that of a typical squamous cell carcinoma (epithelioma), often well differentiated with a good deal of keratinization. Very rarely, carcinoma may arise in Bartholin's gland. Secondary infection of any ulcerated growth is usual.

Although multiple primary cancers of the vulva may occur, multiple foci, even on both sides of the vulva, are most commonly due to lymphatic spread. Lymph node involvement is present in more than half of the cases when first seen, usually on the side of the lesion but often on both sides because the lymphatics cross the midline in the anterior part of the vulva. The superficial inguinal glands and the gland of Cloquet in the femoral canal are involved first; later the iliac glands are involved. Glands may be palpable because they are enlarged from infection of the growth rather than from malignant involvement, and conversely glands which are involved in growth may not be palpable.

*Symptoms and diagnosis*
Early signs are the formation of an ulcer or swelling on the vulva, with soreness or irritation. Slight bleeding may occur, and later there is a purulent discharge which becomes very offensive. In the late stages of the disease enlarged inguinal glands may break down and ulcerate, and occasionally severe haemorrhage occurs from erosion of the femoral vessels.

The diagnosis is made by biopsy. Since the tumour arises in dysplasic skin, malignant change may occur at any point and multiple biopsy is often necessary. A fissure or a persistent red area in leukoplakic skin must always be regarded as a possible site of carcinoma.

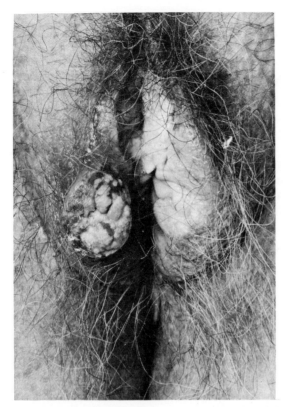

**Fig. 19.1** Squamous cell carcinoma of the right labium majus. There is leukoplakia on the left side.

*Treatment*
The treatment is radical excision of the vulva with the inguinal and femoral glands on both sides (see p. 344).

Recurrences are commonly local, and follow-up examinations may permit further surgery or irradiation. Radiotherapy has little place in primary treatment because the surrounding tissues have a low tolerance, but it may be used to treat local recurrences.

*Prognosis*
The prognosis depends on the stage at which the growth is first treated, and is very much worse if glands are involved. The size of the lesion affects the outcome; lesions less than 2 cm in diameter have twice as good a prognosis as that of larger tumours. If the growth is small when first seen and there are no palpable glands, after complete excision with removal of the glands about 75 per cent of the patients will survive 5 years.

**Malignant melanoma.** As a result of irritation or perhaps after incomplete excision a pigmented naevus may become malignant. Pregnancy will accelerate its growth.

The tumour forms a raised smooth swelling, which may become pedunculated and may ulcerate. Pleomorphic cells containing melanin spread into the underlying dermis. Invasion of the lymphatics and blood stream may lead to metastasis to the lung, brain and liver.

The prognosis is extremely bad. Treatment is by wide local excision; radical vulvectomy with dissection of the lymph nodes is inappropriate. Chemotherapy is not recommended for primary treatment but may be considered for any recurrence.

**Basal cell carcinoma (rodent ulcer)** of the vulva is a rare tumour which grows slowly and does not metastasize, although it infiltrates locally. It is removed by local excision with a good margin of skin.

## Lesions of the urethra

**Urethral caruncle.** This name is applied to a small swelling, usually bright red in colour, which presents at the urethral orifice. It is always single and arises from the posterior wall of the urethra, reaching a size of 0.5 cm. A caruncle consists of vascular granulation tissue, in which a few glandular structures may be seen; it is covered by thin stratified epithelium.

Caruncles usually occur in postmenopausal women. Some cause no symptoms, but most of them are very tender, causing pain on micturition or dyspareunia. Slight bleeding may occur.

They are not neoplastic, but probably result from chronic infection of the paraurethral glands in the floor of the urethra.

Caruncles are treated by excision or destruction with diathermy.

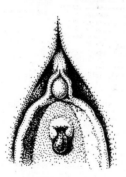

**Fig. 19.2** Urethral caruncle.

**Urethral cysts and diverticula.** Small cysts may occur in the floor of the urethra from blockage of the paraurethral glands.

A urethral diverticulum may present as a cystic swelling under the epithelium of the anterior vaginal wall. The diverticulum often becomes infected and causes dysuria and frequency, sometimes with intermittent discharge of pus or blood into the urethra. Occasionally a probe can be passed into such a diverticulum from the urethra, or it can be shown on a urethrogram. During excision any communication with the urethra must be carefully sutured; otherwise a urethral fistula may develop.

**Prolapse of the urethral mucosa.** This may occur in both children and adults. It presents as a vascular swelling which is distinguished from a caruncle because it surrounds the urethral orifice. It is treated by excision.

**Carcinoma of the urethra.** This is a rare tumour. It is usually a squamous-cell carcinoma arising near the meatus, but sometimes an adenocarcinoma arises in the paraurethral glands. The lymphatic drainage from the lower urethra passes to the inguinal glands, but that from higher levels passes to the obturator and internal iliac glands.

The growth may appear as a nodule or indurated ulcer around the urethral orifice. If it arises more deeply there is only thickening of the urethra to be felt. There is soon bleeding from the meatus, and retention of urine may occur. The diagnosis is made by biopsy.

If the lesion is near the meatus the treament is that described for carcinoma of the vulva. For lesions higher in the urethra an extensive excision of the urethra and bladder, with transplantation of the ureters into an ileal loop, may be necessary. Alternatively, teleradiation may be given, but with either method the prognosis is poor.

## Vaginal cysts

The vagina is lined with stratified squamous epithelium and normally does not contain glands. Occasionally, aberrant mucus-secreting glands occur in the upper vagina (*adenosis vaginae*).

Vestiges of the Wolffian ducts may give rise to cysts on the lateral aspect of the vagina (*Gartner's cysts*). In the lower vagina such cysts tend to lie more towards the midline of the anterior vaginal wall. They are lined with low columnar epithelium and contain serous fluid. Such cysts do not need treatment unless they are very large or become infected, when they can be excised or marsupialized.

Inclusion cysts lined with stratified epithelium may occur in the lower vaginal wall after childbirth or surgical procedures.

## Vaginal tumours

**Fibromyomata** occasionally arise in the vaginal wall. A hard, smooth tumour is felt under the epithelium and can easily be enucleated.

**Condylomata acuminata** may occur in the vagina (see p. 98).

**Endometriosis** of the rectovaginal septum may involve the posterior vaginal fornix.

**Carcinoma.** Primary squamous-cell carcinoma of the vagina is rare, but carcinoma of the cervix very commonly spreads to the vaginal vault, and in cases of endometrial carcinoma isolated vaginal metastases may occur, usually in the lower third of the anterior wall. Endometrial cancer may also recur in the scar in the vaginal vault after removal of the uterus.

Primary squamous-cell carcinoma of the vagina usually occurs after the menopause and most commonly affects the upper posterior wall. It occasionally follows the chronic ulceration which accompanies complete uterovaginal prolapse, or which may result from a long-retained pessary.

If an adenocarcinoma is found this is likely to be metastatic from the ovary or uterus, and the endometrium must be examined by curettage.

In the United States a number of cases of adenocarcinoma of the vagina have been found in teen-age girls whose mothers were treated during pregnancy with large doses of stilboestrol. The carcinoma is usually preceded by vaginal adenosis. The condition appears to be almost unknown in Britain, but if a woman carrying a female fetus has had such treatment during pregnancy the child should be followed up in her teens with regular vaginal cytological smears and colposcopic examination.

A patient with carcinoma of the vagina complains of bleeding, especially after coitus, and later an offensive watery discharge appears. The growth may ulcerate deeply to form a fistula into the rectum or bladder.

Treatment is very unsatisfactory. Most cases will be treated by local application of radium or caesium and teleradiation to the lymphatic glands of the pelvis.

The only alternative is an extensive operation involving removal of the whole vagina and the uterus, and the pelvic lymphatic glands. If the rectum is involved this must also be removed, and a colostomy established.

**Choriocarcinoma.** This rare form of malignant disease (at least in Britain) may occur as a secondary growth in the vagina. It forms a vascular nodule, dark purple in colour, which bleeds easily and resembles a localized haematoma. The appearance of such a nodule soon after abortion or delivery, and especially after the expulsion of a hydatidiform mole, should excite suspicion. High blood levels of chorionic gonadotrophin make the diagnosis relatively simple, but biopsy is also required. For treatment, see p. 192.

# 20

# Benign tumours of the uterus

## Fibromyoma of the uterus

Fibromyomata are the commonest new growths of the uterus and one of the most common tumours of the human body. They arise in the muscular wall of the uterus and vary in size from minute seedling growths to enormous masses occupying nearly the whole abdomen. They are often multiple.

To begin with they are interstitial and lie in the substance of the uterine wall. Those developing near the peritoneal or endometrial surfaces tend to project more and more towards these surfaces and to become subperitoneal or subendometrial. The projection towards the surface or the cavity of the uterus may continue until the covering of uterine muscle becomes so thin that the tumour is extruded through it and then is covered only by peritoneum or endometrium. Further extrusion will result in a polyp with a narrow pedicle in the uterine cavity, or a pedunculated tumour on the peritoneal surface.

## Structure

*Naked eye appearance*
On section the fibromyoma is paler, harder and more fibrous than the uterine wall. It has a silky, glistening cut surface, which shows a characteristic whorled arrangement of the tissue bundles. On comparing an interstitial tumour with the surrounding false capsule of uterine wall the difference is well marked. The muscle fibres of the uterine tissue are pinker, have a more parallel arrangement, and are separated from the growth by a thin plane of loose cellular tissue containing blood vessels. This layer offers a plane of cleavage and allows the tumour to be shelled out at the operation of myomectomy. The most active growth of the tumour takes place at the periphery. There is a tendency for the centre of the tumour to show degenerative changes.

*Microscopial structure*
These growths are composed of unstriped muscle and fibrous tissue. Although they are often referred to as 'fibroids' this is an inaccurate designation; the essential part of the tumour is the smooth muscle, and they should be described as fibromyomata or myomata.

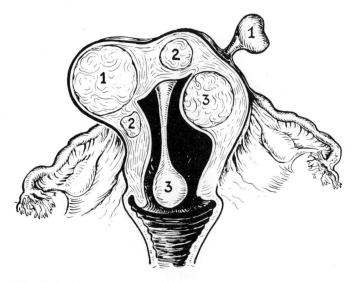

**Fig. 20.1**　Diagram to show positions which fibromyomata may occupy.
1, subperitoneal; 2, interstitial; 3, subendometrial.

In young and rapidly growing tumours the nuclei of the muscle cells are short fat rods with rounded ends. The nuclei of the fibrous tissue cells are not so uniform in shape, and are thinner and spindle shaped. The fibrous tissue lies between the muscle bundles.

Fibromyomata receive their blood supply from the vessels in the surrounding capsule. Within the tumour itself there are few vessels; they run in the connective tissue stroma between the muscle bundles.

## Aetiological factors

Clinical evidence suggests that the development of fibromyomata is related to the action of oestrogens. They arise during the period of menstrual activity, although they rarely give rise to symptoms before the age of 25. They do not originate as a new formation once menstruation has ceased.

Fibromyomata are more often found in nulliparous women or in women who have not been pregnant for some time. On the other hand, once developed they tend to favour infertility and miscarriage, possibly by distorting the uterus and by producing changes in the endometrium. During pregnancy fibromyomata hypertrophy and become more vascular and softer, and the oestrogenic contraceptive pill has a similar effect.

Fibromyomata occur three times more frequently in negresses than in white women, and occur at an earlier age. The reason for this is not known.

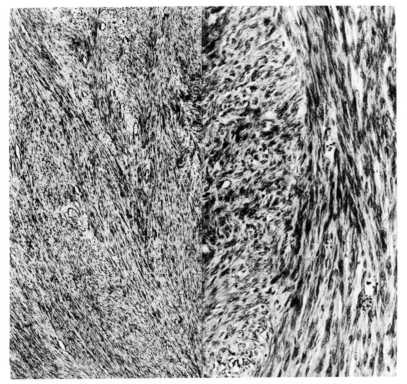

**Fig. 20.2** Microscopical sections of fibromyoma. × 40 and × 140.

## Varieties

### Corporeal fibromyomata

Fibromyomata arise far more often in the body of the uterus than in the cervix.

   **Interstitial fibromyomata.** Fibromyomata begin as small nodules in the myometrium. With increasing size they tend to be extruded towards the peritoneal surface or into the uterine cavity. With interstitial fibromyomata enlargement of the uterine body usually occurs, often with distortion and elongation of its cavity so that there is increased menstrual loss.

   **Subperitoneal (subserous) fibromyomata.** These vary greatly in size and are usually multiple. They range from small nodules on the surface of the uterus to enormous masses of 20 kg or more in weight. Subperitoneal tumours tend to grow up into the abdomen, and may become pedunculated so that on bimanual examination the tumour seems to be separate from the uterus and simulates an ovarian tumour. Rarely, torsion may occur, resulting in interference with the blood supply to the tumour. Adhesions to the omentum may occur from which a fresh circulation to the tumour develops, so that a tumour may become completely detached from the uterus and obtain its blood supply from these secondary attachments. Such tumours are spoken of as parasitic.

A fibromyoma may be extruded from a part of the uterus which is not covered with peritoneum — from the anterior wall below the peritoneal reflection or from the lateral wall between the layers of the broad ligament. Such tumours may cause considerable displacement of the pelvic viscera, including the ureter, which may then be endangered at operation.

**Subendometrial fibromyomata.** Some interstitial tumours are extruded towards the uterine cavity. At first they are still encapsulated in a layer of muscle, but this becomes progressively thinner until eventually the tumour is covered only by endometrium. The uterus contracts in an attempt to expel the tumour and it may be extruded until it becomes polypoid. The stalk of the polyp contains the few blood vessels which nourish it. Uterine contractions dilate the cervix and expel the polyp through it. The result is further elongation of the pedicle so that the blood supply of the tumour becomes inadequate, with liability to necrosis and infection of the tumour.

Small fibromyomata may sometimes be completely extruded through their capsule and overlying endometrium.

### Cervical fibromyomata

Only 2 per cent of fibromyomata arise in the cervix. Cervical tumours are usually single, although there may be other tumours in the body of the uterus. They cause distortion and elongation of the cervical canal and displace the body of the uterus upwards (see Fig. 20.5). A large cervical fibromyoma may cause retention of urine from elongation and distortion of the urethra.

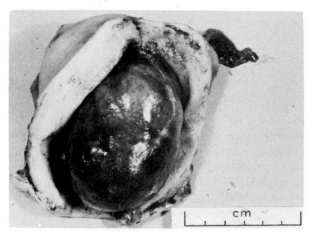

**Fig. 20.3** Uterus opened from in front to show subendometrial fibromyoma growing from the posterior wall and becoming polypoid.

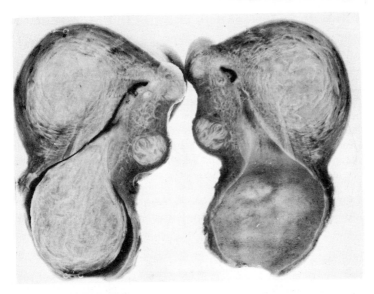

**Fig. 20.4** Fibromyomatous polyp. The tumour has been extruded into the cervical canal, which is expanded.

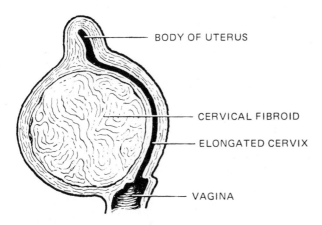

**Fig. 20.5** Diagram to show relationships of a cervical fibromyoma.

Cervical tumours may grow downwards into the rectovaginal septum, laterally into the broad ligament, or forwards between the cervix and bladder. Interstitial growths may displace the cervix or expand it so as to obliterate its projection into the vagina, making the os uteri difficult to recognize.

## Rate of growth and secondary changes in fibromyomata

Fibromyomata grow slowly; in some cases there may be no evident change in size for many years. In a few cases growth is more rapid and secondary changes may also cause swelling of the tumour. Pregnancy may result in increased growth. After the menopause the tumour ceases to grow, and may atrophy, sometimes becoming calcified.

Secondary changes often occur:

1. **Hyaline degeneration** is caused by a gradual inadequacy of the blood supply. Naked-eye examination shows irregular areas of homogeneous appearance which contrast with the fibrillary appearance of the areas which have not degenerated. Microscopical examination reveals that both the muscle fibres and fibrous tissue have undergone hyaline change, the cells being fused together in a structureless eosinophilic mass.

*Cystic degeneration* is not uncommon, especially after the menopause, and is due to liquefaction of the areas of hyaline change. Spaces develop which contain clear fluid and are lined by irregular ragged walls.

2. **Red degeneration (necrobiosis).** In this variety of degeneration the affected area is stained red and resembles raw meat. The freshly cut surface has a faint fishy odour, due to fatty acids. In some cases the process goes on to cystic degeneration in the centre of the tumour, the ragged cavity being filled with greasy brown debris. Thrombosed blood vessels can be seen, especially in the capsule. Fibromyomata less than 5 cm in diameter are seldom affected.

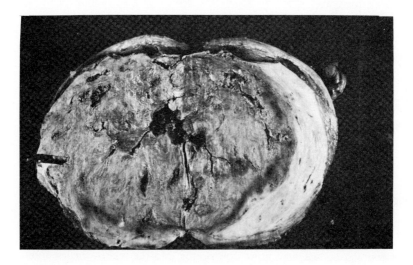

**Fig. 20.6** Red degeneration. The cut surface of this fibromyoma was purplish-red in colour. There is central necrosis.

It is probable that the initial change is fatty degeneration brought about by diminishing blood supply. If the blood supply to such a tumour is renewed, and especially if it takes place rapidly as in pregnancy, varying degrees of haemolysis occur, due to the action of the lipoids in the degenerated areas, producing the characteristic colour of raw meat. It is not certain whether the colour is derived from blood pigment or from a constituent of muscle cells.

3. **Fatty degeneration** is seen most commonly at and after the menopause. Fat globules are deposited mainly in the muscular elements. It is an essential precursor of calcareous degeneration.

4. **Calcification** is most frequently seen in fibromyomata in the aged. After the deposition of fat globules in the tumour cells, fatty acids are formed and these undergo saponification. Carbonates and phosphates in the blood react upon the soapy mass, resulting in the deposition of calcium carbonate and calcium phosphate. In the early stages calcareous deposits may only be recognized by a grittiness on section, or as a thin peripheral shell which is readily seen in an x-ray. Later the whole tumour is converted into a calcareous mass, the so-called 'womb stone'.

5. **Atrophy.** Fibromyomata atrophy after the climacteric as does the rest of the uterine muscle, but it is not to be expected that a large tumour will vanish; there is only a slight reduction in size.

6. **Torsion of the pedicle** of a subperitoneal fibromyoma has already been mentioned. The venous congestion causes the tumour to become dark red in colour from extravasation of blood. Acute symptoms like those due to torsion of an ovarian cyst are produced.

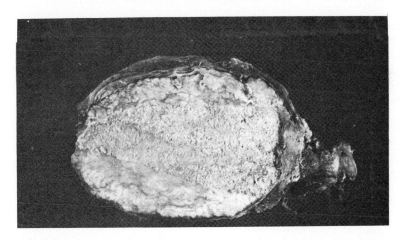

**Fig. 20.7** Calcification of fibromyoma. This tumour had to be cut with a bone-saw. The cut surface was greyish-white.

7. **Infection.** A polypoid tumour may undergo necrosis as a result of interference with its blood supply; the tissue is then invaded by organisms from the vagina.

A subendometrial fibromyoma may become infected after labour or abortion, or after too vigorous curetting. The tumour becomes necrotic and there is an offensive discharge with pyrexia.

8. **Malignant change.** Fibromyomata may become sarcomatous, but the change is extremely rare, being found in less than 0.2 per cent of tumours removed at operation. It is most likely to be seen in large tumours. The growth is usually a spindle-cell sarcoma. Metastasis occurs rapidly by the blood stream in these cases. Cases which have been described as recurrent fibromyomata were probably sarcomata.

Carcinoma of the endometrium may be associated with fibromyomata, but this is probably fortuitous, the fibromyomata being of long standing and unrelated to the carcinoma. Statistics are of little assistance because they relate only to cases in which surgery has been performed and do not include the large number of women with symptomless and untreated fibromyomata. Without denying that there may be common factors in the causes of fibromyomata and endometrial cancer, there is no justification for the removal of all symptomless fibromyomata on account of the risk of carcinoma.

However, it is stressed that haemorrhage after the menopause is always of significance, and it must never be attributed to fibromyomata until thorough exploration of the uterine cavity has excluded malignant disease of the endometrium.

### Changes in the uterus and other organs associated with fibromyomata

The enlargement of the uterus and its cavity caused by the growth of fibromyomata has been mentioned. There is often considerable hypertrophy of the myometrium.

Except with cervical and subperitoneal tumours, there is often hyperplasia of the endometrium; indeed it is possible that both fibromyomata and endometrial hyperplasia are related to hyperoestrinism. The ovaries are often enlarged and may contain follicular cysts.

Pelvic endometriosis (including adenomyosis of the uterus) is not infrequently associated with fibromyomata, and may be discovered unexpectedly at operation. Particularly in negresses, fibromyomata and salpingitis often occur together, but probably only because both conditions are common in these women.

## Pressure effects of fibromyomata

Bladder function may be affected. If the uterus is enlarged by the tumours and lies on the fundus of the bladder, there may be frequency of micturition, particularly on standing.

More serious pressure symptoms are caused by tumours which fill the pelvic cavity, displace the neck of the bladder upwards and elongate the urethra. Cervical fibromyomata are especially liable to have this effect, but it may also occur with tumours of the posterior wall which fill up the sacral hollow and push the cervix and body of the uterus upwards and forwards, or with tumours of the fundus which retrovert the uterus and occupy the rectovaginal pouch. Difficulty in micturition and retention of urine are produced, which may be of gradual or sudden onset. Retention may occur at the onset of a menstrual period, when slight engorgement of the pelvic structures may be just sufficient to cause it; after establishment of the menstrual flow the retention may disappear, to return again with the succeeding period.

Pressure on the ureter sufficient to obstruct it and cause hydronephrosis is extremely rare; the ureter may be displaced but is seldom obstructed.

The rectum is not often affected by pressure from fibromyomata; the bowel may be pushed to the side and flattened out, but intestinal obstruction from this cause is almost unknown. Constipation, haemorrhoids and varicose veins may occasionally occur, especially if the tumours remain confined to the pelvis, and with very large tumours gastrointestinal symptoms can arise.

The effects on pregnancy and labour are described on p. 162.

## Symptoms

Uterine fibromyomata may not cause any symptoms. It is not uncommon for tumours extending half way to the umbilicus to be discovered in the course of a routine examination.

**An abdominal tumour** is sometimes the first thing that the patient notices. It is so hard that it often attracts attention before any general abdominal enlargement is observed. The tumour is not tender (unless there is some complication) and rarely gives rise to pain, but occasionally causes local discomfort and a feeling of weight.

**Menorrhagia** is another frequent reason for patients to seek advice. The periods increase in amount and duration; they may be accompanied by the passage of clots. Intermenstrual bleeding is unusual, except if polypoid subendometrial fibromyomata are in the process of extrusion. Subperitoneal growths do not affect the menstrual loss; interstitial tumours may increase the loss; with subendometrial fibromyomata menorrhagia is nearly always present, and quite small tumours can lead to severe anaemia.

Severe bleeding may occur during extrusion of a fibromyomatous polyp, sometimes from tearing of a vessel at the neck of the polyp. If sloughing of the tumour occurs there will be an offensive discharge.

Fibromyomata are often associated with a late menopause, but haemorrhage after the menopause and any irregular loss should always suggest the possibility of carcinoma of the endometrium or cervix.

**Pain** is not a common symptom. When it occurs it is generally an indication that there is associated endometriosis or pelvic inflammatory disease, or of some complication of the tumour such as red degeneration or torsion. There may be colicky pain while a fibromyomatous polyp is being extruded through the cervix by uterine contractions.

**Frequency and retention of urine** may be caused by pelvic tumours, as described above.

**Effects on childbearing.** Although pregnancy associated with sub-peritoneal and interstitial fibromyomata is common, subendometrial tumours may cause sterility. Should pregnancy occur, subendometrial and interstitial tumours (if large or multiple) tend to cause abortion. Pelvic tumours may obstruct labour (p. 162).

## Physical signs

The physical signs vary with the size, position and number of the tumours. A symmetrical enlargement of the uterus is found with a submucous growth projecting into and distending the uterine cavity, and with interstitial growths of small or medium size. The uterus feels harder than when the enlargement is due to pregnancy, unless degenerative changes have occurred. More often the enlargement is asymmetrical; the tumour does not occupy a median position; it is often nodular on the surface because there are multiple tumours.

With subperitoneal fibromyomata the body of the uterus may be unaffected. If the pedicle is well formed the connection of the tumour with the uterus may be difficult to establish. Subperitoneal tumours with little myometrial covering often feel particularly hard. In large tumours the consistency may vary if degeneration has occurred.

Fibromyomata are not tender on palpation, with the uncommon exception of a tumour undergoing red degeneration.

A uterine souffle, similar to that of pregnancy, may occasionally be heard on auscultation.

In any case of doubt or difficulty an ultrasonic examination should be made.

On pelvic examination the cervix may be found to be pushed down or displaced to one side. Its projection may be obliterated if it is expanded by an intracervical tumour, or it may be dilated with the lower pole of a tumour felt within it. If a uterine sound is passed, the cavity of the uterus is often found to be enlarged; it may measure 12 cm or more.

During extrusion of a fibromyomatous polyp the cervical canal may be sufficiently patulous to allow the lower pole of the tumour to be felt. Later a hard growth surrounded by the dilated cervical lips is felt, or a rounded mass in the vagina with a pedicle which can be traced up through the cervix into the uterus. If the tumour is sloughing the surface will be soft and break away readily under the finger, and the discharge will be foetid; then the distinction from cervical carcinoma may not be easy. The size of the tumour may make it difficult to decide whether it comes through or arises from the cervix. The diagnosis is confirmed by examina-tion under anaesthesia so as to permit the finger being passed above the growth to explore its relations, and then by microscopial examination of non-necrotic portions of the tumour.

## Symptoms and signs caused by secondary changes in fibromyomata

**Degeneration.** No symptoms are caused by hyaline or cystic degeneration but the tumour may become so soft that diagnosis from an ovarian cyst may be difficult. In the case of a calcified tumour extreme hardness is characteristic, and the fibromyomata can be seen in a radiograph.

Red degeneration occurs most frequently during pregnancy. It is associated with increase in size of the tumour, pain and tenderness. There is often fever, and there may be vomiting.

**Torsion** may affect a pedunculated subperitoneal fibromyoma, or sometimes a whole mass of fibromyomata, including the uterus itself. Acute abdominal pain, vomiting and shock occur.

**Infection** of a fibromyoma after delivery or abortion causes high fever, uterine tenderness and foul discharge.

**Sarcomatous change** may be suspected if there is pain, with a rapid increase in size of the tumour, especially if this occurs after the menopause. There may be irregular bleeding.

## Differential diagnosis

**Other conditions which cause menorrhagia** may have to be considered. In dysfunctional bleeding there is, at most, slight enlargement of the uterus and at diagnostic curettage the cavity of the uterus is found to be symmetrical. The endometrium may show histological changes of endometrial hyperplasia.

Fibromyomata, except in the case of polypoid tumours in the process of extrusion, do not cause irregular bleeding. In all cases of irregular bleeding the possibility of carcinoma must be considered. Carcinoma of the cervix should be discovered by cytological examination and biopsy. Even if fibromyomata are present, in women near or past the menopause diagnostic curettage is essential to exclude endometrial carcinoma.

In the case of a sloughing fibromyomatous polyp with bleeding and foul discharge diagnosis can be difficult. Similar symptoms can arise with carcinoma of the cervix, uterine sarcoma, septic incomplete abortion or chorioncarcinoma. Exploration of the uterus and histological examination of the material removed is essential.

**Other conditions which give rise to a swelling in the pelvis** may also have to be considered.

*Uterine endometriosis (adenomyoma)* causes only slight enlargement of the uterus, unless fibromyomata are also present. If menorrhagia is accompanied by menstrual pain endometriosis may be suspected but a definite diagnosis of the nature of the tumour may only be made after its removal and histological examination.

*Ovarian tumours.* Ovarian cysts are not usually accompanied by disturbances of menstruation. They are generally obviously cystic, and are not usually attached to the uterus. The rate of growth of fibromyomata is slow; in ovarian cysts it is comparatively rapid.

A fibroma of the ovary is as hard as a uterine fibromyoma, but it is often accompanied by ascites, a very rare occurrence with subperitoneal fibromyomata.

Ovarian endometriomata may be mistaken for fibromyomata because they are usually adherent to the uterus, and ovarian carcinoma may also become fixed to the uterus and simulate a fibromyoma.

*Inflammatory swellings* in the pelvis may be attached to the uterus and so be confused with fibromyomata. In these cases there may be a history of septic abortion, a febrile puerperium or of recurrent attacks of pelvic peritonitis. Menorrhagia may be present, but it is generally accompanied by congestive dysmenorrhoea. The uterus is not enlarged; its fixity and that of the mass adherent to it, and the tenderness on palpation suggest the diagnosis.

*Abdominal and pelvic carcinoma.* Ovarian carcinoma may form a hard mass which is adherent to the uterus. There is often a history of pain, with increase in the size of the abdomen from ascites. Carcinoma of the bowel (and also diverticulitis) may have to be considered. Sigmoidoscopy and radiological examination after a barium enema assist in diagnosis, and laparotomy is often justified.

*Pregnancy* is more often confused with an ovarian cyst than with a fibromyoma. Fibromyomata never cause amenorrhoea. The pregnant uterus is soft and elastic, and contracts from time to time. Fibromyomatous enlargement of the uterus is harder and generally more irregular. Immunological tests for pregnancy will be positive and ultrasonic examination will show the presence of a fetus from about the 7th week, and the movements of the fetal heart can be detected from about the 8th week. Greater difficulty arises with a pregnancy in a uterus with many fibromyomata. Amenorrhoea will always suggest pregnancy, and call for a pregnancy test.

## Treatment

Small tumours that are not causing symptoms do not require any treatment. Patients with such tumours should be re-examined regularly so that treatment can be given if the tumour increases in size or symptoms arise. Once the menopause is reached, fibromyomata cease to grow.

Surgical treatment is indicated in cases with:

1. Heavy or prolonged bleeding.

2. Tumours of large size, even if these are not causing symptoms. In young women further growth is probable, and even in older women large tumours often undergo complications and ultimately cause symptoms.

3. Possible malignant change, such as a tumour which grows after the menopause.

4. Retention of urine.
5. Tumours which obstruct labour.
6. Tumours which have undergone torsion.

Myomectomy is occasionally performed for infertility when no other cause for it can be found, but no benefit is to be expected except in cases in which the tumours are closely related to the uterine cavity.

In cases of red degeneration, even though there is severe pain, surgical treatment is not required because the symptoms usually resolve spontaneously.

Fibromyomata may be removed by themselves (myomectomy) or together with the uterus (hysterectomy). For patients over 40 years of age hysterectomy is generally advisable, but for a younger woman, unless she already has the number of children she wants, myomectomy is to be preferred — not only because it leaves the possibility of childbearing, but also because some women resent the loss of the uterus.

The risks of straightforward myomectomy and hysterectomy are about equal, but if a large number of fibromyomata are present the risk of myomectomy exceeds that of simple hysterectomy. After myomectomy there is a risk that new tumours may develop in the conserved uterus, but this may be accepted by the patient if she is young and wants children.

*Abdominal myomectomy.* By abdominal exploration the surgeon can determine the number, size and position of the tumours and the condition of the uterine appendages. The presence of a large number of tumours is not necessarily a contraindication to myomectomy, but it is obvious that a solitary tumour is more easily dealt with than multiple tumours.

*Vaginal myomectomy.* A tumour which protrudes into the uterine cavity can be removed through the cervix, provided that the cervical canal can be dilated sufficiently to gain access to the tumour. Vaginal removal is contraindicated if the uterus is felt to contain fibromyomata other than the one in the cavity, unless the latter is septic and sloughing, in which case it alone may be removed by the vaginal route and the other tumours left *in situ* to be dealt with later by laparotomy.

The polyp is removed by grasping it with a volsellum to apply traction and then cutting through the pedicle with scissors. A sound should be passed above the tumour to define its extent before dividing the pedicle, to make sure that partial uterine inversion has not occurred; otherwise the peritoneal cavity might be opened. If the pedicle cannot be reached, the tumour has to be removed piecemeal. Serious haemorrhage from the pedicle does not usually occur since the bleeding is controlled by retraction of the muscle fibres.

*Abdominal hysterectomy.* In practice this is the commonest procedure. The operation may be subtotal, when only the body of the uterus is removed, or total, when both body and cervix are removed. Most surgeons believe that the cervix should always be removed during hysterectomy unless there are really exceptional operative difficulties. The possibility of subsequent cervical cancer is thus prevented.

Both ovaries, if healthy, should be conserved unless the patient has reached the menopause.

*Vaginal hysterectomy* is only suitable for tumours which do not make the uterus bigger than it is at the 10th week of pregnancy. It has the advantages that there is less postoperative pain and no abdominal scar. It has the disadvantage that adhesions may be very difficult to deal with. With large tumours which may have to be removed piecemeal the operation can be dangerous even in practiced hands.

## Treatment of fibromyomata complicating pregnancy

In the vast majority of cases pregnancy will go to term and labour will occur naturally, but the following difficulties sometimes occur.

There is an increased risk of abortion. If red degeneration occurs in a fibromyoma there may be pain during pregnancy or for a few days after delivery, but this does not call for surgical treatment. The patient is put to bed and given morphine or pethidine, and the symptoms usually resolve in about a week.

In the majority of cases the fibromyomata are in the upper segment of the uterus and normal labour is to be expected. When the tumours are in the lower segment there is some risk that they will remain below the presenting part and obstruct labour, but it is remarkable how often they will rise up out of the pelvis towards the end of pregnancy or even early in labour as the lower segment begins to stretch. When the tumour is truly cervical and fills an appreciable part of the pelvic cavity, it will certainly obstruct delivery. The patient should be allowed to go to term, and if there appears to be a chance that the fibromyoma may be pulled up, labour may be allowed to begin. If it becomes evident that normal delivery is impossible, Caesarean section is performed. It is occasionally possible to perform myomectomy at the same time, but it is usually safer to leave this until later. In the case of a patient who is unlikely to become pregnant again, Caesarean hysterectomy may be the best treatment; the operation is usually not difficult.

## Cervical adenomatous polypi

These develop from the endocervix as red or pink soft tumours, seldom larger than 1 cm in diameter, which come to project from the external os. The pedicle is occasionally long enough for the polyp to reach the vaginal orifice. They are rounded or tongue-like, and often contain spaces distended with mucus — hence the term 'mucous polyp'. On microscopial examination they are found to consist of glandular tissue similar to that of the cervix. The surface is covered with columnar epithelium, which often undergoes squamous metaplasia. Cervical glands, many of which are distended with mucus, lie in the soft connective tissue stroma. Sometimes the stroma is more dense, when the term fibroadenomatous polyp is used. The dependent part of the polyp is often congested and is the site from which bleeding occurs. The stroma may be infiltrated with inflammatory cells.

Multiple small polypoid tags of proliferating columnar epithelium may be found in association with chronic cervicitis, but with the ordinary type of cervical polyp there is no cervical infection.

There may be no symptoms, but in most cases slight bleeding occurs from the polyp, often after intercourse or examination. There may be a mucoid discharge, but if there is profuse mucopurulent discharge it comes from the cervical glands rather than from the polyp itself. Large polypi are easily felt on digital examination, but small soft polypi are easily missed if a speculum is not used.

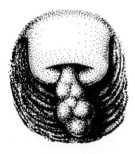

**Fig. 20.8** Cervical polyp.

It is easy to twist off a polyp without an anaesthetic, but there may be recurrence if the base is not cauterized. If the polyp recurs the patient should be admitted to hospital and given an anaesthetic, so that the cervical canal can be dilated and the stalk of the polyp properly cauterized. The uterine cavity should be explored with ring forceps and curetted to exclude the presence of endometrial polypi or of malignant disease which may be the real cause of the bleeding. Although adenomatous polypi are benign, it is essential to examine all polypi histologically to confirm their nature.

## Endometrial adenomatous polypi

Polypoid proliferation of the endometrium occurs in some cases of endometrial hyperplasia (p. 241), and such diffuse change may be indistinguishable from a solitary endometrial polyp on histological examination. However, the term endometrial polyp is confined to a condition in which one or at most a small group of polypi are found, usually in the upper part of the uterine cavity near the cornu, without other endometrial abnormality. They are soft red tumours, usually less than 1 cm in diameter, and often flattened to fit the cavity of the uterus. The pedicle is usually short, but is occasionally long enough for the polyp to project from the cervix.

On histological examination they are found to have a covering of endo-

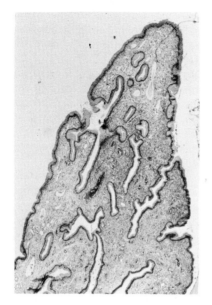

**Fig. 20.9** Histological appearance of endometrial polyp.

metrium and the soft stroma contains endometrial glands. The endometrial tissue may show the usual cyclical response to the ovarian hormones, but in many cases the response is incomplete and the polyp contains hyperplastic glands with cyst formation. Malignant change is rare but polypi may occur in association with endometrial carcinoma.

With solitary polypi there may be excessive menstrual loss or irregular bleeding. Uterine enlargement seldom occurs. Diagnosis is only possible after dilating the cervix and exploring the uterine cavity with ring forceps. Curettage without exploration with ring forceps may result in polypi being left behind. All endometrial tissue must be histologically examined.

## A note on uterine polypi

It may be helpful for the student to have a list of these. The word polypus means many-footed, but has come to mean any mass of tissue attached by a stalk. The following varieties of uterine polypi occur:

1. **Cervical adenomatous polyp.** See p. 162.
2. **Endometrial adenomatous polyp.** See p. 163.
3. **Fibromyomatous polyp.** See p. 152.
4. **Malignant polypi.** A carcinoma of the cervix may form a large polypoid mass in the vagina, and an endometrial carcinoma may project into the cavity of the uterus. A sarcoma or mixed mesodermal tumour of the uterus often forms a large polypoid mass which fills and enlarges the cavity of the uterus. The cervix may become dilated so that the lower pole of the

tumour can be felt through it. The rare botryoid sarcoma of the cervix of children presents as a multitude of grape-like soft polypi.

5. **Placental or fibrinous polypi** consist of a core of chorionic tissue covered with layers of fibrinous blood clot, which may be found in the uterus after delivery or incomplete abortion. The uterine contractions mould the mass into a polypoid form. There is continued bleeding, and the history will suggest that products of conception are retained. After dilatation of the cervix the polypoid mass is removed with sponge forceps and a blunt curette. Microscopical examination will reveal chorionic villi in the centre of it. In every such case the possibility of choriocarcinoma must be excluded.

6. **Nabothian polyp.** Occasionally a small cervical retention cyst is extruded so far that it becomes polypoid. It is of no importance.

# 21

# Malignant tumours of the uterus and Fallopian tube

Cancer may arise in the cervical epithelium or in the endometrium. There is considerable geographical variation in the relative incidence of these two types of cancer. In developing countries and in poor socio-economic conditions cervical cancer is much more common than that of the uterine body. In the United Kingdom the incidence of the two types is now about equal.

## Carcinoma of the cervix

### Aetiological factors

Carcinoma of the cervix occurs almost exclusively in women who have had sexual intercourse, and the incidence is higher in those who begin sexual relations at an early age or have several sexual partners. It has been suggested that cancer may follow infection with herpes virus type II, which is sexually transmitted, but this is far from proven. Recently an association between human papillomavirus (HPV) and carcinoma has also been reported, but it is uncertain whether this is causal or casual. Cervical cancer is less common in Jewesses; this was at one time attributed to the effect of male circumcision, but is more likely to be related to social behaviour.

There is a wide age distribution. Cervical cancer occurs most commonly between the ages of 45 and 55, but cases occur in much younger women (even in their 20s) and in older women of any age. The patients are usually parous, but it is some factor related to coitus rather than pregnancy which is the cause.

### Changes in the cervix that precede invasive cancer

Invasive cancer is frequently, but perhaps not invariably, preceded by dysplastic changes in the cervical epithelium. At the normal squamo-columnar junction there is an irregular and unstable *transformation zone* between two different types of epithelium — columnar epithelium which secretes mucus and squamous epithelium which forms keratin. Patches of small cells, known as reserve cells, are present immediately beneath the columnar epithelium and may also be seen around some of the glands.

On colposcopic examination the normal squamous epithelium on the

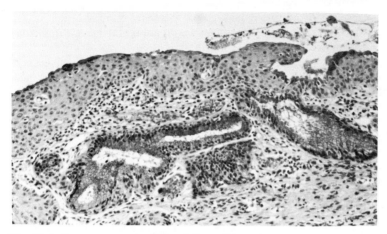

**Fig. 21.1** Squamous metaplasia of the endocervix.

vaginal surface of the cervix looks white, opaque and smooth. The normal columnar epithelium of the cervical canal and of the surface of the cervix near to the external os shows many fine folds, which when magnified appear as small translucent villous processes.

## Metaplasia

Metaplasia of the columnar epithelium into squamous epithelium frequently occurs, and results from proliferation and transformation of the reserve cells. The reserve cells form new squamous epithelium, and for a time degenerating remains of the columnar epithelium overlie this. Metaplasia may be patchy and partial, but in some cases it is widespread and also involves the cervical glands, when squamous epithelium may be seen deep to the surface in a histological section. The term epidermidization has been applied to this appearance, which must not be confused with carcinomatous infiltration. In metaplasia the cells are arranged regularly, without atypical nuclei and with few mitoses. Metaplasia is a reversible change and is not thought to be premalignant.

When metaplasia occurs in the transformation zone the new stratified epithelium looks white and opaque like normal stratified epithelium on colposcopy, but may be recognized as it is perforated here and there by the mouths of cervical glands which it has covered. (Fig. 21.1)

In a smear the cells shed from metaplastic epithelium consist of normal squamous cells, although a few degenerate columnar cells may be seen.

## Dysplasia

Dysplasia is a pathological change in the stratified epithelium which may be of varying degree.

Mild dysplasia may be seen with inflammatory conditions, for example trichomoniasis, and it will regress if the infection is treated and the inflammation resolves. However, it may go on to severe dysplasia which is less likely to be reversible and which sometimes progresses further to carcinoma-in-situ and invasive cancer.

In mild dysplasia the normal stratification of the epithelial cells is maintained, but the nuclei of the cells are large, slightly irregular and hyperchromatic. Degenerative changes may occur in the cytoplasm, giving halo-like clear zones around the nuclei. A cervical smear shows cells with these features but without the gross changes seen in malignant cells.

In severe dysplasia stratification of the epithelial cells is barely discerniable. The nuclei of the cells are enlarged, misshapen and hyperchromatic, and the distinction from carcinoma-in-situ may be very difficult. The smear shows cells with the nuclear features which have just been mentioned, although the outlines of the cells are normal.

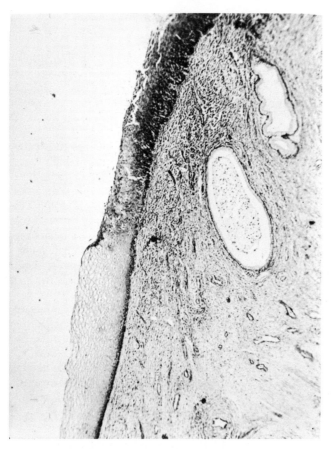

**Fig. 21.2** Squamous carcinoma-in-situ. Note the junction of healthy epithelium (below) and abnormal epithelium, and the absence of invasion.

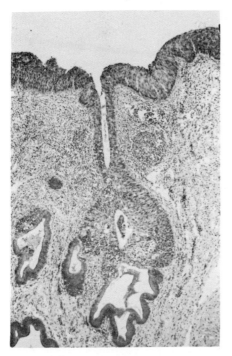

**Fig. 21.3** Carcinoma-in-situ. The surface epithelium is replaced by pleomorphic cells without orderly arrangement and with many mitotic figures. The abnormal epithelium extends down into a cervical gland. The basement membrane is intact but there is lymphocytic infiltration of the adjacent stroma. × 40.

### Carcinoma-in-situ

In carcinoma-in-situ (preinvasive carcinoma) there is complete loss of stratification of the cells. The whole thickness of the epithelium consists of closely packed undifferentiated cells, but the basement membrane is intact and there is no infiltration. The lesion occurs in one or more localized areas, and there is often a sharp line of demarcation between normal epithelium and the carcinoma. The smear shows basophilic cells which vary a good deal in size, but are characteristically rounded, with the nucleus enlarged to occupy more than half the cell. The nuclei show frequent mitoses, with hyperchromasia and coarse clumping of the chromatin.

Neither dysplasia nor carcinoma-in-situ produce symptoms. They cannot be recognized by naked-eye inspection, but in both conditions desquamated abnormal cells can be found in a cervical smear, and with the colposcope areas of suspicious change can be seen, with epithelium showing a mosaic pattern and prominent intra-epithelial capillaries, which appear in a punctate pattern (see Figs. 21.4, 21.5 and 21.6). Larger irregular vessels may suggest invasive cancer.

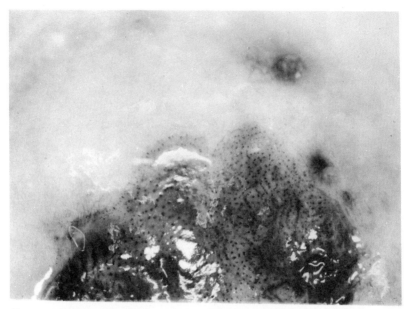

**Fig. 21.4** Colpophotograph of CIN III. The abnormal epithelium is darker, shows a capillary punctate pattern and is sharply demarcated from the normal epithelium above.

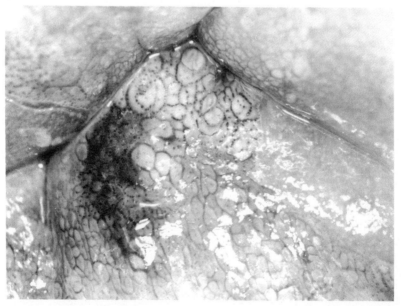

**Fig. 21.5** Colpophotograph of CIN III showing a mosaic capillary pattern.

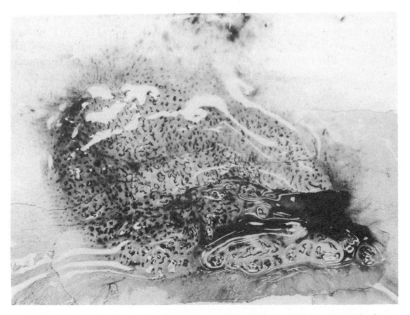

**Fig. 21.6** Colpophotograph showing capillary punctation and atypical vessels. Such irregular vessels raise the possibility of micro-invasive or even invasive carcinoma. (We thank Mr. J.A. Jordan for colpophotographs).

The term *cervical intracellular neoplasia (CIN)* has recently been introduced to include both cervical dysplasia and carcinoma-in-situ. The term denotes a continuum of disorders ranging from mild dysplasia (CIN I), through moderate dysplasia (CIN II) to severe dysplasia and carcinoma-in-situ (CIN III). Cases of CIN I can return to normal, but those of CIN II are more likely to persist, while CIN III is undoubtedly pre-malignant. The older terms were said to be unsatisfactory because they depended on the uncertain judgement of the particular pathologist; it is hard to see how the new terms avoid this difficulty.

The proportion of cases of dysplasia and carcinoma-in-situ that progress to invasive cancer is uncertain, and is now hard to assess because recognized cases are treated, but it is probably about 10 per cent over a time span of 10 years.

## Diagnosis and treatment of cervical intracellular neoplasia

If abnormal cells are found in a cervical smear histological examination is essential. In the past this was usually done by conization of the cervix (cone biopsy), which often also served for treatment. The base of the cone included the entire squamo-columnar junction, and the apex of the cone was at the internal os. This extensive procedure was sometimes accompanied by severe bleeding, and occasionally followed by cervical stenosis or incompetence. It is claimed that with the colposcope suspicious areas can be identified and small pieces of tissue taken for histological examination without the need for cone biopsy. Areas of abnormal epithelium can then be locally destroyed with heat (diathermy cauterization), cold (cryosurgery) or with a laser.

Conization is still required for diagnosis when the whole lesion cannot be seen, for instance if it extends up the cervical canal. It is also required when micro-invasion has been diagnosed by target biopsy. The term micro-invasion is used when there is an early invasive lesion, up to 5 mm in depth, but no clinical sign of disease.

Hysterectomy is advised if histological examination of the cone of tissue shows that the lesion has been incompletely removed. If the vaginal vault is involved hysterectomy with removal of a vaginal cuff is performed.

Pregnancy has no effect on the disorder or its management, except that control of bleeding from a cervical biopsy may be difficult. After colposcopy it is often possible to defer definitive operative treatment until 12 weeks after delivery.

Widespread use of exfoliative cytology can reduce the death rate from cervical cancer, but the number of women with cervical dysplasia is increasing, and so is the death rate from cervical cancer in women under 35 years of age. There is evidence to suggest that when dysplasia progresses over some years to invasive cancer most of the tumours are slow growing, and therefore more curable. On the other hand an invasive growth arising without evident preceding cervical changes tends to be biologically aggressive, with a high mortality rate.

## Pathology of invasive carcinoma

Carcinoma may arise from the vaginal surface of the cervix (*ectocervical carcinoma*) or from the cervical canal (*endocervical carcinoma*). The former occurs five times more often than the latter.

Ectocervical carcinoma may appear as a fungating cauliflower-like growth which may completely fill the vagina, or more commonly as an ulcer on the cervix. This type of carcinoma is almost invariably of the squamous cell variety.

Endocervical carcinoma arises from the columnar epithelium of the cervical canal or from the cervical glands. It may expand the cervix into a barrel shape. The surface epithelium remains intact for a time but is eventually eroded; infection occurs, and the growth sloughs away to produce a large cavity. Contrary to what might be expected, the majority of endocervical cancers are of squamous type, because the epithelium has previously undergone metaplasia. Adenocarcinoma of the cervix is uncommon, and is found in only 4 per cent of cervical cancers.

Carcinoma of the cervix spreads by direct infiltration and by the lymphatic vessels. Infiltration goes on all round the growth; it may spread

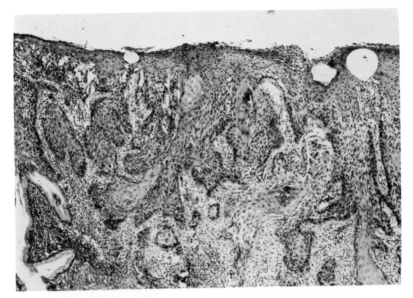

**Fig. 21.7**  Squamous cell carcinoma of cervix.

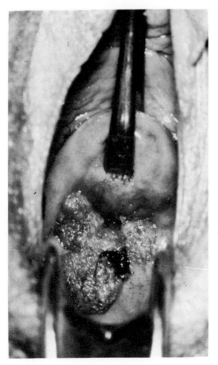

**Fig. 21.8**  Carcinoma of cervix.

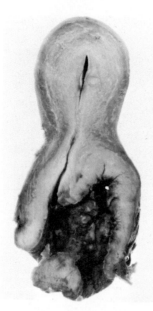

**Fig. 21.9**  Endocervical carcinoma.

downwards into the vaginal wall, forwards into the bladder, laterally into the parametrium and backwards along the uterosacral ligaments towards the rectovaginal pouch and the rectum. Upward extension may also occur to the body of the uterus.

Lymphatic spread occurs outwards and backwards in the parametrium and in the uterosacral ligaments to the internal iliac and external iliac nodes, including those in the obturator and presacral regions, and sometimes directly to the common iliac and para-aortic nodes (Fig. 1.14).

Metastasis to distant organs by the blood stream or lymphatics is relatively uncommon; the patient usually dies from the results of local invasion before these distant metastases become clinically manifest. They are therefore more likely to be seen in treated cases in which the local tumour has been irradiated or removed.

Generally speaking, the more differentiated a carcinoma is, the slower it grows. On the other hand, the more differentiated growths are less responsive to treatment by irradiation. Thus there are two opposing factors affecting prognosis – the less well differentiated growths spread faster, but are more sensitive to radiation. In practice the prognosis depends more on the extent of the growth at the time of diagnosis than on the histological type. When the lymph glands contain a metastasis the prognosis is worse, no matter what the histological type or what treatment is given.

## Cytological diagnosis of cervical cancer

Pre-invasive and very early invasive cervical cancer can be detected by exfoliative cytology before there is any clinical evidence of disease. The appearance of the nucleus of the cell is more important than that of the cytoplasm in deciding whether a suspicious cell is malignant. The nucleus of a malignant cell may be abnormally large, hyperchromatic, or have an irregular shape or chromatin pattern. There may be multiple nuclei and abnormal mitotic figures. The cell as a whole may be of bizarre shape, and show cytoplasmic vacuolation. If a group of cells can be seen, the boundaries between them may be indistinct.

However, the diagnosis of malignant disease by cytological methods is not as reliable as by histological sections, because the observer is only looking at a single cell or small groups of cells, and there is no possibility of determining whether there is invasion, which is an essential criterion of malignancy. A cytological diagnosis of malignant disease must always be confirmed by histological examination of biopsy material, which is fortunately easy to obtain from the cervix.

Despite much effort in screening programmes during the last 25 years the mortality from cancer of the cervix in Britain has hardly changed, and the effectiveness of screening has been questioned. The present screening programme in the National Health Service concentrates on women over 35 years of age. In the population as a whole many women escape being examined, and those of lower social class, in whom the risk is greatest, tend to make least use of the procedure. In other countries, and in more circumscribed groups in Britain such as those at Aberdeen, it has been certainly shown that when screening is intensive and efficient the mortality is reduced. It is possible that the limited success in Britain is also because there has been an increase in frequency of the disease in younger women among whom there is an increase in cervical dysplasia. The best use of limited financial resources for screening is currently being debated.

## Symptoms

Carcinoma-in-situ causes no symptoms.

In most cases of invasive carcinoma the earliest symptom is bleeding, at first irregular and brought on by coitus or noticed after micturition or defaecation. Later it becomes continuous, although varying in quantity. Unfortunately, women sometimes regard irregular bleeding at the time of the menopause as normal, and if the patient is still having periods the bleeding may be attributed at first to irregular menstruation.

When the growth ulcerates and becomes infected, a thin blood-stained discharge appears, and later becomes offensive.

Pain develops late, and indicates extension of the growth beyond the limits of the cervix.

In advanced cases bleeding may be very heavy, although it is seldom the immediate cause of death. The discharge becomes copious and exceedingly

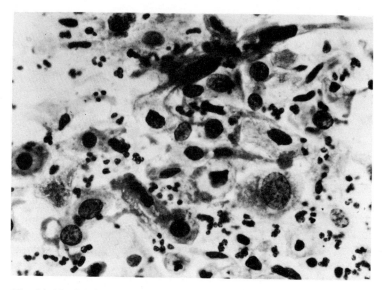

**Fig. 21.10** Cervical smear. × 530. Squamous carcinoma of cervix. Large cells with abnormal nuclei.

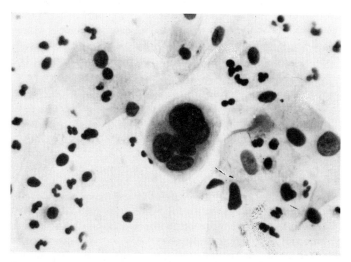

**Fig. 21.11** Cervical smear. Squamous carcinoma of cervix. × 600. Multinucleated malignant cells with altered nuclear/cytoplasmic ratio, nuclear hyperchromasia and variation in nuclear size.

foul. There may be lower abdominal pain when there is a large pelvic mass, or pain may be felt over the sacrum if there is extension along the utero-sacral ligaments. Very severe and intractable sciatic pain may result from involvement of lymphatic nodes which have become adherent to the sacral plexus. Vertebral metastases will also cause back pain.

Finally, incontinence of urine, and sometimes of faeces, may occur following ulceration into the bladder or rectum. The patient is in constant distress and becomes cachectic. Sepsis and pain are important contributory factors. Death is most commonly due to uraemia following the blockage of both ureters or to ascending pyelonephritis, but it sometimes occurs from haemorrhage or the effects of metastases.

## Physical signs of invasive cancer

Carcinoma arising on the vaginal surface of the cervix when seen early (which unfortunately is unusual unless the discovery follows cytological examination) presents either as a nodule, a small ulcer or a diffuse patch not unlike an exuberant erosion. Whichever form it takes, the examiner may be struck by the amount of bleeding which very light touch provokes. When the growth is more advanced it presents either as a crater-shaped ulcer with high and everted edges or as a friable warty-looking mass which may give the impression of being partly pedunculated. The term 'friable' means that small fragments of the growth may break away on touch, or that a probe will sink easily into the growth. There is free bleeding on examination, and more or less watery discharge which is often very offensive.

Endocervical carcinoma in the early stage is more difficult to recognize. Examination with the speculum may shown no abnormality, and the condition may only be discovered when curettage is performed for irregular bleeding. Later the cervix becomes much enlarged, hard and barrel shaped. When the growth has broken through the cervical surface, a deep excavation with indurated edges is felt.

The mobility of the cervix varies with the stage of the growth. When the parametrium is involved in growth or infection the cervix becomes fixed. Rectal examination, which is essential in every case, will show whether the growth has spread to the parametrial tissues and uterosacral ligaments.

Pyometra occasionally occurs and causes uterine enlargement.

## Differential diagnosis

Irregular bleeding at any age must always be promptly investigated. Many cases of cancer of the cervix are missed for a time because of a failure to make a vaginal digital and speculum examination. Any lesion on the cervix that bleeds on gentle examination should be regarded with suspicion, and the diagnosis must be settled by taking a biopsy.

It is worth mentioning that normal squamous epithelium covering the cervix and lining the vagina contains glycogen and stains a dark brown colour if it is painted with Lugol's solution (iodine and potassium iodide in water). Areas of abnormal epithelium may fail to stain and are possible sites for carcinoma. This is known as Schiller's test.

The fungating type of growth can hardly be mistaken. The friable growth can hardly be confused with a sloughing fibromyomatous polyp, which is harder and not friable. A septic abortion has only a superficial resemblance to a cervical cancer; the products of conception are seen to be in process of extrusion through a dilated cervix, not growing from it.

Carcinoma has occasionally been confused with a cervical erosion, which also sometimes causes postcoital or intermenstrual bleeding. The surface of an erosion is velvety, with an underlying firmness. It is never friable, and when rubbed with the finger oozes from many points, unlike a carcinoma which bleeds from a definite vessel. Rare causes of error are tuberculosis, syphilitic chancre, schistosomiasis and choriocarcinoma.

## International classification of stages of carcinoma of the cervix

The selection of treatment and the prognosis depend on the extent of the growth. The International Federation of Obstetrics and Gynaecology (FIGO) is now responsible for the system of staging. It was originally devised as a purely *clinical* method of assessment, so that the results of surgery and radiotherapy could be compared. The classification has since been extended to include the result of preoperative biopsy, but for statistical purposes the staging should never be revised after treatment, for example, in the light of operative findings. The stages may be summarized as follows.

*Preinvasive carcinoma*
Stage 0. Carcinoma-in-situ.
*Invasive carcinoma*
Stage I. Carcinoma confined to the cervix (except that extension up to the body of the uterus may be disregarded). Cases in which the diagnosis cannot be made clinically, but only by histological examination, are termed Ia; all other cases of stage I are then Ib.
Stage II. The carcinoma extends beyond the cervix but not to the pelvic wall. The carcinoma involves the vagina but not the lower third. The cases may be subdivided into IIa with no obvious parametrial involvement, and IIb with parametrial involvement.
Stage III. The carcinoma has extended to the pelvic wall, or the tumour involves the lower third of the vagina.
Stage IV. The growth has extended beyond the true pelvis, or has involved the mucosa of the bladder or rectum.

Staging is best done when the patient is anaesthetized for cervical biopsy. Rectal examination is essential for proper assessment.

Before a decision about treatment is made other investigations are required. Some surgeons perform cystoscopy routinely, although extension to the bladder is very unlikely to be found at the time of first diagnosis. Bullous oedema of the mucosa is the first sign. In every case an intravenous pyelogram should be obtained. If there is hydronephrosis or evidence of ureteric obstruction, this indicates parametrial involvement. It is also advantageous to discover any congenital anomaly such as a double ureter before surgical treatment. A radiograph of the chest is obtained in every case.

## Treatment

The treatment of carcinoma-in-situ has already been described on p. 174.

If invasive cancer of the cervix is left untreated, the average course of the disease from the onset of the first symptom to death is about 2 years.

It may be treated by surgery or by irradiation, or by a combination of these. In the past there has been a tendency to treat the disease entirely by surgery (in operable cases, which are those in stages I or IIa) or entirely by radiotherapy. The exponents of these two lines of treatment have not been entirely free from bias in assessing the results, but it may be said that for comparable cases the final results have been about equal. However, the two methods are not mutually exclusive, and the best results are obtained when treatment is planned by a gynaecologist and a radiotherapist working in close co-operation. The clinical staging should be done by them together, when agreement can be reached about treatment.

Radiotherapy will cure many patients who cannot be treated surgically, because of the advanced stage of the growth, old age or coincidental ill health. It may also be argued that radiotherapy is the method of choice for early cases, although in such cases there is no certain means of knowing whether the lymphatic glands are involved or not; lymphography for this purpose has not yet given reliable results. Even if the glands are involved it does not follow that surgical treatment is superior; the surgeon cannot cure all such cases by dissecting out the glands, and teleradiation can cure a few of them.

Radiotherapy is contraindicated in cases with pelvic sepsis or large fibromyomata, and the local application of caesium or radium may be difficult if there is vaginal stenosis. If the patient is pregnant, special problems arise (see p. 182).

**Radiotherapy.** With the increasing complexity of apparatus, and the greater accuracy of dosage which is possible, the treatment of carcinoma of the cervix with ionizing radiation has become a specialized subject. There is as yet no universally accepted method of treatment, and little more can be given here than an outline of the basic principles.

The aim is to deliver a lethal dose of radiation to the cervix, the lower part of the uterus, the upper vagina, the parametria and the proximal parts of the uterosacral ligaments. This calls for a zone of irradiation shaped like an inverted pear (see Fig. 21.13), but flattened anteroposteriorly so as to minimize the reaction of the bladder and rectum. If these organs receive

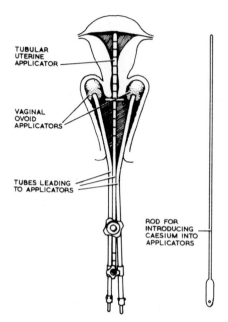

TUBULAR
UTERINE
APPLICATOR

VAGINAL
OVOID
APPLICATORS

TUBES LEADING
TO APPLICATORS

ROD FOR
INTRODUCING
CAESIUM INTO
APPLICATORS

**Fig. 21.12** Intrauterine and vaginal applicators for caesium.

excessive irradiation, severe cystitis or proctitis will ensue, even leading to necrosis and fistula formation.

To provide a local source of $\gamma$ radiation, sealed containers (usually called applicators) holding caesium ($^{137}$Cs) or radium ($^{226}$Ra) are placed in the uterine cavity and vaginal vault. Several methods of treatment are in use. In the Manchester method, which is typical of many, the aim is to deliver an appropriate dose of radiation at a point (A) situated 2 cm lateral to the midline and 2 cm above the vaginal fornix. This was chosen as a good index point in considering the tolerance of the normal tissues as well as the tumour dosage (Fig. 21.13).

Two applications are usually made, separated by an interval of about 6 weeks during which external radiation is given. The radiation from the sources in the uterus and vagina rapidly decreases with distance according to the inverse square law, so that the dose delivered to any involved nodes on the pelvic wall would be inadequate without additional external radiation. A typical total dose would be 7000–8000 cGy to point A and 5000–6000 to the pelvic side wall.

For the insertion of the local sources the anaesthetized patient is placed in the lithotomy position and the cervix is exposed. A uterine sound is passed to measure the uterine cavity, and the cervix is dilated to allow the insertion of an intrauterine applicator of appropriate size. One or two ovoid applicators are placed in the vaginal vault, depending upon the extent of the disease and the capacity of the vagina. A self-retaining catheter

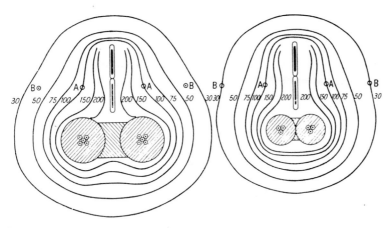

**Fig. 21.13** Manchester technique. Isodose curves with dose at point A as 100 per cent *(a)* Standard applicators for large vagina. *(b)* Standard applicators for small vagina.

is inserted into the bladder, and the vaginal fornices are packed with gauze to keep the bladder and rectum as far away as possible. Some applicators are designed to be attached to a colpostat, an adjustable intravaginal device which holds them in their correct relative positions; otherwise the applicators are kept in place with vaginal gauze packing. They remain in place for 40—60 hours at each application.

Doctors looking after patients in whom radioactive sources are inserted must ensure that proper safety precautions for staff and for other patients are carried out. To reduce the radiation risk most units now employ after-loading techniques. With the patient anaesthetized, empty applicators are inserted in the theatre, and these can be correctly positioned without haste or danger to theatre staff. An x-ray examination is made to check the position of the applicators, and to help the physicist calculate the time needed to give the required dose of radiation. The patient is then removed to a treatment room which has appropriate radiological protection and the radioactive sources are quickly introduced into the applicators. She is kept in a bed shielded to secure the best possible radiation safety until the sources are removed.

Some centres use the Cathetron, a machine which is designed to administer a high local dose of radiation in a very few minutes. Flexible tubular ducts lead to the applicators, and when these are correctly positioned, with the patient in a protected cubicle, very potent radiocobalt sources of radiation are passed directly from a protected store along the ducts by mechanical means. Because of the high intensity of the sources they need be in place for only a short time.

*Complications of radiotherapy.* The risk of radiotherapy is less than that of surgical treatment, but there is a small mortality, mostly associated with sepsis.

However, other complications can occur, such as proctitis which may lead to rectal stricture, radiation cystitis and even fistula formation, and severe vaginitis and vaginal stenosis leading to apareunia. The last complication can be prevented by regular use of vaginal dilators during treatment. Irradiation damage to adherent loops of small intestine may occur, and in premenopausal women ovarian function is destroyed, leading to severe menopausal symptoms. Many gynaecologists prefer to treat young women with early disease surgically, conserving the ovaries to avoid this abrupt menopause.

**Surgical treatment.** Radical hysterectomy can be performed by the abdominal or vaginal route; the former method usually carries the name of Wertheim, the latter that of Schauta.

Wertheim's operation consists of the removal of the uterus, tubes and ovaries, together with most of the vagina, the pelvic cellular tissue lying laterally to the uterus and vagina, and the lymphatic glands in the obturator fossae and along the internal and external iliac vessels. It is a difficult operation and should not be attempted except by those who have been trained in its performance. It has the drawback that the ureter has to be dissected freely, so that it is deprived of part of its blood supply, with a risk of necrosis and fistula formation.

Surgical treatment is suitable for cases in Stages I and IIa. The immediate mortality has been much reduced in recent years by selection of cases and improvements in technique; it should not be higher than 1 or 2 per cent.

Radical vaginal hysterectomy (Schauta's operation) also demands special skill. It has been performed in large series of cases with a low mortality, but it is seldom carried out in Britain because it is not possible to remove the pelvic lymphatic glands by this route.

**Combinations of irradiation and surgery.** Combined methods may be suitable for some cases. Some surgeons use local irradiation as a preliminary measure before surgery. Local sepsis is cleared up and the growth becomes more mobile; a few apparently inoperable growths become operable after irradiation.

Cases that prove refractory to radiation may be extirpated surgically, provided that the primary growth is not too extensive to permit this.

A few surgeons routinely dissect the lymph nodes 3 months after a full course of intracavitary irradiation.

However, so far such combined methods of treatment have not produced results that are strikingly superior to those achieved by surgery or irradiation alone.

**Carcinoma of the cervix and pregnancy.** Difficult problems arise. In early pregnancy external irradiation may be given; abortion of a dead fetus will follow and then local irradiation with caesium can be given. Later in pregnancy the uterus must be emptied by hysterotomy or Caesarean section before caesium can be inserted. Many surgeons prefer to treat these cases by Wertheim's hysterectomy, even at the time of Caesarean section.

**Pelvic exenteration.** In a few selected cases of advanced disease which has spread into the bladder or rectum, but in which clinical evidence of distant metastases is absent, pelvic exenteration may be considered. The operation is of great magnitude and consists of removal of the uterus, vagina and bladder, with implantation of the ureters into the sigmoid colon or into an artificial bladder made from an ileal loop. If the rectum also has to be removed, the ureters are implanted into an end colostomy or an ileal loop. The operative mortality is about 20 per cent, but a 5-year survival rate of 10 per cent in advanced cases has been claimed.

**Carcinoma of the cervical stump after hysterectomy.** The stump of cervix left after subtotal hysterectomy is just as prone to the development of carcinoma as that of the intact uterus. The results of treatment of stump carcinoma are much worse than when the uterus is intact. Intra-cavitary radiotherapy is prejudiced because an intrauterine container cannot be used, and vaginal irradiation may not deliver a dose sufficient to destroy the growth without risk of damage to the bladder or rectum. Surgical treatment is prejudiced by the previous operation.

Stump carcinoma is an avoidable disaster. With very rare exceptions there is no justification for the performance of subtotal hysterectomy in any patient who has had intercourse.

**Palliative treatment** is required for the distressing symptoms which may arise in the advanced stages of the disease. Patients with growths that are too advanced for curative treatment, and also those with recurrent disease, must be kept free from pain and as comfortable as possible. Expert nursing is necessary, especially when incontinence compels frequent changing of pads and sheets. For the pain codeine, pethidine and similar analgesic drugs may at first be sufficient. At a later stage opium and its derivatives are required, and the pain may call for progressively larger doses, which may cause nausea and vomiting. A combination containing a phenothiazine may then be effective. Anaesthetists skilled in this field may be able to help with nerve-blocking procedures involving thecal injection of phenol or alcohol. Surgical division of the spino-thalamic tract (cordotomy) will also give relief.

Surgical measures will sometimes be required for the unpleasant com-plication of a vaginal fistula. While a few surgeons will transplant the ureters or perform a colostomy, such procedures may only prolong the act of dying. The more local operation of *colpocleisis* may be preferable; this means surgical closure of the lower vagina, so that if there is both a vesicovaginal and a rectovaginal fistula the urine and discharge from the growth will be passed through the anus.

## Prognosis

The prognosis of invasive cervical carcinoma varies greatly in reported series of cases according to the method of treatment chosen, the experience of the radiotherapist or surgeon, and from country to country. An illustra-tive general statement might be that the expectation of surviving for 5 years is over 85 per cent in Stage I, 50 per cent in Stage II, 25 per cent in

Stage III and 5 per cent in Stage IV. In cases of Stages I and IIa there is little difference between the results of surgery and radiotherapy.

About 10 per cent of recurrences occur after the fifth year, but a patient who is well at 10 years can nearly always be regarded as cured.

# Carcinoma of the body of the uterus — endometrial carcinoma

## Aetiological factors

The peak incidence of endometrial carcinoma is between the ages of 50 and 65 years, but it may occur before the menopause and in advanced age. Unlike carcinoma of the cervix, the disease has no relation to coital behaviour, and nearly half the patients will be nulliparous.

Many of the patients are obese, and it has often been stated that there is some association with diabetes, although statistical evidence for this is questionable.

Evidence of prolonged or unbalanced action of oestrogens is found in some cases. There may be preceding endometrial hyperplasia or a delayed menopause. Although they are rare events, cases of endometrial carcinoma arising after prolonged administration of large doses of oestrogens, and cases associated with oestrogen-secreting tumours of the ovary, may be mentioned in support of this aetiological theory. The risk of endometrial carcinoma with the administration of oestrogens for menopausal symptoms may be reduced if progestogens are also given in cyclical doses.

Fibromyomata may coexist with endometrial carcinoma, but there is no evidence that they predispose to it.

## Pathology

The growth is nearly always an adenocarcinoma resembling the tubular glands of the endometrium. Occasionally an adenocarcinoma may show squamous metaplasia, the so-called adenoacanthoma.

Endometrial carcinoma so commonly arises in an atrophic senile uterus that there will usually be no evident enlargement of the uterus; any increase in size is often difficult to recognize because the patient is obese. If the uterus is greatly enlarged, the increase in size is usually due to associated fibromyomata or a pyometra, and is caused by the growth itself in only a few cases.

The growth invades the muscular wall, and in advanced cases may reach the peritoneal covering. Secondary growth occurs in the ovaries, omentum and other intraperitoneal organs, and it is from this that the patient usually dies. The growth may extend downwards into the cervix. Isolated secondary nodules are sometimes found under the epithelium of the vagina. Such nodules may also occur in the vaginal vault after hysterectomy, and may be due to direct implantation at the time of operation, or possibly to

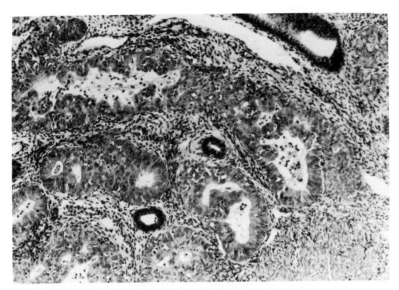

**Fig. 21.14** Adenocarcinoma of endometrium.

previous lymphatic or venous embolism. Suburethral metastases are not uncommonly found about 2 cm from the urethral meatus.

Carcinoma cells have been found lying free in the lumen of the Fallopian tube, and may implant themselves on the surface of the ovary or the pelvic peritoneum.

Lymphatic spread is later and less frequent than in cases of cervical carcinoma. It usually follows the route of the lymphatics accompanying the ovarian vessels; the glands first invaded are those along the aorta. When the growth arises in or extends into the isthmus of the uterus the glands in the obturator fossa and along the iliac vessels are invaded.

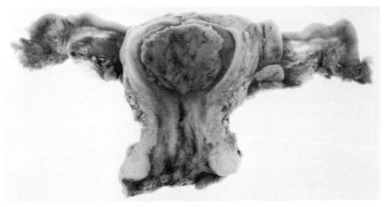

**Fig. 21.15** Carcinoma of endometrium.

Remote metastases in the lungs, bones or elsewhere are not common, but occur more often than with cervical carcinoma.

## Symptoms

The classic symptom is bleeding some years after the menopause. At first the haemorrhage is slight and intermittent, and the intervals between the episodes of bleeding are occasionally long. Later the bleeding may become continuous and heavy, producing severe anaemia. In women who have not passed the menopause irregular intermenstrual bleeding occurs, sometimes following after bleeding caused by endometrial hyperplasia.

In the early stages there may be a watery discharge, and later when infection ensues this becomes offensive.

Pain is a late symptom and denotes extensive spread of the disease.

## Physical signs

Enlargement of the uterus is usually only moderate in extent. In old women when the growth is freely ulcerating no enlargement may be detected. On the other hand, when the growth is chiefly proliferative the uterus may become as large as it would be at the 12th week of pregnancy. Greater degrees of enlargement are caused by the coincident presence of fibromyomata or a pyometra. Fixation of the uterus does not occur until a late stage of the disease.

Endometrial carcinoma cells are sometimes discovered by cytological examination of aspirate from the posterior vaginal fornix, but it is strongly emphasized that a negative cytological report does not exclude endometrial cancer.

Occasionally the diagnosis is made by biopsy after discovery of a vaginal nodule.

## Diagnosis

Postmenopausal bleeding can occur from several causes other than endometrial carcinoma. Atrophic endometritis and vaginitis may cause slight bleeding but the characteristic symptom is purulent discharge. Adenomatous endometrial and cervical polypi, and fibromyomatous polypi, can cause intermittent bleeding. Uncommon oestrogen-secreting tumours of the ovary such as granulosa-cell tumour and thecoma may give rise to endometrial bleeding.

Today many women are given oestrogens at or after the menopause to alleviate menopausal symptoms, and this is a common cause of bleeding.

The possibility that one of these innocent conditions is giving rise to the bleeding must never be allowed to operate against the rule that postmenopausal haemorrhage should be investigated immediately by examination under anaesthesia and curettage, for this is the only way to make a certain diagnosis. It must not be forgotten that an innocent and a malignant source of haemorrhage may coexist, such as an adenomatous cervical polyp and an endometrial carcinoma.

Cases in which the growth develops while the patient is still menstruating and the menopause is expected are those most likely to be the subject of diagnostic error or delay, for the woman herself will attribute the irregular loss to the menopause. Continuous or irregular bleeding is abnormal, whatever the age, and demands investigation. Even if the uterus is enlarged, and fibromyomata can be felt, exploratory curettage should still be carried out, for endometrial carcinoma is quite commonly coexistent with fibromyomata.

Curettage should always be carried out gently for fear of perforating an already thin uterus. In some cases the curette brings away large pieces of obvious carcinomatous tissue; in others the curettings are scanty, but they should always be sent for histological examination.

Patients in whom no evidence of carcinoma is found on curettage should be seen at intervals over the next 3 months and be advised to report if bleeding recurs. If bleeding recurs and it is certain that it is coming from the uterus and not from the bladder or bowel, hysterectomy is probably wise. It is not impossible to miss an early cancer at first curettage, while carcinoma of the Fallopian tube and oestrogenic tumours of the ovary, though rare, may be the cause of bleeding.

## International classification

This is less useful for endometrial cancer than it is for cervical carcinoma because 80 per cent of the cases are assigned to stage I, but it is as follows.

Stage 0. Histological findings suspicious of malignancy, but not proven.

Stage I. The carcinoma is confined to the corpus.

Stage II. The carcinoma involves the cervix as well as the corpus.

Stage III. The carcinoma has extended outside the uterus, but not outside the pelvis.

Stage IV. The carcinoma has involved the bladder or the rectum or has extended outside the pelvis.

## Treatment

Endometrial carcinoma may be treated by operation, by irradiation or by a combination of these methods. Until recently it was generally agreed that endometrial cancer could be adequately treated by total hysterectomy with removal of both Fallopian tubes and ovaries, and that there was no need for a procedure as extensive as Wertheim's hysterectomy. The 5-year survival rate from hysterectomy in many series reaches 70 per cent, but this figure relates only to the cases that were operated upon; if all patients, including those too advanced or unfit for operation, are considered, the figure is about 60 per cent.

There has recently been a tendency to extend the operation by removal of a cuff of vagina in the hope of avoiding vaginal vault metastases. Some operators also remove the obturator and iliac glands during the operation, especially if the lower part of the uterus is affected by the growth and if the patient is well enough for the more extensive procedure. The incidence of lymph node involvement is of the order of 10 per cent.

Improved results are claimed for a combination of irradiation and surgery, and a 5-year survival rate of 90 per cent has been reported for cases so treated. Preoperative treatment may be given with caesium or radium in the uterus and vaginal vault, or by teleradiation. Alternatively, postoperative external irradiation may be given.

It is possible to treat the growth by irradiation alone, but the results of surgical treatment are better. If there is recurrence in the vaginal vault this is best treated by the local application of caesium or radium.

Recently, large doses of progestogens have been found to be effective for palliative treatment in advanced cases, especially those with pulmonary metastases. Radiological examination shows that such metastases may undergo a temporary remission, or at least fail to progress, and there may be clinical evidence of regression of growth in the pelvis. Progesterone inhibits mitosis in endometrial cells, and with large doses increased differentiation or even necrosis may occur. The dosage of progestogens must be high; for example, 5 g of hydroxyprogesterone hexanoate weekly by intramuscular injection, or 250 mg of medroxyprogesterone acetate daily by mouth. Treatment can be continued indefinitely; apart from fluid retention, which may be undesirable if the patient is hypertensive, there are few adverse affects.

All the tumours described in the rest of this chapter are rare.

## Sarcoma and mixed mesodermal tumours of the uterus

**Leiomyosarcoma** may arise in the uterine muscle. Very rarely, such a tumour may arise by transformation of a previously benign fibromyoma; this occurs in less than 0.2 per cent of fibromyomata. Sarcoma also occasionally arises in the stroma of the endometrium.

Tumours of this group grow more rapidly and are softer than fibromyomata. They may increase in size after the menopause, when fibromyomata remain unchanged or shrink. On naked-eye inspection the tumour may be seen to have invaded the uterine wall or the capsule of the fibromyoma, and the cut surface often shows small haemorrhages and areas of degenerative softening. Microscopically they consist of spindle-shaped or rounded cells, many of them pleomorphic, with little stroma and primitive blood vessels. Distant metastasis by the blood stream and direct spread to adjacent structures often occur.

These tumours occur in adults, who usually complain of uterine bleeding. Rapid growth of the tumour with pain may give rise to suspicion of its nature, but in many cases the diagnosis is made only after the tumour has

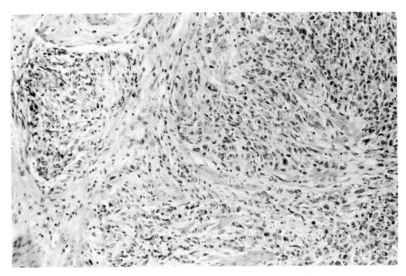

**Fig. 21.16** Leiomyosarcoma of the body of the uterus. The sarcomatous cells are infiltrating between normal muscle cells. The nuclei vary in shape and staining reaction, and many mitoses can be seen.

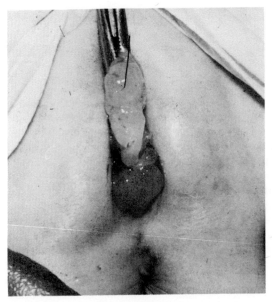

**Fig. 21.17** Sarcoma botryoides. The patient was a child aged 2 years. Grape-like material can be seen protruding through the vaginal introitus.

been removed. In rare cases a sarcoma may be slow-growing, and its nature discovered only when it recurs after operation.

**Mixed mesodermal tumours.** Tumours which contain heterologous mesenchymal elements are given this title. They may occur in adults, when a large fleshy mass protrudes from the uterine wall into the uterine cavity. Histological examination shows that it contains some elements resembling sarcoma and others resembling carcinoma, together with bizarre components such as cartilage and striped muscle. Metastasis by the blood stream is common, as well as local recurrence after removal. The patient complains of bleeding from the uterus, and sometimes pain. Tumours of this type occasionally follow uterine irradiation.

A variety of the same type of tumour that is seen in infants and young children is *sarcoma botryoides* (embryonal rhabdomyosarcoma). There is a blood-stained watery discharge, and the vagina is found to contain grape-like masses of soft growth, usually arising from the cervix. Among the myxomatous cells of the tumour primitive striped muscle cells (rhabdomyoblasts) can be demonstrated. Local recurrence commonly follows removal, and distant metastases occur.

*Treatment*

In adults if the diagnosis is suspected before operation, total hysterectomy and bilateral salpingo-oöphorectomy is performed, followed by external radiotherapy. In many cases the diagnosis is made only after hysterectomy has been performed for supposed fibromyomata; a decision whether to proceed to additional radiotherapy must then be taken, depending on the extent and nature of the disease. The prognosis is bad, except for leiomyosarcoma arising in a fibromyoma.

In children, as with many other forms of malignant disease, the prognosis with conventional treatment has been very poor. The modern use of a combination of external irradiation and radical chemotherapy has altered the outlook, but radical surgery (exenteration, see p. 182) may still be necessary. Such operations are surprisingly well tolerated by young children, who appear to be able to adapt well to the subsequent disabilities.

# Carcinoma of the Fallopian tube

**Primary carcinoma of the Fallopian tube** may be unilateral or bilateral, and is usually an adenocarcinoma. The patients are usually between 40 and 60 years of age. The growth may obstruct the ends of the tube, giving rise to a hydrosalpinx or haematosalpinx. It is symptomless at first, but then causes an intermittent watery discharge, which is often blood stained. In its early stages the growth is limited to the Fallopian tube, and may be felt as a small mass on one or other side of the uterus. If it perforates the wall of the tube and becomes adherent to adjacent structures such as the ovary, omentum or bowel, it may form a mass which can be felt from the abdomen. Ascites is often present.

The possibility of tubal cancer must be remembered if there is a recurrence of postmenopausal bleeding after the uterus has been curetted and no endometrial cause has been found.

*Treatment*
The treatment is to remove both tubes and ovaries and the uterus. The prognosis is bad, as the diagnosis is usually not made until the abdomen is opened, and not infrequently surgical removal is incomplete. Radiotherapy or chemotherapy may then be considered.

**Secondary carcinoma of the Fallopian tube** is more common than primary carcinoma. The tube may be involved by direct extension of an ovarian or uterine growth, or growth may be deposited on the surface of the tube in cases of carcinomatosis peritonei, whether arising from the genital tract or the intestinal tract.

# Gestational Trophoblastic Disease (Choriocarcinoma)

Choriocarcinoma is a highly malignant growth, but is notable as one for which chemotherapy is very effective. It arises from abnormal fetal trophoblast and is therefore also named *gestational trophoblastic disease.* It is usually a sequel to pregnancy with a hydatidiform mole (see 'Obstetrics by Ten Teachers'), but in rare instances it follows normal delivery or abortion. The tumour produces chorionic gonadotrophin.

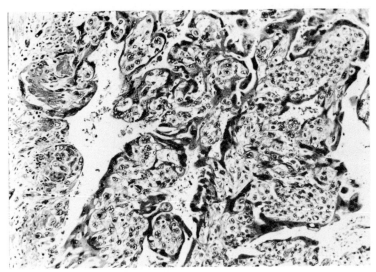

**Fig. 21.18** Microscopical section of choriocarcinoma.

Most cases of choriocarcinoma are now discovered during follow-up of cases of hydatidiform mole by assays of hCG. Recurrence of growth in the uterus after evacuation of a mole, or a growth following abortion or delivery, will cause bleeding which calls for curettage, when the histological report reveals the diagnosis. Vaginal metastases may appear as purplish-red nodules. Symptoms of more advanced cases depend on the site of any metastases. For example, pulmonary metastases cause dyspnoea, haemoptysis, cough and pleural pain, and will be seen in a radiograph. Cerebral metastases will cause headache and neurological signs.

*Treatment*

This tumour was the first for which effective chemotherapy was discovered. With modern chemotherapy the prognosis, which was formerly hopeless, has been transformed, so that in Britain death from trophoblastic tumour has become rare. The main indications for chemotherapy after evacuation of a mole are high blood levels of $\beta$ hCG persisting in the first 2 months, the presence of detectable levels of hCG after 6 months, or persistent uterine bleeding. Various combinations of drugs are used. The folic acid antagonist methotrexate is usually given together with actinomycin D, but these are often combined with other drugs such as vincristine. Repeated courses of chemotherapy are given until the hCG level becomes and remains normal.

These drugs cause severe damage to the bone marrow, with thrombocytopenia and agranulocytosis, and consequent risk of anaemia, haemorrhagic complications and infections. If alopecia occurs it is temporary, but is none the less upsetting to some women. Special nursing precautions, antibiotic cover, and administration of folinic acid after methotrexate, may all be required. Surgery has little place in treatment, save for unusual complications such as a localized deposit which persists in spite of chemotherapy.

# 22

# Cysts and tumours of the ovary

Ovarian enlargement may be cystic or solid. Some ovarian cysts, such as those of the follicle or corpus luteum and endometriomatous cysts, are not neoplastic. Solid ovarian tumours are almost invariably neoplastic. Regretfully we must start with a long classification; detailed elucidation of this will follow.

A. Non-neoplastic cysts:
    Follicular cysts.
    Corpus luteum cysts.
    Theca-lutein and granulosa-lutein cysts.
    Polycystic ovarian disease.
    Endometriomatous cysts.

B. Primary ovarian cysts and tumours:
  1. Tumours originating in the surface epithelium:
    Mucinous.
    Serous, simple and papilliferous.
    Endometrioid.
    Mesonephroid (clear cell tumour).
    Brenner tumour.
  2. Germ cell tumours:
    Benign cystic teratoma (dermoid cyst)
    Malignant germ cell tumours:
      Malignant change in cystic teratoma.
      Solid teratoma.
      Disgerminoma.
      Non-gestational choriocarcinoma.
      Endodermal sinus (yolk sac) tumour.
  3. Sex cord or gonadal stromal tumours:
    Granulosa cell and theca cell tumours.
    Androblastoma.
    Fibroma.

C. Secondary (metastatic) tumours.

It may be helpful to state that, in spite of this formidable list, apart from follicular and lutein cysts and endometriomata (which are not regarded as neoplasms), only six types of tumour account for the great bulk of ovarian tumours — benign and malignant serous tumours, benign and malignant mucinous tumours, malignant endometrioid tumours and benign teratomata.

## Cysts of the ovarian follicle or corpus luteum

### Follicular cysts

These are so common that when they are small they cannot be considered abnormal. They are thin walled, lined by granulosa cells and filled with clear fluid. Multiple cysts of this kind are found in cases of cystic glandular hyperplasia of the endometrium (p. 241), although they may not be clinically palpable.

It is rare for a follicular cyst to exceed 5 cm in diameter, when it may be palpable on vaginal examination. It would be impossible to distinguish such a cyst from a new growth without laparoscopy or laparotomy (Fig. 22.1).

Uncomplicated follicular cysts do not cause symptoms and are entirely benign. They resolve spontaneously, and for this reason any patient thought to have a small cyst should be re-examined after about 4 weeks. Laparotomy should only be performed if the cyst persists or increases in size during this time.

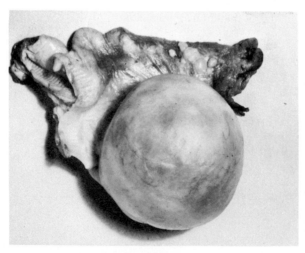

**Fig. 22.1** Follicular cyst of ovary.

### Corpus luteum cysts

At the time of formation of the corpus luteum there is always a little bleeding into the follicle which has discharged its ovum. If the bleeding is excessive, the corpus luteum becomes distended with blood. Strangely such blood-filled cysts seem to keep up their secretion of progesterone beyond the normal life of the corpus luteum and to maintain the secretory endometrium and delay the onset of menstruation, which when it occurs is frequently heavier than usual. If the corpus luteum haematoma causes pain in one or other iliac fossa and the period is delayed, the symptoms may be mistaken for those of an ectopic pregnancy, especially if the haematoma is felt lying in the region of the Fallopian tube.

## Theca-lutein and granulosa-lutein cysts

Multiple bilateral lutein cysts (called theca-lutein or granulosa-lutein cysts according to the supposed parent epithelium) occur in association with hydatidiform moles or choriocarcinoma. They are caused by the high output of gonadotrophin from the chorion, and may reach a diameter of 10 cm. After treatment or removal of the abnormal chorionic tissue the cysts resolve.

Similar cysts may be formed if excessive doses of gonadotrophins or of clomiphene are given during attempts to induce ovulation.

## Polycystic ovarian disease

This condition was originally described by Stein and Leventhal. The patients are usually obese and complain of infrequent or absent periods, infertility and hirsutism. The ovaries are enlarged and smooth (oyster ovaries). The tunica albuginea is thickened and beneath it are numerous small cystic follicles, varying in size but seldom exceeding 0.5 cm in diameter. There is failure of the ovarian enzyme systems which are necessary for the normal production of oestrogens. (see p. 232).

## Endometriomatous cysts. See chapter 23, p. 223.

## Blood cysts (chocolate cysts)

At operation many ovarian cysts are found to contain blood. Bleeding may occur into a follicular cysts, a corpus luteum or a neoplasm of the ovary. Periodic bleeding takes place into endometriomatous cysts (see p. 223). If the blood has been present for some time, it will become thick and dark; the term 'chocolate cyst' (or 'tarry cyst') is then used. Such altered blood can be found in any type of cyst. It is not diagnostic of endometriosis, although that is the commonest cause of bilateral chocolate cysts.

When any cyst or tumour undergoes torsion and becomes strangulated it becomes infiltrated with blood.

# Tumours arising from the surface epithelium

The modified peritoneal cells which cover the surface of the ovary are the most common source of ovarian neoplasms. This layer of epithelial cells was formerly called the germinal epithelium in the mistaken belief that it was the origin of the germ cells. It is densely adherent to the underlying gonadal stroma and it follows the corrugations of the ovarian surface. Sometimes parts of it become buried beneath the surface as germinal inclusions which give the impression of tumours arising within the substance of the ovary. Since the epithelial covering of the ovary and the Müllerian duct (from which the tubal epithelium, endometrium and endocervical epithelium are derived) are both formed from coelomic epithelium, comparable metaplastic transformation into different types of epithelium is theoretically possible. According to this view, tumours with tubal (serous) endometrial (endometrioid) or endocervical (mucinous) epithelium may arise. The mesonephroid clear cell tumour is also derived from Müllerian epithelium, and the Brenner tumour may have the same origin.

## Mucinous tumours (mucinous cystadenoma)

Mucinous tumours, whose epithelium resembles that of the endocervix, are the commonest large ovarian tumours. If left untreated, some of them become enormous, extending well above the umbilicus. They can occur at any age but are uncommon in childhood.

The tumours are multilocular, being composed of several cysts separated from each other by septa. The cysts vary in diameter from 1 mm or so to several centimetres. The larger cysts arise when the septum between two adjacent loculi breaks down. All the cysts contain viscid mucin. It was formerly believed that the mucin in these cysts was different from mucin found elsewhere, and the tumours were called pseudomucinous cysts. It is now recognized that there are many varieties of mucin. Mucins are glycoproteins which differ only in the amount of amino-sugar they contain.

Histological examination shows that the cyst wall mainly consists of fibrous tissue and that the loculi are lined with tall columnar epithelium. The nuclei of the epithelial cells are all at the base of the cells, and secretory vacuoles are frequently seen in the cytoplasm. In areas of rapid proliferation papillary processes with a central core of connective tissues and blood vessels may project into the cavity of the cyst. In benign cysts the epithelial layer is only one cell thick.

Although the view has been expressed that these tumours usually arise from the surface epithelium of the ovary, it is not uncommon for a benign teratoma to be found in association with a mucinous cystadenoma, and it is possible that a few of these tumours arise in teratomata in which one type of epithelium, perhaps of endodermal origin, has overgrown other kinds. There is also an association with Brenner tumours (see p. 210).

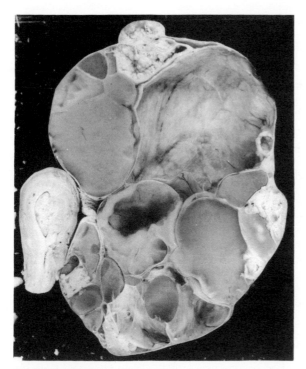

**Fig. 22.2** Mucinous ovarian cyst.

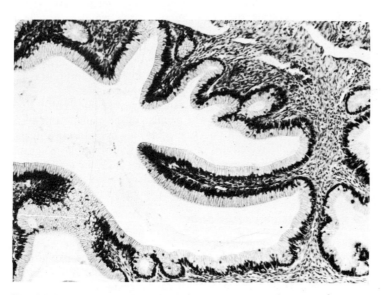

**Fig. 22.3** Microscopical section of mucinous cystadenoma of ovary.

*Myxoma peritonei.* If a mucinous cystadenoma bursts spontaneously or is ruptured during operative removal, epithelial cells may seed themselves on the surface of the peritoneum and grow there, continuing to secrete mucin so that the abdominal and pelvic cavities are slowly filled with a gelatinous mass of mucin and tumour. It is an interesting but unexplained fact that a similar condition may occur after rupture of a mucocele of the appendix or gall-bladder, both of which are lined by endodermal epithelium.

## Malignant mucinous cysts (mucinous carcinoma)

About 10 per cent of ovarian cancer is classified as mucinous. Some 5 per cent of mucinous cysts are found on histological examination to be malignant. Sometimes there is doubt about the nature of a mucinous tumour; a diagnosis of low-grade malignancy should then be made, and a guarded prognosis given. If compared by stage of growth and the grade of histological malignancy, the prognosis for malignant mucinous tumours is the same as that for other epithelial carcinomata; but the preponderance of growths of early stages and low grade among these tumours accounts for the favourable outlook for the group as a whole. These tumours are relatively resistant to radiotherapy and chemotherapy.

## Serous papilliferous cystadenoma

This is a common type of ovarian new growth. There is a range from the benign to the highly malignant. At the benign end of the scale the single cyst has a smooth lining, and may be called a simple serous cyst. At the malignant end of the scale the cyst contains many papillary processes which have proliferated so much that they almost fill the cavity, ultimately perforating the capsule (see below).

These cysts contain thin serous fluid, and can be of any size up to about 25 cm in diameter. They are often bilateral. They occur most commonly during late reproductive and early postmenopausal life.

The simple serous cysts are lined with a single layer of cubical epithelium on a vascular connective tissue base. The papillae of the papilliferous cysts have a similar surface epithelium on a branching core of connective tissue. If the epithelium is multilayered it is probable that the growth is malignant (see next section). The appearance of the epithelium has some resemblance to that of the Fallopian tube, the cells being ciliated.

## Serous papilliferous carcinoma

The malignant serous tumour is the commonest variety of primary ovarian cancer. The tumours are bilateral in about 50 per cent of cases. The growth often penetrates the capsule and projects on the external surface, with dissemination of cells into the peritoneal cavity giving multiple seedling metastases and ascites. With a few well differentiated tumours of relatively

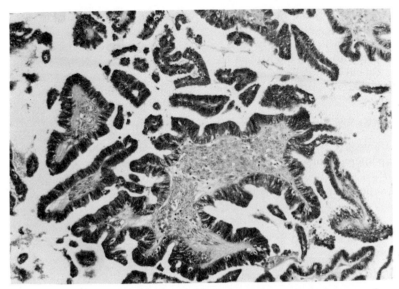

**Fig. 22.4** Microscopical section of serous papilliferous cystadenoma of ovary.

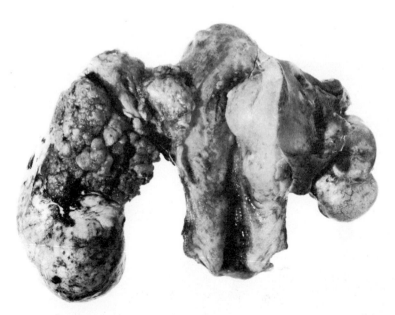

**Fig. 22.5** Serous papilliferous carcinoma of the ovary. The growth has penetrated the cyst wall.

low malignancy the patient may live for years in apparent symbiosis with peritoneal deposits which do not progress or may even disappear after removal of the primary tumour, but in most cases there is rapid spread in the peritoneal cavity beyond the scope of surgical cure.

On microscopical examination the cells of the tumour are no longer in a single orderly layer, and can be seen infiltrating the normal tissues.

## Epithelial tumours of borderline malignancy

Pathologists will report on the histology of most mucinous and serous papilliferous tumours as being either benign or malignant, but in up to 20 per cent of tumours the report will be of borderline malignancy, meaning that some of the features of malignancy are present, such as the multilayering of cells and nuclear atypia, but there is no stromal invasion. Providing that treatment is radical in such cases the prognosis should be less gloomy than with an indisputably malignant tumour of similar extent.

## Endometrioid tumours

A few cases of carcinoma arising in endometriosis of the ovary have been described, but this is very rare.

A much more common tumour arises from the surface epithelium of the ovary in which the histological pattern closely resembles that of an adenocarcinoma or adenoacanthoma of the uterine endometrium.

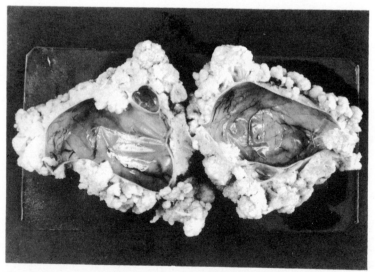

**Fig. 22.6** Serous papilliferous carcinoma of the ovary.

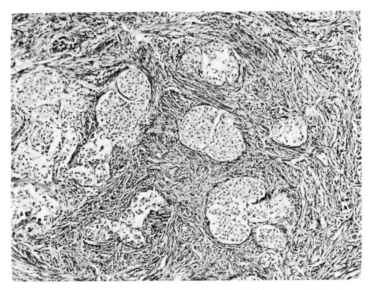

**Fig. 22.7** Brenner tumours, showing epithelial nests in a fibrous stroma.

## Mesonephroid (clear cell) tumours

These are uncommon tumours with a variable histological pattern characterized by tubules, small cystic spaces with papillae projecting into them,
and solid sheets of cells with clear cytoplasm. The small cysts and tubules
are often lined by 'hobnail cells', which have scanty cytoplasm but large
nuclei which project into the lumina. They were originally thought to arise
from the mesonephric apparatus, but are now believed to be a variant of
surface epithelial metaplasia and allied to endometrioid tumours.

## Brenner tumour

These are relatively uncommon benign tumours, varying in size up to
about 15 cm in diameter, and commonly unilateral. They occur mainly
during the reproductive period of life. They do not secrete hormones and
are usually recognized only by histological examination. Some mucinous
cystadenomata contain localized areas resembling a Brenner tumour.

   Macroscopically a Brenner tumour resembles a fibroma, being a solid
tumour with a white cut surface. Histologically, numerous islands of
epithelium are seen embedded in a fibrous stroma. The nests of epithelial
cells are rounded, and look like transitional or squamous epithelium, but
without keratinization. Sometimes the nests show central liquefaction.

   The origin of these tumours is uncertain. They may arise in Walthard
rests, which are groups of embryonic cells found just beneath the surface

of nearly all normal ovaries. An alternative view is that the tumours are of germ cell origin.

# Germ cell tumours

The commonest germ cell tumour is the benign cystic teratoma or dermoid cyst. Also included in this group are the disgerminoma, the non-gestational choriocarcinoma, the endodermal sinus (yolk sac) tumour and the solid teratoma.

Comparable germ cell tumours may arise in either sex, but the relative frequency of occurrence of the several varieties is very different. Dermoid cysts are common in the ovary but very rare in the testis; disgerminoma is seen more often in the testis (seminoma) than in the ovary.

## Benign cystic teratoma (dermoid cyst)

This is a common cystic tumour containing a variety of tissues derived from two or more of the primary germ layers, endoderm, mesoderm and ecto-derm. When the cyst is cut open it is usually found to be unilocular, and at one part of the wall there is a hump of tissue called the mamillary process or embryonic rudiment from which hairs spring, and which is covered by skin with sweat and sebaceous glands. The cavity of the cyst contains greasy yellow material secreted by the sebaceous glands, mixed with hairs, and it is lined with skin or granulation tissue within a capsule of fibrous tissue.

In the mamillary process a variety of tissues may be found, including well formed teeth, bone, cartilage, muscle, bronchial or alimentary epi-thelium, thyroid tissue and nervous tissue. A rare curiosity is a benign teratoma consisting almost entirely of thyroid tissue, called struma ovarii, which may be associated with hyperthyroidism.

Dermoid cysts are almost invariably benign, although malignant change can occur in one or other component of the teratoma (see below).

These tumours are believed to arise from the aberrant division of unfertilized oöcytes, but the stimulus to this variant of parthenogenesis is unknown. Similar tumours rarely occur in other sites, such as the medi-astinum or retroperitoneal tissues.

A dermoid cyst may occur at any age, but is commonly found during reproductive life, particularly between the ages of 20 and 30. About 20 per cent of them are bilateral, and at operation the opposite ovary must always be carefully inspected, and if necessary incised, to make sure that a small teratoma is not present there.

## Malignant germ cell tumours

Although malignant change in the tissue components of a benign cystic teratoma is uncommon, it is sometimes seen in patients of the older age

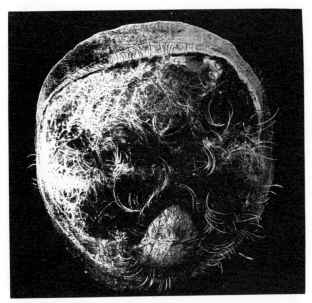

**Fig. 22.8**  Benign cystic teratoma of ovary, showing hair and sebaceous contents.

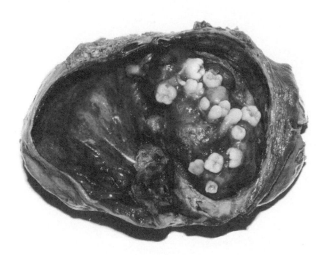

**Fig. 22.9**  Benign teratomatous ovarian cyst, containing teeth. The cavity contained sebaceous material and hair.

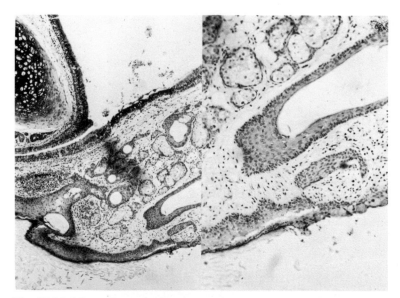

**Fig. 22.10** Microscopical section of benign teratoma. Cartilage, squamous epithelium and sebaceous glands are present.

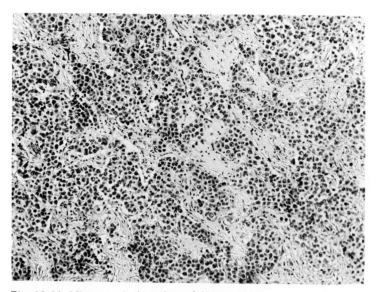

**Fig. 22.11** Microscopical section of disgerminoma.

groups, nearly always as a squamous cell carcinoma of the skin lining the cyst.

Totipotent germ cells in the ovary can give rise to tumours composed of either embryonic or extra-embryonic tissues, or both. Thus we find in this group solid teratomata, choriocarcinomata and endodermal sinus tumours, sometimes combined. Undifferentiated germ cell tumours are disgerminomata.

*Solid teratomata* are uncommon tumours, with a peak incidence of occurrence in the second decade. If they are composed of mature structures they may be benign, but if they contain embryonal tissues they are highly malignant.

*Non-gestational choriocarcinoma* generally arises as a component of a solid teratoma. It consists of syncytiotrophoblast and cytotrophoblast and secretes gonadotrophin, a diagnostic feature.

*Endodermal sinus tumour (yolk sac tumour of Teilum)* is a highly malignant tumour that occurs in young people. It is partly solid and partly cystic, and is composed of yolk sac endoderm and extraembryonic mesoblasts. It secretes $\alpha$-fetoprotein.

*Disgerminoma.* Histologically this tumour resembles a seminoma of the testis. There are large round cells separated by fibrous septa. This is a highly malignant tumour, and it soon perforates its capsule. The usual spread is by lymphatics, but it is not uncommon to see tumour cells within the blood vessels and spread can also occur by this route. The tumour occurs mainly in adolescents and young women, and it may arise in the gonad in cases of testicular feminization. It is radiosensitive.

# Sex cord or gonadal stromal tumours

The main substance of the gonad, the stroma of the cortex, is derived from the sex cord mesenchyme. This differentiates into a variety of cells concerned with the support of the germ cells. Tumours arising from this tissue may therefore contain granulosa cells, theca cells, Sertoli cells, Leydig cells or their precursors, alone or in combination. Some of these cells are also concerned with hormone production, and it is hardly surprising that a tumour consisting of granulosa or theca cells may produce oestrogen and progesterone, although the hormone production sometimes differs from that to be expected from the histology.

## Granulosa cell and theca cell tumours

These tumours are usually of moderate size, but they are occasionally large. At first they are solid, but as they grow larger they contain many small cystic spaces. The cut surface has a characteristic yellow tinge because of the lipoid content of the cells.

The histological appearance is very variable, and their recognition is often a matter for the expert. Essentially there are clusters of epithelial cells arranged in varying patterns, embedded in a fibrous stroma. In one

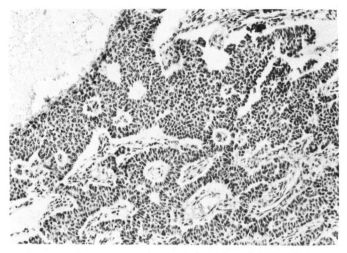

**Fig. 22.12** Microscopical section of granulosa cell tumour.

variety groups of cells seem to liquefy in the centre leaving live cells at the periphery and giving the appearance of rosettes. Some have regarded this as an attempt to form Graafian follicles. In another variety the cells are arranged in trabeculae.

The parent cells of these tumours are those which would have formed the follicle or corpus luteum. Luteal cells arise from the granulosa cells of the normal follicle, and theca cells from the immediately subjacent theca interna, so that it is common to find areas of lipoid-laden luteal and theca cells in granulosa cell tumours. Sometimes the tumour is a nearly pure thecoma.

These tumours must be regarded as malignant, although the malignancy may be of only low grade. Occasionally metastases appear many years after removal of the primary growth. It is not uncommon to find tumour cells in both ovaries.

The tumours usually occur in late reproductive life or after the menopause, but may be seen at all ages. Both granulosa cell tumours and thecomata usually produce oestrogens; only rarely do they produce progesterone. The endocrine effects depend on the age of the patient. If the tumour arises before puberty the oestrogen causes the breasts to grow and endometrial bleeding occurs; the tumour is therefore a rare cause of precocious puberty.

During reproductive life the periods will remain regular if the tumour is producing only small amounts of oestrogen, and it may only be discovered because of some complication such as torsion. If, however, the output of oestrogen is high there will be menstrual irregularity. With very high levels there will be amenorrhoea similar to that of metropathia haemorrhagica; when the level of oestrogen happens to fall, withdrawal bleeding occurs

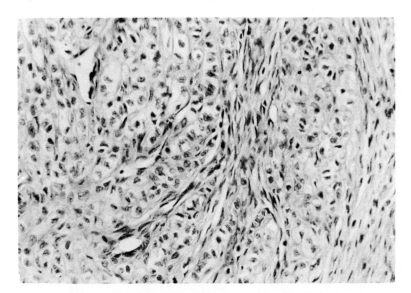

**Fig. 22.13** Microscopical section of thecoma of ovary.

from the hyperplastic non-secretory endometrium. The continuous but fluctuating secretion of oestrogen suppresses ovulation by its effect on the pituitary gland.

After the menopause the outstanding symptom is postmenopausal bleeding. Sometimes the response of the endometrium is so extreme that endometrial carcinoma occurs. There may be some enlargement of the breasts.

## Androgen-secreting tumours

The best known of these rare tumours is the *androblastoma* (formerly known as arrhenoblastoma). One variant of this looks like a testis on histological examination, with tubules but no spermatozoa, and has been called a testicular adenoma. Other variants do not contain tubules but are given names according to their resemblance to various testicular cells, such as Sertoli and Leydig cell tumours. A rare tumour called a *gynandroblastoma* contains a mixture of granulosa and androblastoma cells.

Androgens in large amounts cause amenorrhoea, atrophy of the breasts, enlargement of the clitoris, growth of body hair and deepening of the voice.

## Fibroma

This is a solid benign tumour which consists of fibrous tissue. It may be seen as a small sessile nodule on the surface of the ovary, or as a tumour of up to 10 cm in diameter replacing the ovarian substance. The cut surface of

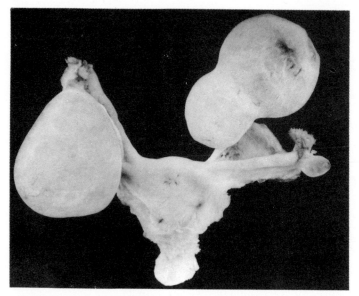

**Fig. 22.14**  Bilateral ovarian fibromata.

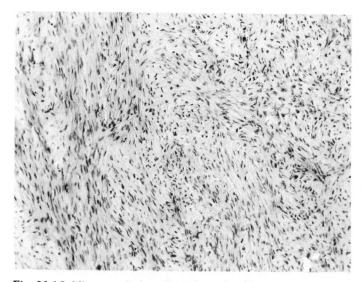

**Fig. 22.15**  Microscopical section of ovarian fibroma.

the tumour is white and the bundles of fibrous tissue can sometimes be seen with the naked eye. It is usually a solid hard tumour, but there may be small cystic spaces due to degenerative changes.

An interesting rarity is Meigs' syndrome in which there is ascites and a pleural effusion with an ovarian fibroma. When the tumour is removed the fluid collections disappear. The fluid is probably exuded from the surface of the tumour, and the pleural effusion does not differ from that which may occur with any large ascitic accumulation.

Ovarian fibromata tend to have relatively long pedicles, probably because of their weight, and may therefore undergo torsion.

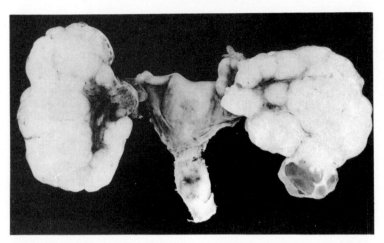

**Fig. 22.16** Metastatic carcinoma of ovary. The primary tumour was in the breast.

## Metastatic tumours

Cancer from other sites may metastasize to the ovaries. There may be microscopic surface deposits or gross solid or cystic enlargement of the ovary. Endometrial carcinoma may spread to the ovary, and other common primary sites are the colon, the stomach and the breast.

The *Krukenberg tumour* is rare. It is a secondary growth in the ovary from a mucus-secreting carcinoma, usually arising in the stomach or colon. Both ovaries are always involved and the interesting question is how these tumours arise, for although they are malignant they are smooth walled and free on their pedicles. This gives rise to the suggestion that the cancer cells gained access to the ovary through the lymphatics of the hilum. Others believe that the cancer spreads from the primary site as cells floating in the peritoneal fluid; if this were so, it might be expected that the tumour would be on the surface of the ovary, which is not the case. Nor will it easily explain spread of cancer from the breast to the ovary.

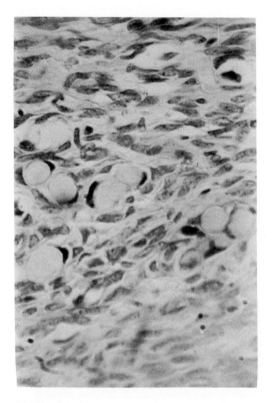

**Fig. 22.17**  Microscopical section of Krukenberg tumour showing signet ring cells.

The tumours are characterized histologically by 'signet ring cells'. These have accumulated a mucoid substance in their cytoplasm so that the nucleus is displaced right to the edge of the cell.

## Malignant ovarian disease

We have so far considered malignant disease of the ovary chiefly on the basis of pathological classification. Some general remarks may be made about the whole group of cases of ovarian cancer.

Malignant disease of the ovary is now the commonest cause of death from cancer of the female genital tract. About 4000 women die each year in Britain from this cause, exceeding the combined total of deaths from cancer of the cervix and endometrium. Unfortunately, the disease may be present for some time before it causes symptoms and in more than half the cases at the time of presentation it has extended beyond the ovary to the peritoneum or adjacent organs.

Ovarian cancer spreads by local infiltration, soon perforating any capsule a cystic tumour may have, or reaching the surface of the ovary to gain attachment to nearby structures such as the uterus, broad ligament, omentum or intestine. Once the peritoneal cavity is invaded, seedling deposits may be implanted on any surface, but especially the omentum.

Lymphatic spread is difficult to disentangle from direct spread, but cancer cells can be demonstrated in subperitoneal lymphatics. The lymphatic drainage of the ovary follows the ovarian vessels to reach the para-aortic glands. Microscopic deposits of growth in these glands and also in the lymphatics under the diaphragm contribute to the poor prognosis. Later the left supraclavicular glands may be enlarged by involvement.

Spread by the blood stream is uncommon, although it does occur in the later stages of disease.

All too often at operation a mass is found in the pelvis together with seedling growths elsewhere in the peritoneal cavity. In this type of growth the abdomen and pelvis may be 'silent' areas for some time and until ascites causes rapid enlargement of the abdomen the patient is unaware that anything is wrong.

### International staging for ovarian cancer

Although staging is usually based on pre-operative clinical examination in this instance the stage is determined at operation. The international staging of FIGO (Féderation Internationale de Gynécologie et d'Obstétrique) may be summarized as follows.

Stage I. Disease limited to one or both ovaries.

Stage II. Growth extending beyond the ovaries but confined within the pelvis.

Stage III. Growth with widespread intraperitoneal metastases.

Stage IV. Cases with other distant metastases.

## Clinical features of ovarian tumours

### Symptoms

Many ovarian tumours cause no symptoms and are only discovered during routine examination for such purposes as family planning, cervical cytology or antenatal care. Even when symptoms are present they are at first non-specific, and many patients are initially referred to specialists other than gynaecologists.

**Pain** is unusual when tumours are uncomplicated. The complications of torsion, rupture, haemorrhage and infection may cause pain. Otherwise any tumour which causes pain should be suspected of being malignant or caused by endometriosis.

**The abdominal girth** may increase rapidly when a large tumour is present, or when there is ascites, which is always a sinister sign.

**Pressure symptoms** may arise with tumours confined to the pelvis. Large tumours escape from the confines of the pelvis into the abdomen, but when a tumour is about the size of a fetal head and lies in the recto-vaginal pouch it will displace the other pelvic structures upwards and may elongate and distort the urethra, causing retention of urine. Conversely, some tumours may press directly on the bladder, reducing its volume and causing increased frequency of micturition.

**Endocrine effects.** Most ovarian tumours, apart from the rare tumours which secrete hormones and endometriomata, do not affect menstruation. Follicular cysts are an unimportant feature of cases of cystic glandular hyperplasia of the endometrium, and with a lutein cyst there may be menstrual irregularity. A few malignant tumours present with postmenopausal bleeding.

**Malignant tumours** will eventually become painful and produce many serious symptoms from such complications as obstruction of the bowel. In the late stages when there is cachexia the general loss of weight contrasts with the gross swelling of the abdomen from ascites and tumour masses.

## Physical signs

**Benign tumours.** While these are small enough to remain entirely within the pelvic cavity they can only be felt on bimanual examination. The essential feature is that a mobile mass can be felt to the side of and behind the uterus, which can be moved independently of the mass. A benign tumour is not usually adherent to any other structure and so will move freely. However, this is not always the case, and a tumour that is infected or caused by endometriosis may become fixed to the uterus. If the tumour distends the rectovaginal pouch, the uterus may be pushed upwards and forwards so that the cervix lies high up behind the symphysis pubis.

Medium-sized cysts may have long pedicles and rise up right out of the pelvis. They then tend to lie in the midline and the rectovaginal pouch is empty, although pressure on the abdomen may bring the lower pole of the tumour within the reach of the fingers in the vagina.

Benign mucinous cysts may be of any size, and may become the largest of all ovarian tumours. Small cysts are freely mobile, but the mobility of large cysts becomes restricted. If the patient is thin, surface lobulation of the cyst may be felt although the general surface is smooth. Very large tumours may cause respiratory embarrassment. In some cases with large cysts and a long history the patient becomes thin and cachectic as though she had malignant disease. However, if such a tumour were malignant it would be improbable that the patient would survive for long, and this is a good reason why all patients with ovarian tumours should be operated upon, for sometimes when the prognosis appears very bad a simple operation will cure the patient.

Serous cysts give rise to signs identical with those just described, but although they do not often attain such a large size they may grow relatively quickly.

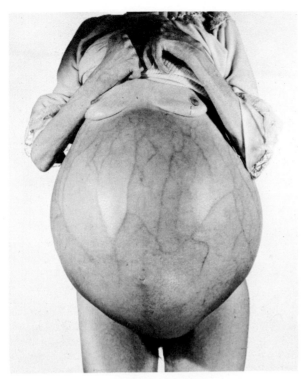

**Fig. 22.18** A large ovarian cyst. It proved to be a benign mucinous cyst.

Benign teratomatous cysts may feel 'doughy' because of their content of sebaceous material. They sometimes have long pedicles which allow them so much mobility that they occasionally lie anterior to the uterus, having risen over the top of the broad ligament to reach the uterovesical pouch. They are seldom larger than 10 cm in diameter, and are the commonest type of cyst to undergo torsion.

Benign solid tumours of the ovary are less common than cystic tumours. They may feel hard and smooth. On the whole they do not grow to more than 15 cm in diameter.

Apart from palpation, percussion will outline ovarian tumours that have risen up out of the pelvis. In every case the flanks should be carefully examined for any evidence of free fluid with shifting dullness on percussion, which might suggest that the tumour was malignant. Auscultation is useful only in the differential diagnosis from pregnancy.

A radiograph of the abdomen is rarely of value except that with a benign teratoma it is diagnostic if teeth or bone are seen in the tumour. Of far more value is ultrasonic screening, which may resolve the diagnosis when signs are equivocal. Unless there is an obvious tumour, careful

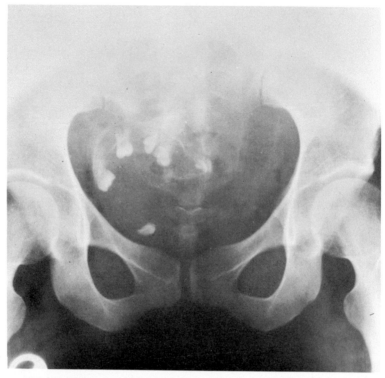

**Fig. 22.19** Radiograph showing several teeth in a teratomatous ovarian cyst.

bimanual examination under anaesthesia should always be performed before the final step of laparotomy or laparoscopy.

**Malignant tumours.** Ovarian malignant disease is insidious in onset, and has the highest mortality of all gynaecological cancers. Early detection would improve the prognosis, and much effort has been directed to the search for effective screening methods, so far with limited success. In the asymptomatic or very early clinical stage pelvic examination still has the chief place. Any woman with even vague abdomino-pelvic symptoms, or any woman attending for cytological examination or contraceptive advice, should have a careful pelvic examination. The ovaries should not be palpable in a postmenopausal woman. In younger women enlargement of the ovary up to about 6 cm in diameter may be caused by cysts of the follicle or corpus luteum which will resolve spontaneously, but any persistent or progressive enlargement must be thoroughly investigated, usually by laparoscopy.

The size of the ovaries can be measured by ultrasonic examination. Such investigation is of great value in any case in which malignant disease is a possibility, but it could also be employed as a screening procedure.

Cytological examination of material from the posterior vaginal fornix may occasionally reveal malignant cells from the ovary, but the method is too uncertain for routine screening. Examination of peritoneal fluid obtained by aspiration through the posterior fornix has also proved to be unreliable in excluding ovarian cancer.

It is often impossible to tell whether an ovarian tumour is benign or malignant before operation, but certain signs give rise to suspicion of malignancy. Malignant tumours may have an irregular surface, and are often partly hard even when there are cystic regions. Ovarian cancer is often bilateral when first discovered. A sign that must always be sought is shifting dullness to percussion in the flanks, for ascites is not found with benign tumours except in the case of a fibroma. If there is free fluid, a sample is taken by paracentesis for cytological examination.

On bimanual examination hard deposits of cancer may be felt in the rectovaginal pouch, especially by rectal examination. These are not tender, unlike nodules of endometriosis which may be felt in the same situation.

If the growth has spread to other organs, there will be symptoms referable to them. Obstruction of the colon or small bowel may occur. The symptoms and signs of bowel obstruction may be summarily listed as colicky pain, vomiting, constipation and tympanitic distension of the abdomen. The dominance of one or other symptom or sign will depend on the level of the obstruction and how complete it is. Occasionally there is bleeding from the uterus or vagina if the growth has eroded through. Obstruction of the ureter may cause hydronephrosis and pain in the loin. Thrombosis of the inferior vena cava or of an iliac vein causing oedema of the leg is an ominous sign.

A barium meal or enema or a pyelogram may sometimes be required. Pulmonary metastases or a pleural effusion may be seen in a radiograph of the chest, which should always be obtained, and a radiograph of the pelvis or vertebrae may show bony metastases. Ultrasonic examination may be very helpful.

## Complications of ovarian tumours

These are, in order of frequency, torsion, rupture, haemorrhage, impaction and infection.

**Torsion**. A tumour can only twist on its pedicle if that is fairly long and the tumour is not fixed to other structures. Large tumours seldom twist because they have no room in which to move freely. The complication is especially common with dermoid cysts and fibromata, but any tumour of moderate size that is not fixed may undergo torsion.

The cause is often not apparent. Some patients say that before the onset of their pain they made some unusual movement, but sometimes the pain of torsion wakes the patient from sleep. It may occur during pregnancy or labour. When torsion has occurred, twisting of the pedicle occludes first the veins and then the arteries. At the stage that the veins are occluded but the arterial supply continues, the tumour fills with blood and becomes plum coloured. Bleeding may take place into the lumen of the cyst, and occasionally there is intraperitoneal haemorrhage. If it is left untreated the tumour will become necrotic.

There is always severe lower abdominal pain. Sometimes this is of slow onset, but usually the torsion occurs rapidly. The patient may vomit repeatedly. There is, in a few instances, a little bleeding from the uterus. The patient sometimes gives a history of one or two lesser episodes of similar pain in the past, presumably because of partial twisting and then untwisting of the tumour.

On examination a firm tender swelling which is separate from the uterus is felt, although tenderness may make definition of the structures difficult without anaesthesia. Most commonly the tumour is palpable in the abdomen, but it may lie entirely within the pelvic cavity.

Urgent laparotomy is required.

**Rupture.** Spontaneous rupture of an ovarian cyst may occur. The wall gives way because of inadequate blood supply to part of it. If a small cyst ruptures there may be little or no pain, but if the cyst is large there may be severe pain with vomiting and a degree of shock. On abdominal examination there is tenderness and rigidity, and on pelvic examination there will be tenderness, but the collapsed cyst cannot be felt. The diagnosis can only be certain if the patient was known to have a cyst, which has become impalpable. Such an event is rare, and in most cases the diagnosis is finally made at laparotomy or laparoscopy.

Apart from the immediate effects, rupture of an ovarian cyst is potentially serious, for spontaneous rupture is most likely to occur with a rapidly growing tumour, which may be malignant, so that the growth is disseminated. Even with a supposedly benign mucinous cystadenoma, the condition of myxoma peritonei (see p. 198) may follow.

Traumatic rupture of an ovarian cyst is rare, although it may occur after a blow on the abdomen. The usual cause of traumatic rupture is bimanual examination under anaesthesia. If the cyst is small, it is then reasonable to do nothing but observe the patient for a few days, for it is likely to have been a follicular cyst; but if the cyst is large, immediate laparotomy should be undertaken.

**Haemorrhage.** Occasionally a massive haemorrhage occurs into an ovarian cyst, particularly a malignant cyst, and causes pain similar to that of torsion.

**Impaction.** It is rare for an ovarian cyst to become impacted in the pelvic cavity and cause retention of urine, because cysts nearly always rise up from the pelvis into the abdomen.

**Infection.** This is an uncommon complication, but a cyst may be involved in any local inflammatory process such as appendicitis, diverticulitis or spread of infection after abortion or delivery. Abdominal rigidity may make definition of the structures difficult, and although a pelvic abscess may be diagnosed its basic nature may not be certain until operation.

## Pregnancy with an ovarian tumour

This is usually diagnosed on routine vaginal examination in the antenatal clinic. The tumour may be of any type, but is most commonly a corpus luteum cyst or a benign cystic teratoma. Rarely, the tumour may be malignant, and it is this possibility which makes it desirable that the cyst be removed without delay. Another reason for early operation is that there is a high incidence of torsion in such cysts during pregnancy, and also in labour. The problem in pregnancy is that laparotomy may precipitate an abortion or premature labour. The chance of causing an abortion is greater in the first 12 weeks of pregnancy; it is therefore usual to defer operation if possible until after the 16th week if the diagnosis is made in early pregnancy. Another reason for delay at this stage is that the tumour may be a corpus luteum cyst or haematoma which is secreting progesterone and maintaining the pregnancy. By about the 16th week the placenta will be secreting sufficient progesterone to maintain the pregnancy without the secretion from the ovary.

If the cyst is found after the 16th week of pregnancy it should be removed forthwith; except that if it is only discovered in late pregnancy it may be better to defer laparotomy until after delivery. When an operation is performed for an ovarian cyst during pregnancy it is not necessary to deliver the fetus by Caesarean section unless the surgeon finds that he cannot otherwise gain access to the cyst.

An ovarian tumour is a rare cause of obstructed labour. See *Obstetrics by Ten Teachers.*

If an ovarian cyst should undergo torsion during pregnancy, immediate laparotomy is required whatever the stage of pregnancy. The risk of miscarriage is high, and if the corpus luteum is removed in early pregnancy, progestogens must be given. In the mid-trimester a β-mimetic drug may be given to inhibit uterine activity.

# Differential diagnosis

### Small tumours lying in the pelvic cavity

While a *full bladder* lying in front of the uterus is unlikely to be confused with an ovarian cyst which lies behind the uterus in the rectovaginal pouch, it is always prudent to make sure that the bladder is empty before trying to interpret physical signs in the pelvis.

An ovarian cyst lying in the pelvic cavity is more likely to be mistaken for a *pregnancy* of about 6–10 weeks. The soft round body of the pregnant uterus feels cystic, and the isthmus of the uterus may be so soft that the body of the uterus feels as if it is separate from the cervix (Hegar's sign). But the history of amenorrhoea, breast discomfort, blueness of the vagina and softening of the cervix should indicate the need for a pregnancy test, or possibly an ultrasonic scan. The latter is especially useful when there is a possibility of both conditions being present.

Multiple hard *uterine fibromyomata,* especially if they are causing menorrhagia, are easily recognized, but a single soft fibromyoma that is not causing menorrhagia may be difficult to distinguish from an ovarian cyst, although careful examination should show it to be continuous with the cervix. Difficulty may also arise with a pedunculated subserous fibromyoma, or one in the broad ligament, and laparoscopy is sometimes helpful.

In *chronic salpingitis* there may be a pelvic mass, but the history of infection, with recurrent attacks of pain, dysmenorrhoea, menorrhagia and sometimes fever, should suggest the correct diagnosis. Both tubes are generally involved and adherent to the back of the uterus. Difficulty arises with a large hydrosalpinx, which may mimic an ovarian cyst until laparotomy is performed.

Similar signs to those of salpingitis may be caused by *endometriosis,* but the history is different.

*Faeces* in the pelvic colon indent on pressure with the finger, but if there is uncertainty an aperient or enema will settle the diagnosis. It is more important not to miss recognition of a mass caused by *diverticular disease, Crohn's disease, or carcinoma of the bowel,* and barium studies and colonoscopy are sometimes essential investigations.

A very rare diagnostic problem is caused by a *pelvic kidney.* While this could be diagnosed with an intravenous pyelogram, this is unlikely to be requested unless there are urinary symptoms.

## Large abdominal ovarian tumours

Distension of the abdomen is often said to be caused by fat, fluid, faeces, flatus, fibroids or a fetus, and these may all require diagnosis from a large ovarian cyst.

To this list might be added a *full bladder.* A patient may fail to empty the bladder because of nervousness or a neurological disease, or because of retention due to an impacted tumour in the pelvis. Doubt whether a swelling is a full bladder can always be resolved by passing a catheter.

*Obesity* can be a real problem in diagnosis. As the examining hand sinks into a fat abdominal wall it is easy to imagine that an ill-defined cyst is present, and the fact that the patient has fat deposits elsewhere is not helpful, because even a fat patient may harbour a cyst. Percussion is not very helpful, for if the fat layer is thick enough there may be dullness. Ultrasonic examination may be very useful.

In differentiating *ascites* from an ovarian cyst, the essential points on abdominal examination are that a cyst occupies a roughly central position with dullness to percussion there, whereas with ascites the dullness is mainly in the flanks. Moreover, with ascites the gut floats on the fluid and causes resonance over the centre of the abdomen. With ascites the site of dullness moves as the patient rolls onto her side, but this shifting dullness may not be present if the fluid is encysted, as it may be in tuberculosis, or when carcinomatous masses are disseminated in the abdomen. Again, ultrasonic examination may be helpful.

If ascites is caused by carcinoma the growth can usually be felt, especially after paracentesis. If it is due to portal hypertension, renal or cardiac failure, this can usually be recognized from the history and general examination.

Only rarely does a *faecal mass* present as an abdominal tumour, but in gross constipation an enema will solve the problem. *Flatus* may fill the bowel with gas, and the abdomen will be resonant on percussion. If the patient declares that an abdominal swelling comes and goes frequently this is usually the diagnosis, although very rarely volvulus of the sigmoid colon may have to be considered.

*Pregnancy* is diagnosed on the history of amenorrhoea, the breast changes, the vascularity and softening of the cervix, and the enlarged soft uterus. Later the fetus can be felt and the fetal heart sounds are heard or fetal heart movements are recognized with ultrasound. The pregnant uterus may be felt to contract; virtually no other abdominal tumour does this.

An immunological pregnancy test will be positive, but it must not be forgotten that pregnancy may coexist with an ovarian cyst. The essential observation is then to demonstrate the separateness of the tumour from the pregnancy by examination under anaesthesia or ultrasonic examination.

*Mesenteric cysts* lie in the abdomen and do not rise out of the pelvis nor return to the pelvis as most ovarian cysts do. Since they lie between the layers of the mesentery their mobility is restricted to a line at right angles to the attachment of the mesentery.

An unusually large *hydronephrosis or hydrosalpinx* has very rarely been confused with an ovarian cyst.


## The treatment of ovarian tumours

There must be times when the clinician is uncertain of the nature of a pelvic tumour. Since such a tumour may be malignant, surgical exploration or laparoscopy is essential. Ovarian tumours in particular should always be operated on, and this is desirable even when it seems likely that the growth will be inoperable, because this does not always prove to be correct.

Another decision must be taken about the extent of surgery once the abdomen has been opened, and here there is much scope for judgement, depending on the nature of the tumour and the age of the patient. The nature of the tumour is assessed by its appearance, whether it is free or adherent, whether it is cystic or solid, whether it has grown through its capsule, whether there is ascites and whether there are seedling deposits. The age of the patient determines her capability for further reproduction. Whilst a malignant tumour in an older woman demands radical surgery, a benign tumour in a younger woman will be treated conservatively. Between these two extremes there are many cases in which decisions are not easy. If an older woman is treated by more radical surgery and the tumour proves on histological examination to be benign, little or no harm is done, whereas if it proves to be malignant the operation will be justified.

The surgeon may excise a tumour from the ovary, remove the whole ovary or both ovaries, remove the ovaries with the uterus and tubes, or remove as much malignant tissue as is safely possible although excision is incomplete, or retreat after taking a specimen for biopsy.

Many benign tumours can be shelled out of their ovarian beds, so leaving behind normal ovarian tissue which will continue to function. Benign teratomata and chocolate cysts caused by endometriosis often shell out surprisingly easily.

Removal of the whole ovary is carried out if all the normal ovarian tissue has been destroyed by pressure of a benign tumour or strangulation after torsion. The Fallopian tube is often stretched tightly over the surface of an ovarian tumour, and as there is little point in preserving it the tube is often removed with the tumour.

If both ovaries have to be removed, the uterus is often also removed at the same time. In patients who are near or have passed the menopause the opposite ovary should always be removed when one ovary shows any pathological change.

The difficult cases are those in younger patients with tumours of doubtful malignancy. In every case the opposite ovary must be carefully examined, as many ovarian tumours are bilateral. If there is any doubt about the nature of a cyst, it should be opened in the theatre so that the surgeon can inspect its contents before he completes the operation. In the case of a young woman who desires further children and in whom there is doubt whether an ovarian tumour is malignant, unilateral oöphorectomy is justifiable provided that the other ovary appears to be normal. Experience has shown that an ovarian tumour which is confined to one ovary has a relatively good prognosis whatever operation is performed. If the tumour is highly malignant and of germ cell origin, the outcome will depend on adjuvant treatment rather than extensive surgery. The decision will be influenced by the likelihood of bilateral disease with the particular type of tumour.

If a malignant tumour has spread to surrounding structures, and particularly if it has spread widely in the peritoneum, it may be impossible to remove it in its entirety. It is then best to remove as much of the growth as possible, in the hope that radiotherapy or chemotherapy will deal with the tumour cells that have been left behind. Such an operation, sometimes described as debulking, is based on the observation that the fewer the malignant cells that are left behind the better is the prognosis with chemotherapy or radiotherapy. The omentum should be removed, because even when it looks normal it often contains small deposits of growth.

The need for hysterectomy is controversial. Once an ovarian tumour has transgressed its capsule, hysterectomy is usually a necessary step in achieving wide local excision, but it contributes little to a grossly incomplete operation, unless the patient is suffering from uterine haemorrhage.

More extensive operations involving the colon, bladder or rectum may occasionally be justified, or resection of an involved loop of small intestine.

## Radiotherapy

Some ovarian tumours are radiosensitive, but many of those which regress reappear, and the cure rate is not closely related to the apparent sensitivity, so there is no place for radiotherapy as primary treatment. It may, however, be important adjuvant or secondary treatment. Although radiotherapy is often given to cases of early disease there is little evidence that it improves the survival rate after complete surgery. Little is to be expected from it in cases of disease in Stages III or IV.

At present its principal role is for patients with disease that is locally extensive, yet has not extended beyond the pelvis or the para-aortic lymph nodes. After incomplete local excision a salvage rate of 25 per cent may still be achieved, and isolated distant metastases may also respond. Tumours which are deemed to be inoperable at laparotomy are sometimes rendered operable after radiotherapy, but the dose should not exceed 3000 rads; otherwise, necrosis of normal tissues may occur after surgery.

An outstanding exception to these remarks is the disgerminoma, which is particularly radiosensitive, and these growths should always be given radical radiotheraphy to the pelvis and lymph nodes.

## Chemotherapy

Cytotoxic chemotherapy has recently altered the dismal prognosis in some cases of ovarian cancer. This is one of the few solid tumours in which benefit may be obtained in otherwise hopeless disease. Although the treatment may be unpleasant and even dangerous, it has advanced beyond the stage of being purely palliative. It is being used increasingly in preference to radiotherapy and has the best hope of success when the tumour mass remaining after surgery is not large.

The best results have been obtained with cisplatin. The drug is given in an intravenous drip over 24 hours. It may cause profuse vomiting, but newer less toxic compounds are being tried. For maintenance therapy alkylating agents such as chlorambucil are given by mouth in doses of 10 mg daily. Various combinations of cytotoxic drugs have been tried, but they tend to be toxic, causing dangerous leukopenia, and alopecia which can be distressing to a woman. Prolonged remission is rare in cases of advanced disease, and the compassionate physician will not wish to prolong the act of dying nor to exacerbate its discomforts. However, with certain tumours, notably those of germ cell origin, combined chemotherapy, using several chemotherapeutic drugs, has revolutionized the results. For example, with the endodermal sinus tumour of young people, hitherto uniformly fatal, major or complete regression may occur. To obtain the best results co-operation with a physician with special experience in this field is desirable.

*Second-look surgery.* Opinion is divided about the desirability of re-inspecting the pelvic organs by laparotomy or laparoscopy in a patient whose growth appears to be in remission on chemotherapy, with a view to further surgery. Even if the growth appears to be quiescent a decision to stop chemotherapy is not lightly undertaken; but it must not be forgotten that the prolonged use of cytotoxic agents has its own dangers.

## The management of terminal complications

Many patients eventually relapse and their terminal care will devolve on the gynaecologist and general practitioner. Ovarian cancer is a little unusual in that it often remains confined to the peritoneal cavity even in the final stages, and so the problems of management are largely abdominal. The cachectic patient seems to be shrivelling around her distended abdomen. Ascites is common and may require repeated paracentesis for relief. Instillation of cytotoxic agents seems to achieve little, but if the disease is controlled by systemic chemotherapy, serous effusions are usually restrained.

Pain is chiefly caused by intestinal obstruction, which may be insidious and subacute at first with distressing vomiting. For this, phenothiazine and morphine alkaloids are required. Surgery is occasionally to be considered. Provided that the large bowel is not obstructed, internal anastomosis of the small bowel and transverse colon may be possible, but if the disease is widespread and progressive it is not in the patient's best interest. Prolonged intravenous infusion of fluid may only prolong the act of dying, but if thirst is a source of distress it must be relieved.

In all cases early and adequate pain relief is essential, progressively increasing the dosage and frequency of administration of analgesic drugs. Nausea or vomiting with morphine may be reduced if chlorpromazine is added.

# 23

# Endometriosis

The term endometriosis is used to describe the condition in which ectopic endometrium is found in situations other than the lining of the cavity of the uterus. Although the word 'endometrioma' is often used, the lesions are not neoplastic in the ordinary sense of the word.

Figure 23.1 shows the sites at which endometriosis may occur. It is discovered most frequently in the ovaries, when it is usually bilateral, and may be associated with deposits in the rectovaginal pouch, rectovaginal septum and uterosacral ligaments. Another common site is in the wall of the uterus, where islets of endometrial tissue are found surrounded by uterine muscle; this is referred to as *adenomyosis.*

Small nodules of endometriosis may occur on the surface of the pelvic peritoneum, and thus involve the wall of the bowel or bladder. It may involve the peritoneal coat of the Fallopian tube, but the tubes are usually found to be patent. More rarely, endometriosis is found in the umbilical region, in lower abdominal scars, in the inguinal canal and in the vulva in relation to the round ligament.

The ectopic endometrial tissue responds to the ovarian hormones. Endometriosis never appears before puberty and regresses after the menopause. Microscopically the lesions show typical endometrial tubular glands and stroma cells, although sometimes the glands are not easy to find. Although the ectopic endometrium may exhibit the characteristic changes of the menstrual cycle, it may not always show the full response to progesterone and there may be cystic glandular hyperplasia.

Bleeding may occur in the islets of endometriosis, forming small blood cysts, and in the ovary these cysts can become quite large, up to about 10 cm in diameter. Adhesions form round endometriotic lesions, probably because of the bleeding. Endometriomatous cysts of the ovary are usually adherent to the back of the uterus and broad ligament, and to the rectum or bowel. Sometimes the uterus becomes retroverted and fixed by dense adhesions to the rectum as a result of endometriosis in the rectovaginal pouch and rectovaginal septum.

Endometriosis is associated with infertility, but if the patient becomes pregnant the decidual changes characteristic of pregnancy are seen in the ectopic endometrium.

## Aetiology

Numerous theories have been put forward to account for endometriosis, and it is possible that it may arise in different ways in different sites.

Adenomyosis arises by downgrowth from the endometrium of the uterine cavity into the underlying myometrium, as a result of some unknown stimulus. Serial sections may show direct continuity between endometrial tissue deep in the wall of the uterus and the normal endometrium.

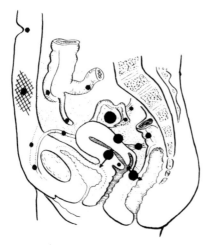

**Fig. 23.1** Diagram to show the sites at which endometriosis may occur. The sizes of the circles give an indication of the incidence at various sites.

Direct extension from the endometrium cannot possibly explain the occurrence of extrauterine endometriosis, and to account for this the implantation or cellular spill theory was introduced. This suggests that minute fragments of endometrium pass along the Fallopian tubes during menstruation and spill into the pelvic part of the peritoneal cavity, becoming implanted on the surface of the ovary, in the rectovaginal pouch or in some other situation, and developing into endometriosis. Although the endometrium shed at menstruation is mainly necrotic, living fragments have been found at operation in the lumen of the tube and in the peritoneal cavity. Direct transplantation of endometrial fragments into the tissues of the abdominal wall is thought to have occurred during operations on the uterus during pregnancy, such as hysterotomy, later giving rise to endometriosis in the abdominal scar.

An alternative theory is that of serosal metaplasia. The Müllerian ducts are originally derived from an infolding of the embryonic coelom, and it is suggested that endometriosis may result from metaplasia of the peritoneal endothelial cells in the peritoneal cavity.

In extremely rare instances endometriosis has been described in situations that could not be explained by either implantation or serosal metaplasia, such as the thigh and the pleura. It is possible that these tumours were synoviomata and not endometriomata.

## Clinical features

The frequency of occurrence of endometriosis is difficult to assess. There are geographical and racial variations. The disease is relatively common in Europe and the United States and almost unknown in Africa and the West Indies. It is common in women who marry late and limit the size of their families. Small symptomless deposits of endometriosis, unsuspected clinically, are often found when laparoscopy or laparotomy has to be performed for some other condition.

Endometriosis may give rise to symptoms at any time during the childbearing period. The commonest symptom is pain, which is usually premenstrual but can occur at other times. Pain may be absent even in the presence of extensive endometriosis. Deep dyspareunia occurs when the uterosacral ligaments or the rectovaginal pouch or septum are involved. Menorrhagia may occur, especially with uterine adenomyosis but also with extrauterine lesions. Endometriosis is associated with some degree of infertility, but the disease regresses if the patient happens to become pregnant. Regression certainly occurs after the menopause, whether occurring naturally, induced by removal of the ovaries or irradiation, or temporarily mimicked by hormone treatment.

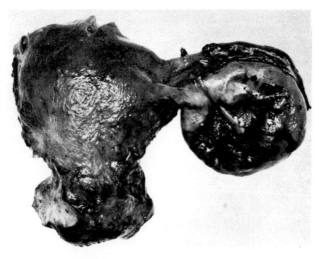

**Fig. 23.2** Endometriomatous cyst of the right ovary.

The pathology and clinical features of endometriosis vary somewhat with the anatomical site of the lesions, as follows.

**Uterine endometriosis or adenomyosis.** The uterus is usually uniformly but not grossly enlarged. Adenomyosis causes a localized thickening of part of the uterine wall, but this is not encapsulated and cannot be shelled out of the surrounding normal muscle. Close examination of the cut surface shows a trabeculated appearance with numerous small dark areas, these being cystic spaces containing thick, tarry menstrual blood. Histological examination shows interlacing muscle bundles and fibrous tissue, together with numerous islets of endometrial tissue. Stromal cells are found surrounding typical endometrial glands; occasionally the glands are few or completely absent. The cervix is rarely involved.

Fibromyomata sometimes coexist with adenomyosis, and then the uterus is considerably enlarged and of irregular outline. Extrauterine endometriosis is sometimes also present.

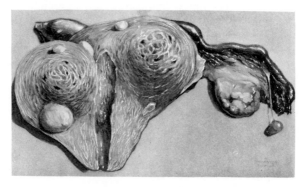

**Fig. 23.3** Adenomyosis of the uterus. There are also several small uterine fibromyomata and a Kobelt's tubule on the broad ligament.

**Ovarian endometriosis.** This may occur as small dark-red superficial deposits, often associated with similar blood spots on various parts of the pelvic peritoneum. Alternatively, it may occur apparently in the substance of the ovary as the characteristic 'chocolate cyst'. It is believed that a nodule of endometriosis begins as a surface lesion, and as it expands owing to periodic stimulation and bleeding it gradually displaces the ovarian cortex, which becomes part of the cyst capsule.

Endometrial cysts of the ovary may be single or multiple, and usually both ovaries are involved. Leakage of menstrual blood from the endometrial cyst excites an inflammatory reaction so that the cyst nearly always becomes adherent to the back of the uterus and broad ligament, and to the rectum. Surgical removal of the cyst is almost invariably accompanied by rupture when the attachments of the cyst are separated, and there is a gush of thick dark blood like liquid chocolate.

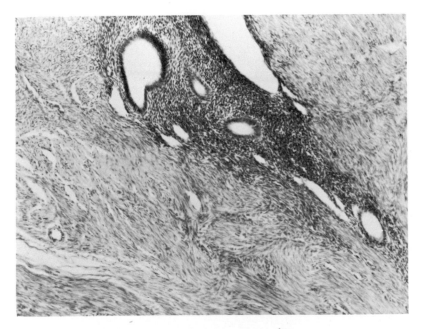

**Fig. 23.4** Microscopical section of adenomyoma of uterus.

Microscopical examination of the cyst wall usually shows areas of typical endometrium, having the same cyclical changes as normal endometrium. In some chocolate cysts endometrial tissue is difficult to find; as a result of repeated menstrual bleeding into a small closed cavity, the endometrium may degenerate and completely disappear, and it may then be difficult to distinguish between an endometrial cyst and a follicular haematoma. Large phagocytes, laden with blood pigment, are often seen beneath the degenerating endometrial lining. The cyst wall is composed of fibrous tissue and compressed ovarian cortex, from which the endometrial lining can often be enucleated.

Endometriosis of the ovary may present with the classic symptoms of pain, menorrhagia, deep dyspareunia and infertility, but in a few cases the condition is unsuspected until laparoscopy or laparotomy is performed for some other reason.

On examination a relatively fixed cystic tumour may be felt in the rectovaginal pouch, and it may be difficult to identify the uterus separately. The physical signs resemble those of chronic salpingo-oöphoritis, but there is no history of a preceding attack of acute infection.

Occasionally an endometrial cyst leaks, either spontaneously or as a result of comparatively minor trauma. The escape of tarry menstrual blood into the peritoneal cavity causes acute abdominal pain, and the diagnosis from acute salpingitis or torsion of the pedicle of an ovarian cyst may be

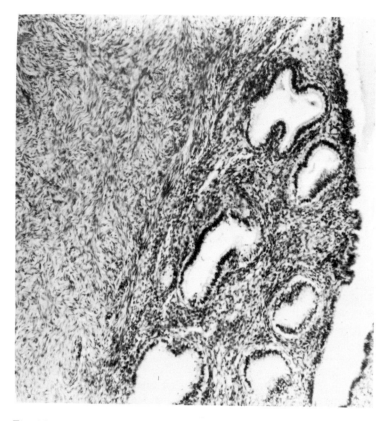

**Fig. 23.5** Microscopical section of ovarian endometriosis. The cavity of the chocolate cyst is to the right and endometriomatous tissue can be seen lying on ovarian stroma.

impossible until laparoscopy or laparotomy is undertaken. The finding of a tender mass in association with severe lower abdominal pain may also suggest the diagnosis of ectopic pregnancy, but there will be no evidence of pregnancy and the history will be longer than in ectopic pregnancy.

**Endometriosis of the rectovaginal septum.** Small nodules of endometriosis are frequently found in the rectovaginal pouch, and they may invade the uterosacral folds and the rectovaginal septum, giving rise to an indurated mass with considerable fibrosis. The uterus is often held in retroversion by dense adhesions. Occasionally the endometriosis penetrates the vaginal wall in the posterior fornix, presenting there as small dark haemorrhagic nodules. The rectal mucosa is not as a rule affected, although after a considerable time this can occur, with bleeding from the bowel at the time of menstruation.

The patient usually presents with deep dyspareunia or rectal pain, but there may be other symptoms because of ovarian lesions, as described above. The induration of the rectovaginal septum, and the local tenderness, should suggest the diagnosis, but the condition has to be differentiated from carcinoma of the bowel. On sigmoidoscopy the rectal mucosa is nearly always free, whereas in carcinoma an ulcer will be seen.

**Endometriosis in other sites.** *The intestine.* Endometriosis can occur in the bowel, particularly the pelvic colon, either alone or with other lesions of endometriosis. Small haemorrhagic nodules may be found on the peritoneal surface, and occasionally endometriosis involves the muscular wall, causing dense fibrosis, and rarely intestinal obstruction. The lesion closely resembles, and is often mistaken for, an annular scirrhous carcinoma of the colon. Endometriosis occasionally occurs in the caecum or appendix, but the small intestine is rarely affected.

*The bladder.* Endometriosis of the bladder is very rare. It may cause frequency of micturition or haematuria at the time of the menstrual period. On cystoscopy small bluish-red cysts may be seen under the vesical mucosa.

*Endometriosis in an abdominal scar* may follow an operation for endometriosis, myomectomy if the uterine cavity is opened, and particularly hysterotomy in mid-trimester pregnancy. It is almost unknown after lower segment Caesarean section but in the past was sometimes seen after upper segment operations.

*Umbilical endometriosis.* Small nodules are found, which increase in size and become tender in each menstrual cycle. Bleeding from the umbilicus is very rare, but has been recorded.

# Treatment

If symptomless endometriosis is an incidental discovery there is no need to insist on any treatment, although the patient should be re-examined periodically. If there are symptoms a diagnosis of intraperitoneal endometriosis has to be confirmed by laparoscopy or laparotomy; if the lesions are not extensive, treatment by diathermy cauterization or excision of localized disease may then be carried out.

In most cases a choice has to be made between hormonal treatment and surgery; in relatively young patients treatment with hormones is tried first.

**Hormonal treatment.** Progestogens are given in large doses for 9-12 months to suppress ovulation and the endogenous production of oestrogens and progesterone and consequently menstruation. The ectopic endometrium is converted into 'decidua' resembling that of pregnancy, and the monthly bleeding from it ceases. After some months the endometrium undergoes atrophy and the lesions regress.

Many progestogens may be used. Oral norethynodrel may be given in doses of 2.5 mg daily for 2 weeks, then the dose is doubled every 2 weeks until the patient is receiving 40 mg daily. This dose is maintained for at least 9 months. During treatment there will be amenorrhoea and there may be breast enlargement, abdominal distension, water retention and sometimes nausea.

An alternative is dydrogesterone, given in gradually increasing doses orally up to 200 mg daily.

A different method of treatment is to give danazol, which is a very weak androgen and has some inhibiting action on the ovary, but its main effect appears to be on the endometrium, causing atrophy. It is given in doses of 200–800 mg orally daily. The drug is very expensive.

Analogues of GnRH which inhibit the production of pituitary gonadotrophins are now under trial (p. 261).

The results of hormone treatment are disappointing in the sense that, although the symptoms are controlled, the lesions remain and seldom regress permanently. Although the uterus and the ovaries are conserved, pregnancy obviously cannot occur during the treatment, and there is no certainty that the patients are more likely to conceive after the treatment than before.

**Surgical treatment.** Many patients eventually come to surgical treatment and, as has already been mentioned, it may be applied at the time of diagnosis of early and localized lesions. For women who no longer wish to become pregnant, surgical treatment may be preferable to prolonged and uncertain hormonal treatment. Even in younger women who hope for pregnancy, surgical treatment can be conservative. For example, enucleation of chocolate cysts of the ovary is often possible, leaving sufficient ovarian tissue on one or both sides to maintain normal ovulation. The knowledge that she has some hope of having children is most important to a young woman, and may compensate for the risk that endometriosis may recur and eventually necessitate further, more radical, surgery.

Small endometriomatous deposits on the surface of the ovary, or on the peritoneum over the bladder or bowel, or in the rectovaginal pouch, may be coagulated with diathermy.

For women who no longer wish to become pregnant more radical treatment may be preferable to prolonged and uncertain hormone treatment. If both ovaries are involved and there are widespread deposits, it is best to perform total hysterectomy with bilateral salpingo-oöphorectomy; removal of both ovaries will ensure that residual areas of endometriosis no longer remain active.

Endometriosis of a scar or the umbilicus is treated by local excision. Endometriosis of the colon or small bowel may need resection if it is causing obstruction or is judged likely to do so. Lesions of the bladder can be treated by cystoscopic diathermic cauterization. Deposits in the rectovaginal septum may be excised during the course of hysterectomy, although there may be difficulty in separating the rectum without damage.

Treatment by irradiation of the ovaries in cases with extensive bowel or bladder involvement is rarely appropriate as pain may not be relieved, and modern surgical methods can overcome most technical problems of excision.

# 24

# Amenorrhoea

Absence of menstruation is called amenorrhoea. Amenorrhoea is a symptom and not a disease in itself; in fact it is often physiological, as in pregnancy. The term *primary amenorrhoea* refers to a patient of any age who has never menstruated. *Secondary amenorrhoea* refers to cessation of the periods after menstruation has been established.

The term *cryptomenorrhoea* is sometimes used in cases in which menstruation is occurring, but is concealed because the vagina is occluded by a congenital septum or atresia.

Amenorrhoea may be classified as follows:

**Physiological**
1. Before puberty.
2. During pregnancy.
3. During lactation.
4. After the menopause.

**Pathological**
1. Uterine lesions.
2. Ovarian lesions.
3. Pituitary disorders.
4. Disorders of the other endocrine glands.
5. Psychiatric illness and emotional stress.
6. Severe general illness.
7. Drugs causing amenorrhoea.
8. Amenorrhoea following surgical operations or radiotherapy.

## Physiological amenorrhoea

### Before puberty
Menstruation normally begins between the ages of 11 and 14, but this will be affected by heredity and the nutritional state of the patient. Oestrogenic activity of the ovary begins some years before the menarche, but at first the oestrogen levels are not sufficient to cause bleeding from the endometrium.

### During pregnancy
Amenorrhoea is present throughout pregnancy. There is a space between the decidua capsularis and the decidua vera until the 12th week of preg-

nancy when these layers fuse, but any bleeding should be regarded as potentially pathological.

### During lactation

The average time between delivery and the first subsequent period is 6 weeks in the case of patients who do not feed their infants and 10 weeks in those who do. Ovulation may start again at about the same time. During lactation prolactin is secreted in large amounts by the anterior lobe of the pituitary gland and there is partial, but not complete, suppression of secretion of luteinizing hormone, so that ovarian follicles may mature but fail to rupture.

### After the menopause

Microscopical examination of the ovaries of a woman who is well past the menopause shows no active Graafian follicles. Cessation of oestrogen production from the ovary is temporarily associated with overproduction of gonadotrophic hormone from the pituitary gland.

## Pathological amenorrhoea

### Uterine lesions

Amenorrhoea occurs when the uterus is rudimentary and only represented by a nodule of fibromuscular tissue at the top of the vagina. In such cases the vagina may also be absent, but the ovaries and the secondary sexual characteristics are usually normal.

Except with these severe congenital defects of the uterus it is rare for amenorrhoea to be due to uterine hypoplasia. If there is any endometrium present it will respond to stimulation by oestrogens.

Destruction of the endometrium by advanced pelvic tuberculosis is not now seen in Britain, although such cases still occur in some developing countries.

### Ovarian lesions

Primary amenorrhoea occurs with ovarian dysgenesis.

Secondary amenorrhoea may be caused by failure of the enzyme systems in the ovary which are necessary for the production of oestrogens. There is a spectrum of such disorders, of which the *polycystic ovary (Stein-Leventhal) syndrome* is the one most commonly recognized. In this, secondary amenorrhoea is associated with bilateral enlargement of the ovaries, which have thickened capsules and contain multiple small follicular cysts in a dense stroma. Many of these patients are obese, and have an excessive growth of facial and body hair. The secretion of FSH is within the normal range, and some oestrogen is produced, but not enough to cause uterine bleeding. Because of the enzyme block, one of the precursors of oestrogen, androstenedione, which has a weak androgenic effect, is found in the follicular fluid, and this may explain the hirsutes. A surprising thing about this condition is that a fairly extensive wedge-resection of both ovaries is often followed by a return of normal menstruation and even pregnancy. However, such surgical treatment is not now usually employed, because ovulation and menstruation may often be induced with clomiphene (see p. 270).

Secondary amenorrhoea from ovarian failure may occur without evident cause. The serum level of oestrogens is very low, while the level of gonadotrophins is raised, hence the disorder is sometimes called hypergonadotrophic amenorrhoea. If ovarian laparoscopic biopsy shows that follicles are present the term *resistant ovary syndrome* is used, and in these cases ovulation may sometimes be induced with clomiphene, or with LHRH (GnRH) if it is obtainable. If ovarian follicles are not present the case is described as *premature ovarian failure* (premature menopause) and treatment is not possible. However, ovarian biopsy is not always conclusive as only a small part of the ovary is examined, and both spontaneous and induced ovulation may unexpectedly occur.

Inflammatory disease or neoplasms of the ovaries seldom cause amenorrhoea. To do so all the ovarian tissue in both ovaries would have to be destroyed – an unlikely event.

### Pituitary disorders

Rare cases of *pituitary infantilism* (Levi-Lorain syndrome) occur; the cause is unknown. The patients are of child-like stature and proportions, with primary amenorrhoea. Secretion of FSH is absent or low, and no oestrogens are found in the urine.

*Ischaemic necrosis of the pituitary gland* (described by Simmonds, but often known as Sheehan's disease) is the result of thrombosis of the pituitary blood vessels after profound hypotension and hypovolaemia, most commonly caused by severe postpartum haemorrhage. The production of gonadotrophic, thyrotrophic and adrenotrophic hormones ceases or is very inadequate. The patients are lethargic, gain weight and have a low metabolic rate, hypotension and amenorrhoea. Treatment with hormones is disappointing. Thyroxine, cortisone and methyltestosterone (for its anabolic effect) are usually given. Oestrogens may produce cyclical bleeding, but this can only be of psychological benefit.

*Adenomata of the anterior lobe of the pituitary gland* (prolactinomata) may cause an excessive secretion of prolactin and consequent amenorrhoea. The tumour may be very small and difficult to demonstrate by radiography of the sella turcica, even with the aid of computerized tomography. Hyperprolactinaemia may be diagnosed if the prolactin level exceeds 1000 m.i.u./l. Prolactin release is increased by thyroid-releasing hormone, and levels may be high in cases of hypothyroidism. Stress will cause a temporary increase in secretion of prolactin.

Galactorrhoea can occur, and if the tumour is large enough there may be pressure on the optic nerves. The other cells of the pituitary are usually unaffected.

If a tumour is found it is treated by radiotherapy or surgery, but if no tumour is evident bromocriptine will inhibit the output of prolactin.

## Disorders of other endocrine glands

### The adrenal gland

The adrenogenital syndrome is caused by a tumour or hyperplasia of the adrenal cortex. There is excessive production of androgens and the urinary excretion of oxosteroids is increased. The symptoms and signs are those of virilism, with deepening of the voice, hirsutes, acne, amenorrhoea and enlargement of the clitoris.

In Cushing's syndrome hyperplasia, or less commonly a tumour, of the adrenal cortex produces an excess of glucocorticoids which stimulate the conversion of protein into carbohydrate. These patients have amenorrhoea, hypertension, polycythaemia, osteoporosis and diabetes; the abdomen often shows striae like those of pregnancy.

Amenorrhoea occurs in advanced cases of Addison's disease.

### Thyroid gland

In both myxoedema and hyperthyroidism, amenorrhoea occurs in severe cases.

### The pancreas

Amenorrhoea may occur in severe or uncontrolled diabetes.

## Psychiatric illness and emotional stress

The hypothalamus controls the output of gonadotrophins from the pituitary gland, and higher centres in the brain affect the function of the hypothalamus. Starting a new job, being away from home for the first time or emigration are examples of stressful conditions which may cause amenorrhoea until social readjustment has been made. Sudden bad news or severe emotional distress may have the same effect. The periods are likely to return spontaneously and reassurance is all that is required, but the possibility of some other coincidental cause such as pregnancy must not be forgotten.

Amenorrhoea accompanies anorexia nervosa. The girl is often rejecting the imagined burdens of maturity, and the refusal of food is intended to stop progress from childhood to womanhood. Psychiatric help is necessary, and restoration of a diet with adequate proteins and vitamins.

## Severe general illness

Menstrual function may be temporarily suppressed during or after any severe illness, or during a chronic illness such as chronic renal disease.

Secondary amenorrhoea occurs with starvation. This was seen in the inmates of concentration camps during the World War II; there were, of course, severe psychological stresses as well as starvation.

**Drugs causing amenorrhoea**

Sometimes after stopping oral contraception amenorrhoea occurs, and continues for some months. Spontaneous return of menstruation is to be expected within 6 months, but in a few cases treatment by induction of ovulation with clomiphene or gonadotrophins is required. This type of amenorrhoea is more common in women who had irregular periods before starting oral contraception, and some of them are merely reverting to their previous menstrual pattern. The possibility that the amenorrhoea is due to pregnancy must not be forgotten.

Prostaglandin inhibitors occasionally cause amenorrhoea.

**Amenorrhoea following surgical operations or radiotherapy**

Obviously, amenorrhoea will follow hysterectomy or removal of both ovaries. The ovaries may be affected by pelvic irradiation for malignant disease.

# Investigation and treatment of cases of amenorrhoea

## Primary amenorrhoea

If a girl does not begin to menstruate by the age of 17, investigation should be advised. The management of these cases calls for some discretion; to subject an embarrassed child to a barrage of investigations is not always helpful. Some or all of the following investigations may be required, but those which involve discomfort, such as examination under anaesthesia or laparoscopy, should not be made until the other tests show that they are essential.

1. *Observation of stature and body form.* Dwarfism may be the result of some long-standing metabolic disorder; for example, renal disease or a malabsorption syndrome, or lack of growth hormone as in pituitary infantilism. In such cases amenorrhoea is a trivial part of a wider problem.

In some cases of gonadal dysgenesis (Turner's syndrome) the patients are of short stature, but in others (simple gonadal dysgenesis) the patients tend to be tall. Webbing of the neck or wide carrying angles at the elbows suggest Turner's syndrome. Patients with the adrenogenital syndrome may be short and muscular with hirsutes.

2. *Examination of the breasts and pelvic examination.* If breast development has taken place there must have been some oestrogenic activity, and in such cases it is possible that there is some abnormality of the lower genital tract such as haematocolpos causing cryptomenorrhoea, or a rudimentary uterus.

A special type of case is that of testicular feminization (p. 66). In these cases the breasts are well formed, but the vagina may be short and the uterus is absent. There may be a family history of the disease. The diagnosis rests on the discovery that the patient is 'chromatin negative', XY.

Patients without breast development are likely to have gonadal dysgenesis (p. 64), and for such cases chromosomal analysis is essential. There will also be absence of breast development in cases of pituitary infantilism.

3. *Hormone assays.* While it is not at present possible to obtain extensive hormonal assays in all hospitals, in Britain regional laboratories will often assist with difficult problems. The essential distinction to be made is between cases of hypothalamic or pituitary failure in which the levels of both gonadotrophins and oestrogens will be low, and cases in which the ovary fails to respond, when the level of gonadotrophins will be high and that of oestrogens very low.

4. *Chromosomal studies.* A blood film to show polymorphonuclear leucocytes or a buccal smear should be stained and examined for Barr bodies, and in cases of primary amenorrhoea in which the diagnosis is not clinically certain a full chromosomal analysis should be carried out.

5. *Radiological examination.* An intravenous pyelogram is carried out in all cases of uterine or vaginal malformation, as there are often associated abnormalities of the ureters and kidneys in these cases.

A lateral radiograph of the sella turcica (or tomography) may show it to be expanded by a pituitary tumour; this examination should be made in all cases in which there is a raised prolactin level, or clinical reason to suspect such a tumour.

6. *Laparoscopy.* Laparoscopy and biopsy of the gonads is not indicated if the diagnosis can be made by less invasive methods. If the diagnosis is certain after clinical examination, perhaps with the addition of chromosomal or hormonal studies, little purpose is served by proving, in Turner's syndrome for example, that the ovaries are mere streaks. However, laparoscopy is useful in cases in which there is doubt about the nature of the gonads, or if it is uncertain whether there are any primordial oöcytes in the ovary, when ovarian biopsy is performed. Laparoscopy is also occasionally useful in cases of vaginal atresia to determine whether the uterus is present.

Laparotomy is required in cases of testicular feminization to remove the testes after the secondary sexual characteristics have been established, to prevent the danger of disgerminoma arising.

Ovarian dysgenesis and absence of the uterus cannot be altered, but in some girls morale can be improved by intermittent oestrogen therapy. This will cause breast enlargement, and monthly withdrawal bleeding if the uterus is present. A low dose of oestrogen is given, such as ethinyl oestradiol 20 micrograms daily for 21 days, with norethisterone 5 mg daily added on days 14 to 21. After an interval of 7 days the cycle is repeated.

For delayed puberty in girls whose ovaries are shown by laparoscopic biopsy to contain oöcytes, ovulation may be induced with human gonadotrophin. In the near future GnRH or synthetic analogues of it may be available and prove to be a better alternative; it is administered intravenously or subcutaneously in pulses by a special pump.

## Secondary amenorrhoea

A patient who has previously menstruated evidently then had a patent lower genital tract, endometrium which responded to ovarian hormones, ovaries which responded to gonadotrophins, and must then have produced gonadotrophins. In every case pregnancy must be excluded, even if the patient thinks it to be unlikely. This done, a systematic series of investigations are:

1. *Previous menstrual history.* Enquiry about the patient's previous menstrual history is made. If she has had irregular cycles for many years there is little point in investigating or treating a minor abnormality unless infertility is her problem.

2. *Change in the patient's environment.* Enquiry should be made about any recent change in her social and emotional environment, any stress that she has undergone, or any attempt at severe dieting.

3. *General medical examination.* Any history of recent or long-standing illness is sought, and a general examination is made (including observation of the body build and hair distribution) to exclude any general illness. The breasts and pelvic organs are examined. Any appropriate investigations, such as tri-iodothyronine binding capacity and free thyroxine indices for suspected disorder of the thyroid, are performed. Prolactin levels are measured.

If pregnancy is not desired, and if the patient has no evidence of any underlying disease which has caused the amenorrhoea, at this point the doctor must decide whether there is any useful purpose in further investigation. In some cases the further steps will be as follows:

4. *Hormone assays.* Generally, LH levels correspond with those for FSH, although the latter may be a more sensitive index of pituitary function and show earlier change. By assessment of the tests relating to the various levels of the hypothalamic-pituitary-ovarian axis, the patient's problems can be placed at the appropriate level. With hypothalamic or pituitary failure the levels of both gonadotrophins and ovarian hormones will be low; with failure of ovarian response, because of lack of negative feed-back the gonadotrophin levels may be raised.

5. *Radiography and tomography* of the pituitary fossa may be required.

If amenorrhoea is judged to be caused by stress or an emotional problem, spontaneous recovery is to be expected if the problem can be removed or alleviated by the passage of time.

If it is caused by some underlying disease or nutritional deficiency that must be treated or removed.

If no cause is obvious, and it is decided to treat the patient (which is unnecessary if the patient does not wish for a pregnancy and is not anxious about the amenorrhoea) response is to be expected by induction of ovulation with clomiphene or gonadotrophins, or possibly in the future with GnRH.

In cases of polycystic ovary (Stein-Leventhal) syndrome clomiphene often succeeds, but if it fails bilateral wedge-resection of the ovaries may be tried.

Patients found to have high levels of prolactin must have the assay repeated, as temporary rises may occur from stress. Hypothyroidism or the effect of drugs such as phenothiazines must also be excluded. If radiological examination of the sella turcica, using coning and other special techniques, does not reveal a pituitary adenoma the prolactin level can be reduced with the dopamine agonist, bromocriptine. The dose has to be varied according to the prolactin level measured by radioimmunoassay, and this treatment should be employed only in units that have the facilities for the hormone assays. The dose is increased very cautiously, starting with oral tablets of 2.5 mg daily.

From this account it will be realized that women with primary amenorrhoea often receive extensive investigation but treatment is seldom successful, whereas many women with secondary amenorrhoea receive little more than clinical assessment but in them spontaneous recovery often occurs.

Women are often unduly anxious about menstrual abnormalities, and may regard amenorrhoea as a cause of illness or a variety of symptoms. In itself amenorrhoea is not a cause of ill-health, although it may be an indication of impaired fertility or a warning of some general medical disorder. Often the doctor's chief duty in these cases is to give reassurance.

# 25

# Abnormal uterine bleeding (during menstrual life)

Excessive menstrual bleeding is called *menorrhagia*. Strictly, this term should be used only to describe heavy menstrual loss with a normal cycle, but it is often used more loosely. When the cycles are shortened, so that the periods occur more frequently, the term *polymenorrhoea* is sometimes used, and the word *metrorrhagia* refers to any irregular uterine haemorrhage which may occur during menstrual life. Hybrids of these words are sometimes employed, but simple phrases such as excessive, prolonged or irregular bleeding, or frequent or irregular cycles, are much to be preferred.

It is important to realize that abnormalities of menstruation are only symptoms and do not describe pathological entities. Before treatment is given the cause must be determined, and any endocrine treatment without previous investigation is to be condemned.

Excessive or irregular periods may be caused by any of the following:

**Local lesions of the pelvic organs**
These include:
   Uterine fibromyomata, adenomyosis and endometrial polypi.
   Ovarian endometriosis.
   Salpingo-oöphoritis.
   Menstrual loss may be heavy when an intrauterine contraceptive device is used.
   Carcinoma of the uterus may occur before the menopause, and cause irregular bleeding.
   The diagnosis and treatment of all these conditions have been described in previous chapters.

**General diseases**
In some cases of myxoedema menorrhagia occurs, which will respond to treatment with thyroxine. (In other advanced cases there is amenorrhoea.) It is uncertain whether thyroid deficiency affects the pituitary gland or the ovaries.

Blood diseases are very rare causes of uterine bleeding. It may occur in acute leukaemia, thrombocytopenic purpura and hereditary capillary fragility (von Willebrand's disease), but in all these diseases the diagnosis is evident on other grounds. It is strongly emphasized that anaemia is almost invariably the effect and not the cause of menorrhagia.

Hypertension does not seem to affect menstrual loss.

Climatic conditions seem to have some effect; women expatriated from temperate to hot climates may have menorrhagia, but some of these have a stressful environment which is the real cause.

**Emotional causes**
Women suffering from a psychosomatic disturbance may temporarily develop heavy or frequent periods, which resolve when the cause has subsided, just as other individuals may present with peptic ulcers, for example. The menstrual irregularity in these cases is due to disturbance of pituitary function, which arises in turn from hypothalamic response to activity of higher centres. Some, but not all, of the cases of dysfunctional bleeding which are described in the next section have an emotional cause, and this possibility must always be considered.

# Dysfunctional uterine bleeding

The term dysfunctional uterine bleeding refers to those cases in which the bleeding is not due to some local disorder such as new growth or pelvic infection, nor to some complication of pregnancy. It may occur at any age between the menarche and the menopause.

Heavy or irregular bleeding without abnormal physical signs on ordinary examination will always suggest this diagnosis, but this must never be taken for granted because curettage may reveal that there is a local cause for the bleeding after all. An endometrial polyp may be discovered, unsuspected retained products of conception may be found, or even early malignant disease of the endometrium or cervix.

## Causation

Dysfunctional bleeding may be caused by alteration in the output or balance of gonadotrophic or ovarian hormones, and probably also of endometrial prostaglandins.

Bleeding from the endometrium is controlled by vasoconstriction, myometrial contraction, and local aggregation of platelets with deposition of fibrin around them, processes which are all influenced by prostaglandins. The endometrium, and to a less extent the myometrium, is able to synthesize prostaglandins from arachidonic acid by the action of the enzyme cyclo-oxygenase. The endometrium contains:

$PGF_{2\alpha}$, which causes myometrial contraction and vasoconstriction.
$PGE_2$, which causes myometrial contraction but is a vasodilator.
Prostacyclin ($PGI_2$), which causes myometrial relaxation and vasodilatation, and also inhibits platelet activity.

It is believed that $PGF_{2\alpha}$ normally plays the chief part in preventing excessive menstrual bleeding. In theory abnormal bleeding may occur if there is a decrease in production of $PGF_{2\alpha}$, or an increase in production of $PGE_2$ or prostacyclin. In support of this suggestion, a relative decrease in $PGF_{2\alpha}$ against $PGE_2$ has been reported in endometrium in some cases of menorrhagia.

Drugs which block the action of cyclo-oxygenase, such as mefenamic acid, are sometimes effective in checking menorrhagia, but such treatment is non-specific in the sense that in a particular case we do not know which of the prostaglandins is reduced.

In ordinary clinical work, as distinct from a research programme, it is difficult to make frequent estimations of the blood levels of gonadotrophic hormones or of oestrogens and progesterone, and of local concentrations of prostaglandins. Without such estimations the fault in the endocrine physiology must often be uncertain. To add to the difficulty the causes of shortened cycles and of lengthened cycles may overlap the causes of excessive bleeding, as will be seen in following paragraphs.

In some cases of dysfunctional bleeding the cycles are ovulatory, but in others, and perhaps the majority, ovulation is not occurring.

In *ovulatory cycles* excessive bleeding may be caused by corpus luteum insufficiency, with decreased secretion of oestrogen and progesterone in the second half of the cycle. The luteal phase is abnormally short, but at the same time the endometrium shows irregular ripening, with patchy response to the hormones and consequent prolongation of menstrual bleeding.

In some cases, on the other hand, the corpus luteum persists longer than is normal, sometimes with the formation of a luteal cyst. The luteal phase of the cycle is then prolonged, but there is eventual irregular shedding of the endometrium, with prolonged and heavy bleeding.

In women with dysfunctional bleeding with *anovular cycles* the oestrogen secretion rises to high levels, and then the output of FSH is checked by feedback, so that the oestrogen level falls and endometrial shedding takes place. In many women with anovular cycles the loss is not excessive, and unless they are complaining of infertility nothing abnormal may be noticed. But in a few cases the endometrial shedding is irregular and incomplete, which causes excessive blood loss.

In another type of case with anovular bleeding, formerly known as *metropathia haemorrhagica* but now called *cystic glandular hyperplasia*, oestrogen production rises to high levels, but there is no 'feedback' inhibition of the pituitary, so FSH secretion continues and oestrogen levels remain high, perhaps for 6–8 weeks. There is no endometrial bleeding during this time, but the prolonged action of the abnormally high level of oestrogen, without progesterone, causes endometrial hyperplasia. On macroscopical examination the endometrium is very thick, and in places almost polypoid. Microscopical examination shows hypertrophy of the columnar epithelium of the endometrial glands, and many of the glands show cystic dilatation so that the tissue has a 'Swiss cheese' appearance. There are areas of necrosis in the stroma, with small haemorrhages and leucocytic infiltration. The myometrium may also show some hyperplasia. After a time the oestrogen level begins to fluctuate, and when it falls endometrial bleeding ensues. Bleeding may also occur because parts of the grossly hypertrophied endometrium have outgrown their blood supply. Bleeding tends to be heavy, prolonged and irregular.

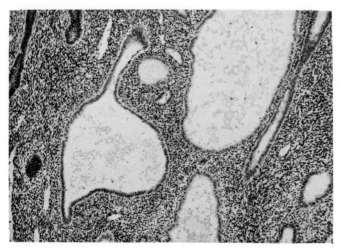

**Fig. 25.1** Cystic glandular hyperplasia of the endometrium.

In cases of dysfunctional bleeding successive episodes may vary in pattern. It is clear that an emotional upset, presumably acting through the hypothalamus, can sometimes precipitate an episode of dysfunctional bleeding, but in most cases no such trigger is evident.

It has been suggested that in dysfunctional bleeding of puberty the output of gonadotrophins is erratic, whereas near the menopause the ovary may be failing to respond. It may be well to repeat that in about half of the cases of dysfunctional uterine bleeding no histological abnormality of the endometrium is found on curetting, and in some of these cases the cause of the bleeding remains obscure.

The cases can be roughly grouped by the ages of the patients into those occurring at puberty, during the childbearing period and near the menopause. Although this classification has little basis in pathology it is useful when considering treatment.

**Abnormal bleeding at puberty**

Menorrhagia for a few periods after the menarche is not uncommon. This cyclical bleeding is anovular in type. Less commonly there may be severe and continuous bleeding with a diminishing haemoglobin level – such cases are similar to those described above as metropathia haemorrhagica, and show endometrial hyperplasia from the effect of oestrogen in the absence of progesterone. Nearly all the cases recover spontaneously in a few months.

A rectal examination should be made to exclude any ovarian tumour, but there is no indication for curettage unless the medical history strongly suggests the possibility of tuberculosis. In a few cases with heavy bleeding norethisterone 5 mg three times daily is given by mouth, gradually reducing the dose over the succeeding 10 days. Iron is prescribed if the child is anaemic.

## Dysfunctional bleeding in the childbearing years

Abnormal bleeding without obvious local cause is not uncommon in women of this age group. The bleeding may be cyclical or irregular. Particularly in parous women the uterus may be slightly and symetrically enlarged. In the past such cases were described as chronic uterine subinvolution. If sections of the myometrium are stained to differentiate the elastic tissue from the plain muscle and fibrous tissue, an increasing deposition of elastic tissue is seen around the arteries in the wall of the uterus with each successive pregnancy. This is a physiological process and part of the normal process of involution; it is not now believed to have any relation to dysfunctional bleeding, which is attributed to a hormonal effect on the endometrium.

Cases of dysfunctional bleeding in this age group may be of any of the types already described.

It is not uncommon for abnormal bleeding of endocrine origin to undergo spontaneous remission; in young women without abnormal physical signs it is worth waiting for a short time to see if normal menstruation returns. However, in any patient with abnormal bleeding that persists for more than 3 months, or in whom the bleeding is severe, diagnostic curettage is performed. In all cases a blood count is done, and if necessary iron is given; in a few cases blood transfusion will be required. Oxytocin or ergometrine are usually of no benefit.

Curettage will exclude local causes of bleeding. If, as in about half the cases, the endometrium looks normal on histological examination, having regard to the day of the cycle on which the curettage was done, the treatment is of necessity empirical. Should the endometrium be obviously non-secretory in the latter half of a cycle a diagnosis of anovular bleeding is made, and in some cases cystic glandular hyperplasia will be found. In about a third of the cases a regular cycle returns after curettage, probably because spontaneous remission would have occurred in any case.

For women who have not reached middle age, or do not already have the number of children they want, hormone treatment may be used. In younger women with unopposed oestrogen activity, progestogens given in the second half of the cycle are helpful, such as norethisterone 5 mg orally twice daily, from days 16 to 25 of the cycle. In the older patient it is easier to take over the control of the cycle with an oral oestrogen-progestogen pill for 21 out of each 28 days. A daily dose of 50 micrograms of oestrogen and a moderately high dose of progesterone will be required; for example, Anovlar which contains 50 micrograms of ethinyloestradiol and 4 mg of norethisterone acetate may be given.

There are a number of other non-surgical forms of treatment which may be considered. Danazol was at one time considered to inhibit pituitary gonadotrophic secretion; this is dubious. However it acts, it can cause endometrial atrophy. It is given orally, 200–800 mg daily in divided doses.

Long-acting analogues of GnRH which inhibit gonadotrophin secretion (see p. 261) are being tried.

Numerous drugs which inhibit the synthesis of prostaglandins in the endometrium are now available and are under trial. Mefanamic acid (Ponstan) and naproxen (Naprosyn) are examples. Unfortunately, they are not specific as to the particular prostaglandin which they inhibit, and it is at present difficult in clinical practice to measure the concentration of the various prostaglandins in menstrual blood. These drugs are effective in an unpredictable but not inconsiderable number of cases of menorrhagia and they deserve a trial, especially for any woman anxious to avoid hysterectomy.

If all these measures fail the final step is hysterectomy, with conservation of the ovaries, which should be considered for women who have some years to wait for the menopause if the amount of blood loss threatens their health, or sometimes because the bleeding is grossly inconvenient and limits their activities.

### Abnormal bleeding near the menopause

At the normal menopause the periods may either stop abruptly, or the cycles may lengthen until the periods cease altogether, or the cycle may remain unaltered but the menstrual loss gradually diminishes at each period.

However, dysfunctional uterine bleeding (including the type known as cystic glandular hyperplasia) may occur, with heavy or irregular bleeding. In this group of patients it is of the utmost importance to exclude malignant disease of the uterus by curettage. No hormone treatment should be given unless malignant disease has first been excluded. In cases of severe bleeding at this age hysterectomy will often be advised.

## Anovular bleeding

By this is meant a blood loss from the endometrium that has not been preceded by ovulation. Confirmation of the diagnosis is made by biopsy of the endometrium in the late cycle. The luteal secretory changes will be absent.

Anovular bleeding may be regular and cyclical, and to all outward appearances it is normal menstruation. The condition would then only be discovered during the investigation of infertility. Women who are taking the oral contraceptive pill have regular anovular bleeding.

It has already been explained that many women with dysfunctional uterine haemorrhage have anovular cycles, and in these cases the cycles may be irregular and the loss may be heavy.

Although anovular bleeding may appear at any age and last for varying intervals, it is commonest in the early cycles after the menarche, or in the years preceding the menopause.

Treatment by induction of ovulation (see p. 270) may be required if the patient complains of infertility, or treatment for heavy or irregular bleeding may be needed as described in the previous section.

## Short menstrual cycles (polymenorrhoea)

A reduction in the length of the menstrual cycle may occur at any age. This type of polymenorrhoea is sometimes seen in the early months of marriage, after abortion, and when menstruation is re-established after childbirth. Although often associated with menorrhagia it may occur alone. If menorrhagia does not accompany the polymenorrhoea the patient is unlikely to suffer from anaemia, and will only be inconvenienced by the frequency with which menstruation occurs.

Although it has been stated that short cycles are caused by overactivity of the pituitary gland, this is far from established; indeed it is more likely that there is inadequate ovarian response with failure of ovulation or an inadequate corpus luteum so that there is a short luteal phase.

If the patient has always had a short menstrual cycle since puberty it may be difficult to alter this, and there is often little point in the attempt. If she is complaining of infertility and has anovular cycles ovulation may be induced, otherwise the cycle may be controlled by use of the combined oral contraceptive pill.

## Intermenstrual bleeding

There is usually a local cause for irregular bleeding between the periods. A urethral caruncle occasionally bleeds. Intercourse may cause bleeding from carcinoma of the cervix, from an adenomatous (mucous) polyp of the cervix, or from a vascular cervical erosion, especially during pregnancy or if the patient is taking the oral contraceptive pill. Endometrial adenomatous polypi may cause intermenstrual bleeding, and sometimes carcinoma of the body of the uterus may occur before the menopause.

Slight bleeding may occur at mid-cycle at the time of ovulation; it only lasts for a few hours. Break-through bleeding may occur with oral contraception.

It must be strongly emphasized that in every case of intermenstrual bleeding at any age the diagnosis must be established before treatment is given, otherwise an occasional carcinoma may be missed, with fatal results. Diagnostic curettage must be performed in all cases in which a local cause is not found on ordinary examination with a speculum.

# 26

# Dysmenorrhoea and premenstrual tension

Although menstruation should be, and often is, painless many women suffer from discomfort or pain in association with periods at some time during their reproductive life.

It has been customary to classify cases of dysmenorrhoea into two main groups:

1. Primary or spasmodic dysmenorrhoea.
2. Secondary or congestive dysmenorrhoea.

These terms are unsatisfactory because they have been used in two senses; to indicate the time of origin of the complaint (at puberty or later) and, alternatively, to express an opinion about the cause of the pain and whether it is secondary to evident pelvic disease. It may be more useful to classify the cases into (1) those due to evident pelvic disease and (2) those without evident pelvic disease.

## Dysmenorrhoea caused by pelvic disease

The type of pain experienced is very variable. It may precede the onset of a period for about a week; such premenstrual pain is common with pelvic inflammatory disease and endometriosis. The pain is often a dull ache in the lower abdomen and back, sometimes extending down the thighs.

An acute colicky pain may occur if a fibromyomatous polyp is being extruded through the cervix, and in some women an intrauterine contraceptive device will cause colicky dysmenorrhoea. It may, rarely, occur with a stricture of the cervix.

Apart from the discovery of abnormal physical signs on examination, two features suggest that there may be underlying pelvic disease. First, the symptoms may appear after some years of painless menstruation, and secondly, there may be other symptoms of pelvic disease such as menorrhagia, dyspareunia or infertility.

The treatment of dysmenorrhoea caused by pelvic disease is described in other chapters according to the cause.

## Dysmenorrhoea without evident pelvic disease

This is the commoner type of dysmenorrhoea and it usually occurs in girls or young women. It is difficult to state its frequency, as most women have occasionally experienced some degree of pain. Severe pain only occurs in a minority, but there is no doubt that it can be incapacitating and often leads to absence from work.

The pain is spasmodic or colicky in nature, usually starting on the first day of the period. It may last for several hours or continue throughout the first and second day. Not infrequently the menstrual flow is scanty at first, and the pain often becomes easier when the flow is properly established. The acute colicky pain may be followed by a dull ache. Nausea and vomiting, and occasionally diarrhoea may occur, and sometimes headache and fainting.

Most women present for advice when they are between 16 and 25 years old. They may say that they have had pain ever since their periods started, but closer questioning will usually show that the periods were painless at first, and only became painful after a few months or even years, sometimes becoming progressively worse.

It is usually said that spasmodic dysmenorrhoea is cured by childbirth; it often is, but in some cases it persists in spite of the birth of children. The continuation of dysmenorrhoea to the age of 30 or more is more common in unmarried than married women.

Examination of a patient complaining of spasmodic dysmenorrhoea usually reveals no general or local abnormality. The patient is physically healthy, although she may be somewhat tense. A vaginal examination, or if the hymen is intact a rectal examination, must always be made to exclude unexpected pelvic pathology. In nearly every case the genital tract is normal.

## The cause of the pain in women without evident pelvic disease

The pain is due to spasm of the uterine muscle, which is sufficiently intense to cause ischaemia. The cause of the muscle spasm is not certain, and several factors have been discussed.

*Cervical obstruction*
Although organic stricture of the cervix can cause menstrual pain this is exceedingly rare, and there is no evidence of obstruction in the ordinary cases. Dilatation of the cervix is still sometimes practised for spasmodic dysmenorrhoea, but seldom effects a cure.

*Hormonal imbalance*
It has been suggested that excessive action of the corpus luteum will cause the formation of a thick menstrual decidua, which separates in large flakes or as a complete cast of the uterus (described as membranous dysmenorrhoea), and that the expulsion of these large endometrial fragments causes excessive colicky contractions of the uterus. However, observation does not support this, and large fragments of endometrium are not found in the menstrual lochia of most cases.

*Prostaglandins*

Dysmenorrhoea occurs only when ovulation has taken place; anovular cycles are painless, as is seen in women using oral contraception. It is probable that necrosis of the endometrium is caused by prostaglandins, especially $PGF_{2\alpha}$, and this also causes spasm of the myometrium. The endometrial content of prostaglandin $F_{2\alpha}$ increases under the influence of progesterone in the second half of the cycle. Administration of prostaglandins to normal women can produce many of the symptoms associated with dysmenorrhoea, and prostaglandin inhibitors will relieve these symptoms.

*Psychological factors*

Although spasmodic dysmenorrhoea is often described as psychosomatic, because of the lack of any recognizable pelvic pathology, it is wrong to state that all these patients are neurotic. Upbringing can have some effect; a girl may have come to expect that menstruation must be painful, while adolescence may bring fears of sex or childbearing. However, the majority of patients are entirely free from any fear or phobia. It is true that they may have an increased sensitivity to painful stimuli, but this may sometimes be the effect of recurrent pain rather than the cause.

*Nerve pathways*

Muscle spasm might be produced by imbalance of the autonomic nerve supply of the uterus. Division of the sympathetic superior hypogastric plexus (wrongly called the presacral nerve) abolishes pain during menstruation by interrupting the sensory pathway, but there is no evidence that there is any motor imbalance.

## Treatment

Attention should be paid to the woman's general health, and it is advisable to enquire about her family and social life so as to discover, and if possible to correct, any cause of emotional stress. It will help to tell her, after examination, that she is normal and to explain that menstruation is a healthy normal function.

During an attack of severe pain many patients take a hot bath and then relax in bed with a hot water bottle. Analgesic drugs such as aspirin, codeine or dihydrocodeine should be prescribed, but the use of habit-forming drugs such as morphine, pethidine or alcohol is unwise. Antispasmodic drugs such as atropine are usually ineffective, although many proprietary preparations containing such drugs are sold.

The most effective medical treatment is to suppress ovulation. The easiest way of doing this is to prescribe one of the combined oral contraceptive preparations, using a pill containing 20 to 30 $\mu g$ of oestrogen. The fact that this is a contraceptive should be mentioned. Alternatively, an oral progestogen such as dydrogesterone (Duphaston) is often used in doses of 10 mg daily by mouth from days 5 to 25 of each cycle. Obviously, hormonal treatment is unsuitable for a patient who wishes to become pregnant.

Drugs which inhibit the production of prostaglandins in the endometrium may diminish myometrial contractions and therefore relieve dysmenorrhoea. These drugs, which are given orally 3 times daily during the period, include mefenamic acid (Ponstan) 500 mg, flufenamic acid 200 mg and indomethacin 50 mg.

Dilatation of the cervix was formerly frequently performed for spasmodic dysmenorrhoea, but few patients were benefited for long. Forcible dilatation of the cervix should be condemned, as it may be a cause of subsequent abortion or premature labour because of incompetence of the cervix.

Sympathectomy is usually reserved for patients who have not obtained relief by other methods. Many gynaecologists consider that it is now seldom necessary. The superior hypogastric plexus conveys afferent fibres from the uterus. It lies immediately behind the parietal peritoneum in front of the fifth lumbar vertebra and between the diverging iliac arteries. After opening the abdomen the posterior parietal peritoneum just below the aortic bifurcation is incised to expose the plexus, which is then divided.

In patients aged over 30 whose symptoms are unrelieved by other measures laparoscopy should always be considered, as small endometriomatous lesions may otherwise be missed.

## Premenstrual tension

The premenstrual tension syndrome is a separate entity from painful periods. It mostly occurs in women over 30 years of age. It is characterized by premenstrual discomfort in the lower abdomen and back, and in the breasts, which is often described as a bloated feeling of distension or pelvic engorgement, which precedes the period by a week or 10 days. Sometimes the onset of the menstrual flow brings relief. It is accompanied by varying degrees of irritability, depression and other emotional disturbance, and not infrequently by headache. Those who employ women on skilled work that requires close concentration may notice a falling off in efficiency, and it is said that there is a relationship between acts of violence and this condition.

Patients suffering from premenstrual tension may show a gain of weight of 1 kg or more in the latter part of the menstrual cycle due to salt and water retention. The retention of fluid is partly due to ovarian steroids, but there is also an increased output of antidiuretic hormone from the posterior pituitary gland. It is held by some that the syndrome is caused by a relative lack of progesterone.

Emotional stress often contributes to the symptoms, and the social relationships of the patient must be reviewed. A pelvic examination to exclude unexpected pelvic pathology is also essential.

## Treatment

Although reassurance and simple psychotherapy will help some of these patients, it is also necessary to treat the symptoms with various drugs. Some women obtain relief with diuretics such as chlorothiazide 500 mg three times daily in the premenstrual week. Oral progestogens, such as norethisterone 5 mg twice daily or dydrogesterone 10 mg twice daily, taken in the latter part of the cycle may also be effective in some cases. For some women progesterone itself is effective. This is inactive by mouth and is given by daily intramuscular injection or as rectal suppositories. Some patients are also helped by mild tranquillizers, such as diazepam 2–5 mg twice daily.

# 27

# Hormone therapy in gynaecology

Treatment with hormones has been mentioned in other chapters but it may be helpful to bring together comments on this form of therapy.

Hormonal therapy is often given without accurate biochemical investigation, and results of treatment are sometimes difficult to assess because of the tendency of some endocrine disturbances to resolve spontaneously. Modern methods of measuring hormone levels in the blood have rationalized treatment to some extent, but the information needed to monitor treatment is the tissue concentration of hormones at the end organs, and this is usually unknown. Another practical difficulty is the complexity and cost of some of the methods of assay.

Chemical formulae given in this chapter are not intended for memorization but for explanation.

## Ovarian steroids

Oestrogens and progesterone from the ovaries, and androgens from the testes, are all derivatives of cyclopentenophenanthrene.

The carbon atoms are given conventional numbers, and for simplicity the hydrogen atoms which complete the valency requirements are not shown.

## Oestrogens

In the natural oestrogens which are secreted by the ovary a methyl group is attached in the thirteenth position:

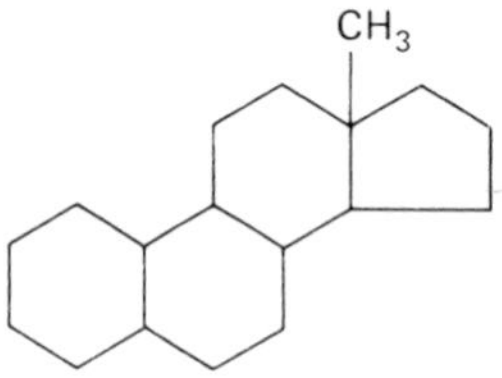

Further chemical modifications show the structure of the three common hormonally active compounds which are found in body fluids and urine. The ovary produces oestradiol 17β, part of which is converted to oestrone and oestriol.

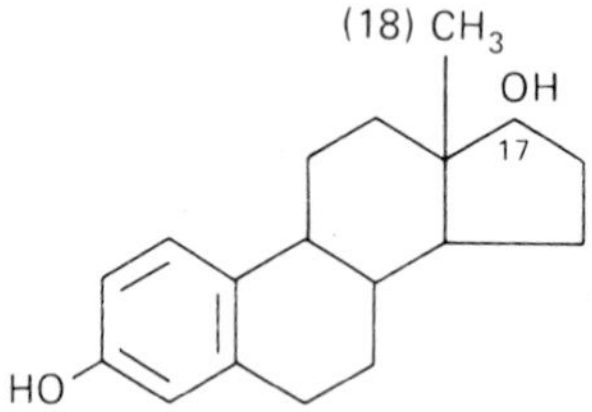

Oestradiol 17β

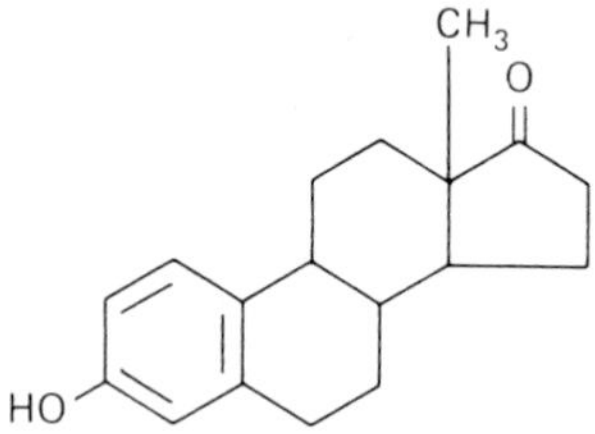

Oestrone

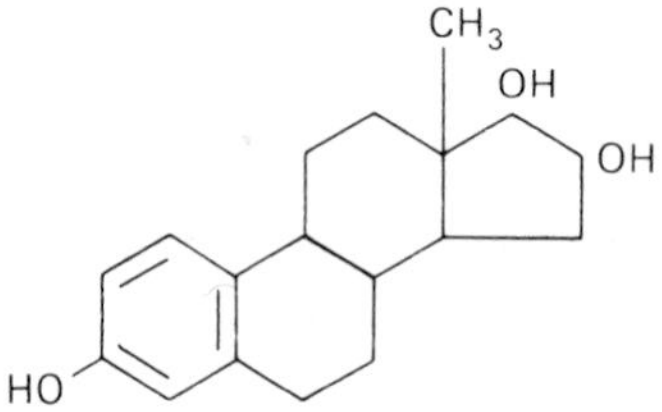

Oestriol

*Oestradiol* can be used therapeutically, but it is only slightly active by mouth and is therefore given by intramuscular injection, usually combined with benzoic or propionic acid in order to prolong its effect.

If oestradiol is modified by attachment of an ethinyl group in the 17α position a very potent synthetic oestrogen is obtained, which is active by mouth:

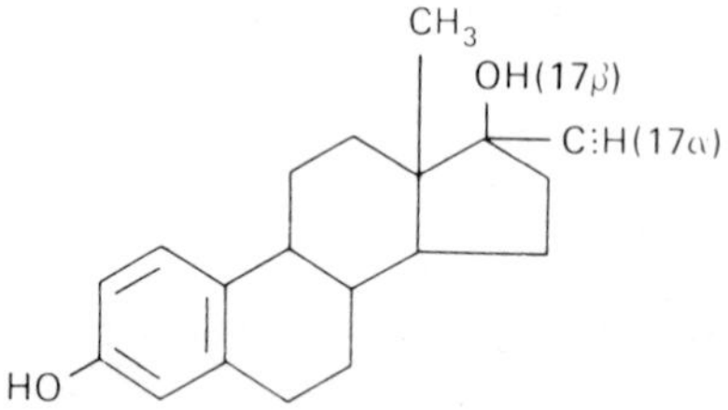

17α-Ethinyloestradiol

The other synthetic oestrogen which is commonly used in oral contraception is mestranol:

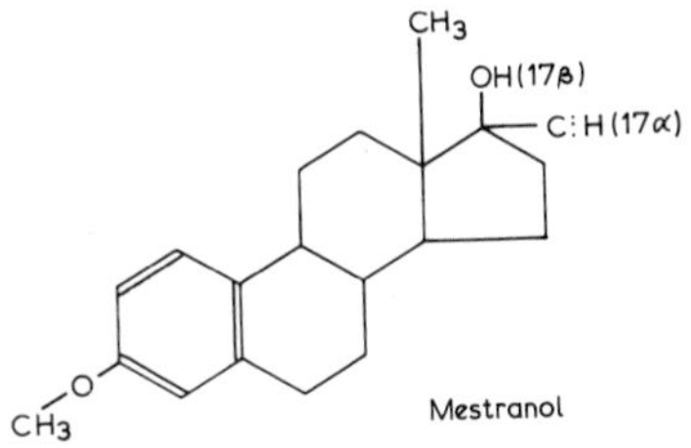

Mestranol

A natural mixture of oestrogens which is active by mouth can be extracted from the urine of pregnant mares, known as *equine conjugated oestrogen* (Premarin). It is relatively free from such side-effects as vomiting, which commonly occurs after administration of other oral oestrogens. It is often used for treatment of menopausal symptoms.

Another group of synthetic oestrogens which are active by mouth includes *stilboestrol, dienoestrol* and *hexoestrol.* The chemical structures of these do not resemble those of the natural oestrogens:

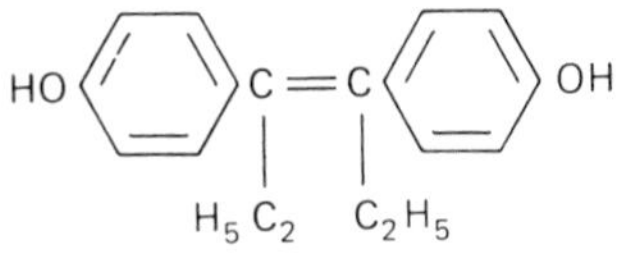

Diethylstilboestrol

*Chlorotrianisene* (Tace) is a synthetic substance which is absorbed when given by mouth, and stored in the body fat, from which it is slowly released and then converted by the liver into an oestrogenic metabolite. It is sometimes used to treat menopausal symptoms, but the statement that it will not cause uterine bleeding is untrue.

**Dosage and administration**
There is no advantage in giving oestrogens by injection in view of the activity of ethinyloestradiol when that is given orally. Oestrogen pellets should not be implanted subcutaneously except in women who have had a hysterectomy. Otherwise the unpredictable rate of absorption may result in severe and uncontrollable uterine bleeding. Vaginal pessaries and ointments containing oestrogen are available for local application, but some of the oestrogen is absorbed into the circulation.

The dose of oestrogen should be the least which produces the desired effect. This dose varies from patient to patient according to tissue susceptibility, age and physiological state at the time; the method should be to

Table 32.1  Hormones by roughly equivalent dosage

|  | *By injection* | *By mouth* |
|---|---|---|
| Oestradiol 17β | 1 mg | |
| Oestrone | 10 mg (100 000 i.u.) | 50 mg |
| Oestriol | 80 mg | |
| Ethinyloestradiol | | 0.05 mg |
| Mestranol | | 1 mg |
| Equine conjugated oestrogen | | 0.625 mg |
| Diethylstilboestrol | | 1 mg |
| Hexoestrol | | 16 mg |

begin with a dose lower than the probable optimum and then to increase it until the effective dose is reached. Furthermore, oestrogens ought to be given intermittently, and the treatment should not be indefinitely prolonged. For most purposes three weeks' treatment should be interrupted by one week without treatment.

Before puberty and after the menopause oestrogens have a greater effect than in the childbearing years. For example, menopausal symptoms can often be controlled with 0.025 mg of ethinyloestradiol daily, whereas an effective dose for most purposes in the childbearing years is 0.2 mg a day. During pregnancy women tolerate large doses of oestrogens without side-effects.

Prolonged oestrogen therapy may cause irregular uterine bleeding, and ill-advised or ill-managed oestrogen treatment after the menopause may cause bleeding which requires diagnostic curettage. There is a risk of endometrial cancer with prolonged oestrogen treatment unless intermittent courses of progesterone are given with it.

Other side-effects of oestrogen therapy are nausea and vomiting, painful breasts, gain in weight and a bloated feeling due to water retention. Oestrogens are powerful drugs that should be used with prudence.

**Principles of oestrogen therapy**

1. *Relation to endometrial bleeding.* If a certain dose of oestrogen is given for two weeks or so to women from whom the ovaries have been removed, endometrial bleeding occurs 2–10 days after stopping the treatment; this is known as *oestrogen withdrawal bleeding.* Larger doses given continuously produce amenorrhoea for a time (6–8 weeks) and then there may be irregular bleeding for as long as the oestrogens are continued. The endometrium shows the changes described as cystic glandular hyperplasia. Bleeding produced in this way can be stopped by discontinuing the oestrogens, but sometimes also by increasing the dose so as to raise the blood concentration still further. It seems that there are limiting thresholds within which the blood concentration must lie when endometrial bleeding is taking place; either a fall in concentration to subthreshold limits or an increase to superthreshold limits will stop the bleeding.

2. *Inhibition of the hypothalamus and pituitary gland.* A rise in oestrogen concentration will inhibit the release of hypothalamic releasing hormones, so that in turn the pituitary gland does not release FSH and LH, and ovulation does not occur. This is part of the basis of action of the oral contraceptives.

Spasmodic dysmenorrhoea only occurs in cycles in which ovulation and formation of the corpus luteum have taken place, and this explains the beneficial effect of the contraceptive pill on dysmenorrhoea.

At the menopause, when the oestrogen levels fall, the amount of pituitary gonadotrophin in the blood rises to such an extent that a false positive pregnancy test may be obtained from the urine. It is doubtful whether this rise in gonadotrophin concentration causes menopausal flushes, but if oestrogens are given to inhibit the output of gonadotrophins the flushes usually become less frequent or stop.

Oestrogens also inhibit the release of prolactin by the anterior pituitary gland during pregnancy, and will inhibit lactation in the puerperium, but because of the risk of thrombo-embolism this method of treatment is not now used.

3. *Action on the lower genital tract.* Oestrogens cause proliferation of the vaginal stratified cells and increase their glycogen content, thereby allowing the formation of lactic acid by Döderlein's bacilli and increasing resistance to infection.

Attempts are sometimes made to make cervical mucus less viscid in cases of infertility by giving oestrogens in the 5 days prior to ovulation, but a dose which is likely to have any effect on the mucus might inhibit or delay ovulation.

**Therapeutic applications of oestrogens**

These are described elsewhere and include oral contraception (p. 300), treatment of menopausal symptoms (p. 44), atrophic vulvovaginal conditions (p. 101), atrophic endometritis (p. 112) and vulvovaginitis in children (p. 112). They may also be used to produce breast development in cases of ovarian dysgenesis (p. 64).

# Progestogens

*Progesterone* is the natural substance produced by the corpus luteum. The chemical structure is:

Progesterone

It is excreted in the urine as pregnanediol (which is biologically inactive) in combination with glycuronic acid.

Progesterone is inactive by mouth, and even when it is given by intramuscular injection its action is transient. However, a very large number of synthetic progestogens have been introduced, many of which are active when given by mouth.

The synthetic progestogens may be divided into four groups.

1. *Esters of 17α-hydroxyprogesterone.* Addition of a hydroxyl group to progesterone in the 17α position yields a compound which is inactive because it is rapidly excreted or transformed, but if hexanoic acid is also attached to this hydroxyl group an active progestogen, *17α-hydroxyprogesterone hexanoate* (Proluton Depot) is obtained.

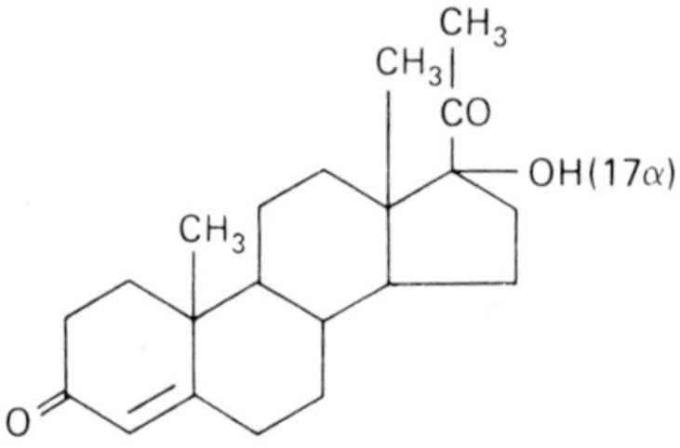

17α-Hydroxyprogesterone

This has a prolonged action when injected intramuscularly in doses of 250 mg once or twice weekly.

2. *Derivatives of testosterone.* The chemical structure of progesterone has some resemblance to that of testosterone. It was found that attachment of an ethinyl group to testosterone in the 17α position yielded a progestogen which was active by mouth, *ethisterone.*

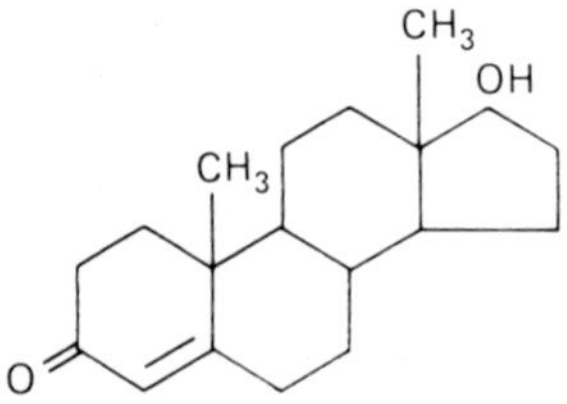

Testosterone

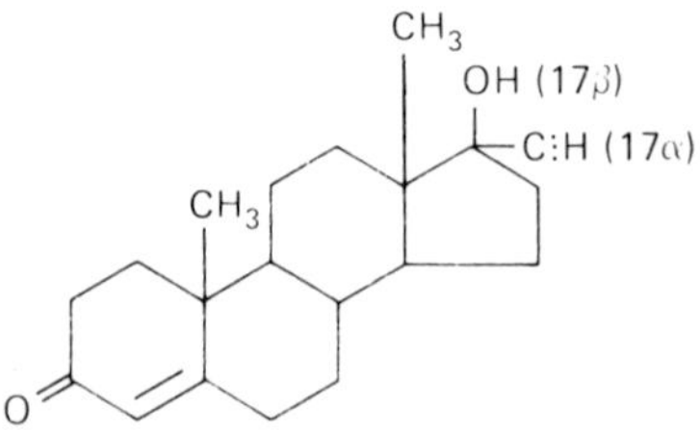

Ethisterone

3. *Derivatives of 19-nortestosterone.* In nortestosterone the methyl group in the 19 position in testosterone is replaced by a hydrogen atom:

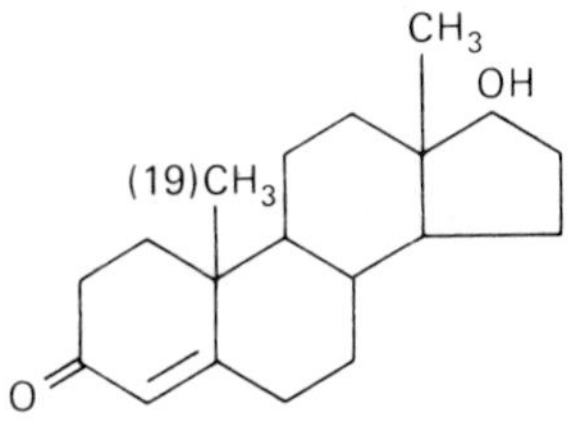

Testosterone

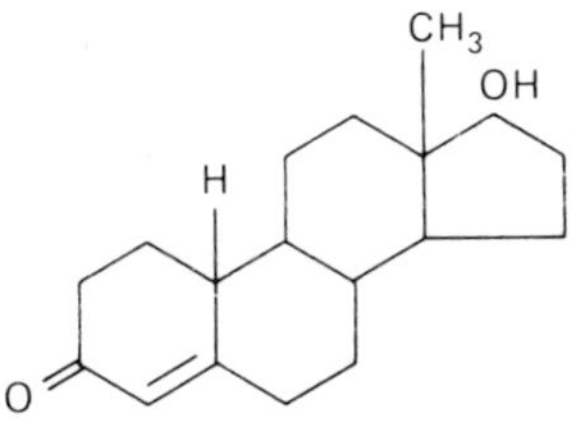

Nortestosterone

Attachment of an ethinyl group to the 17α position in nortestosterone yields a progestogen, *norethisterone,* which is even more active than ethisterone when given by mouth.

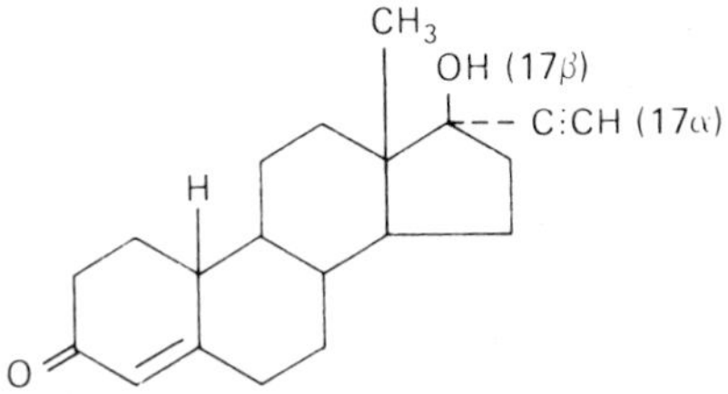

Norethisterone

Many other active progestogens have been derived from 19-nortestosterone, including *norethynodrel* (with a double bond between C5 and C10):

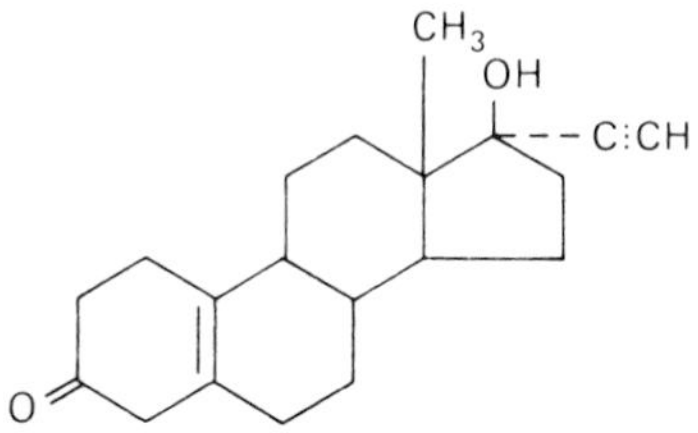

Norethynodrel

These derivatives of 19-nortestosterone differ from progesterone in their strong inhibitory action on pituitary gonadotrophic activity, and because of this they are used in oral contraceptives. They also cause endometrial proliferation of a type which differs from that seen in the luteal phase of the normal menstrual cycle. Daily doses of 10 mg are often used for the treatment of menorrhagia, but for contraceptive purposes very much smaller doses are effective in combination with oestrogens.

4. *Stereoisomers of progesterone.* Another type of synthetic progestogen, whose action more closely resembles that of progesterone itself with little effect on ovulation, is dydrogesterone (Duphaston), often giving in doses of 10 mg daily by mouth. In this compound the progesterone molecule has been modified stereochemically, rather than by attachment of side chains.

### Therapeutic applications of synthetic progestogens

1. *Oral contraception.* Synthetic progestogens are included in the combined pill. Not only do they assist in inhibiting ovulation, but they also control the anovular withdrawal bleeding which is caused by the oestrogenic component. With these progestogens there is more stromal proliferation and less glandular secretory activity in the endometrium than occurs under the influence of progesterone in the normal cycle.

With the progesterone-only pill ovulation may not be inhibited, but the cervical mucus becomes more viscid and prevents the ingress of spermatozoa, and the endometrial changes are hostile to implantation.

2. *Dysfunctional uterine bleeding.* In cases of cystic glandular hyperplasia of the endometrium, progestogens will control the erratic disintegration of the endometrium which is causing the bleeding.

3. *Dysmenorrhoea.* It is claimed that dydrogesterone will relieve spasmodic dysmenorrhoea without inhibiting ovulation, possibly by reducing the strength of uterine contractions.

4. *Premenstrual tension.* Progesterone given by injection or as a rectal suppository or, more commonly, as a synthetic progestogen by mouth, will relieve premenstrual tension in many women.

5. *Endometriosis.* Continuous administration of progestogens in large doses will prevent cyclical bleeding from ectopic endometrium, and so relieve the symptoms of endometriosis.

6. *Endometrial carcinoma.* Progestogens will produce secretory (decidual) change in the tumour, and this may lead to its regression or delay its spread.

7. *Recurrent abortion.* Although often used in the past, progestogens are probably useless for recurrent abortion.

## Androgens

In the female, testosterone is synthesized in small amounts, probably in the suprarenal gland, but a weaker androgen, androstenedione, is formed as a step in the metabolism of progesterone.

Androgens are not often used in gynaecology. Testosterone must be given by injection, but methyltestosterone is active by mouth. It will inhibit the pituitary output of gonadotrophins, but has no advantage over oestrogens for this purpose.

## Prostaglandins

Strictly these are not hormones, as they are produced locally, but it is convenient to mention them here.

The term prostaglandin was first applied in 1936 to a factor in human semen which caused contraction of smooth muscle. Since the original source was the prostate the name has remained to describe a group of biologically active compounds that have since been found in nearly all the tissues of the body. They are long-chain hydroxy fatty acids derived from arachidonic acid, which is released from cell membrane phospholipids and catalysed by the enzymes cyclo-oxygenase and endoperoxidase.

The endometrium, and to a less extent the myometrium, is able to synthesize prostaglandins, including:

$PGF_2\alpha$, which causes vasoconstriction and myometrial contraction.

$PGE_2$, which causes vasodilatation and myometrial contraction.

$PGI_2$ (prostacyclin) which causes vasodilatation and myometrial relaxation, and also inhibits platelet activity.

It is likely that endometrial prostaglandin production is affected by oestrogen and progesterone levels. It has already been mentioned that prostaglandins play a part in causing vasoconstriction and subsequent endometrial necrosis at menstruation (p. 32), and also in controlling menstrual blood loss (p. 240).

Prostaglandins are useful in obstetrics for induction of labour and termination of pregnancy, but are not at present used in gynaecology. Drugs which inhibit the action of cyclo-oxygenase such as mefenamic acid, flufenamic acid and indomethacin are sometimes used for the treatment of menorrhagia and dysmenorrhoea.

## Pituitary protein hormones

The protein hormones of the pituitary gland are long chain molecules of amino-acids linked by peptide bonds. Some, such as follicle-stimulating hormone and luteinizing hormone, have sugar components as well and are glycoproteins. The molecular weights of these hormones range from about 1000 (oxytocin) to about 30 000 (FSH and LH). Those of lower molecular weight have been synthesized but the more complex protein hormones have only recently had their structure elucidated. Three of these hormones are used for gynaecological treatment: FSH, LH and prolactin.

## Follicle stimulating hormone (FSH) and Luteinizing hormone (LH)

These are produced in the basophilic cells of the anterior pituitary gland. Their actions have already been described in Chapter 4.

In treatment the use of hormones from animals has mostly been discontinued because of the disadvantages of anaphylactic reactions. There are at present two chief sources of human gonadotrophins. (1) Human pituitary gonadotrophins (HPG) can be extracted from pituitary glands obtained *post mortem*, but there is much variation in the methods of extraction and presentation of the products. (2) Human menopausal gonadotrophins (HMG) are extracted from the urine of postmenopausal women, where they are found in large amounts. A preparation commonly prescribed is Pergonal, which contains 75 units of FSH and 75 units of LH per ampoule. The responses to these are more predictable than to the extracts of pituitary gland. Doses are stated with reference to an arbitrary international standard preparation.

The main uses of these hormones are in cases of infertility due to failure of ovulation, and in some cases of secondary amenorrhoea. HPG and HMG should be used only when adequate monitoring of hormone response is possible, such as daily plasma or urine oestradiol estimation. Women vary greatly in their response, so the dosage must be tailored to the individual patient if overstimulation and multiple pregnancy are to be avoided.

## Chorionic gonadotrophin

Although this is not a pituitary hormone it may be mentioned here as its physiological actions resemble those of LH, and it is given by intramuscular injection during induction of ovulation (p. 270). It is present in large amounts in the urine of pregnant women and is therefore more easily available than LH. A preparation in common use is Pregnyl.

## Prolactin

This is produced by the acidophilic cells of the anterior pituitary gland. The secretion has no direct relationship to that of FSH and LH. The best known action of prolactin is the maintenance of lactation, as its name implies. The hormone stimulates (1) the growth of mammary glandular tissue (in association with oestrogens and progesterone) during pregnancy and (2) the production of milk. The second action is inhibited during pregnancy by the high level of oestrogens at that time, and lactation begins only when this falls after delivery.

High levels of prolactin (hyperprolactinaemia) are associated with failure of ovulation, and hence amenorrhoea. Prolactin probably acts directly on the ovary, and any associated change in gonadotrophin output is because inhibition of the production of ovarian steroid hormones interferes with the feedback to the pituitary gland.

About 20 per cent of women who are not ovulating are found to have high prolactin levels in blood. This may be associated with a relatively benign tumour of the pituitary gland, and this should be excluded by an x-ray of the skull or tomography. However, most women with hyper-prolactinaemia have no demonstrable tumour and they respond to *bromocriptine*, which often causes a return of normal gonadal function. Bromocriptine is a semisynthetic ergot alkaloid, which is a dopamine receptor agonist. The inhibitory effect on pituitary cells (including tumour cells) is increased, and so less prolactin is produced. Because it has many other effects on the cardiovascular system it should be used very cautiously, starting with doses of 2.5 mg orally at night time, and building up from this if hypotension does not occur.

## Hypothalamic gonadotrophin releasing hormone

Gonadotrophin releasing hormone (GnRH), sometimes described as LHRH, is a decapeptide which is degraded if taken by mouth but is active by in-jection or as a nasal spray. It is secreted in intermittent pulses, and for the induction of ovulation it is given intravenously or subcutaneously by a special pump which delivers the hormone in pulses.

If, however, GnRH is given continuously, it *inhibits* the pituitary output of gonadotrophins and therefore ovulation. Synthetic long-acting analogues of GnRH, in which one or more of the amino acids has been changed, are now under trial for the treatment of endometriosis and dysfunctional uterine bleeding (e.g. Buserelin 400 micrograms subcutaneously daily).

# 28

# Infertility

Most normal couples achieve a pregnancy within a few months of trying. Failure to do so after one year may be arbitrarily defined as infertility provided that normal intercourse is taking place not less than twice a week. *Primary infertility* is the term used for a couple who have never achieved a pregnancy, and *secondary infertility* that for a couple who have previously succeeded in achieving at least one pregnancy, even if this ended in spontaneous abortion. At least 10 per cent of all married couples have an infertility problem.

## Aetiological factors

### General factors affecting fertility

**Age**
In the female conception can occur at any time after the menarche and before the menopause. Conception is rare in the first few cycles, which are commonly anovular, and in the last few cycles before the menopause for the same reason. Fertility in women is at its height in the late teens and early 20s and declines slowly thereafter.

In the male spermatogenesis commences actively at puberty and continues throughout life, but ageing reduces fertility to a variable extent.

**General health and nutrition**
Good general health is associated with fertility, but bad health is not an absolute barrier to conception except when ovulation or spermatogenesis is directly affected. Malnutrition and poor economic circumstances may reduce the general level of fertility, but only in very severely adverse conditions will individuals be rendered infertile and then only temporarily. Women who lose weight deliberately through strict dieting or who suffer from anorexia nervosa are liable to develop amenorrhoea and fail to ovulate when their weight falls to 35 kg or less. At the other end of the nutritional scale obesity and infertility seem sometimes to be associated in women, probably because fat women ovulate and menstruate less frequently. The same explanation for failure to conceive probably applies to alcoholics and drug addicts.

**Psychological factors**
Anxiety and tension are common in modern life and seem to be responsible for infertility in some individuals although no specific effect on the reproductive system can be demonstrated.

## Female infertility

**Ovulatory failure**
Total failure to ovulate causes infertility as long as it persists, but infrequent ovulation is more common and results in relative infertility. Ovulation results from the pulsatile release of follicle-stimulating hormone (FSH) and luteinizing hormone (LH) from the anterior pituitary gland under the influence of releasing hormones secreted by the hypothalamus. FSH brings about maturation of the selected Graafian follicle, while a mid-cycle surge of LH causes the release of the ovum from the follicle, which then becomes the corpus luteum. Any disturbance of this chain of events may cause failure of ovulation. External influences such as those exerted on the hypothalamus by the higher centres in the brain have a similar effect. Prolactin, another of the anterior pituitary hormones, when produced in excess inhibits ovulation (see p. 261). This is a normal occurrence during pregnancy and lactation but if high levels persist after breast feeding has been discontinued or occur at other times, failure of ovulation results. Hyperprolactinaemia may or may not be associated with galactorrhoea.

Failure of the ovary to respond normally to gonadotrophins may result in anovulation, for example in the polycystic ovary (Stein-Leventhal) syndrome.

The oestrogen secreted by the follicle and the oestrogen and progesterone secreted by the corpus luteum have important effects on the rest of the genital tract which influence fertility. In particular, these hormones build up the endometrium to its secretory phase, and at mid-cycle they alter the character of the cervical mucus so as to make it receptive to the sperm.

**Tubal blockage**
Salpingitis caused by infection after abortion or delivery, by gonorrhoea, chlamydia or tuberculosis, or by pelvic peritonitis from acute appendicitis, may damage the tubal epithelium and in severe cases brings about tubal blockage. This most commonly occurs at the outer end where the fimbriae adhere together, or in the very narrow interstitial part of the tube. When the tubes are not completely blocked fertilization of the ovum may still take place in the tube, but because of the damage to the ciliated epithelium it may not be carried down the tube to the uterus, and an ectopic pregnancy results.

**Other factors in female infertility**
**Hypothyroidism** is generally associated with infertility, and mild cases may present for the first time in the infertility clinic. This possibility should

always be considered especially in obese infertile women.

**Hyperthyroidism** is also associated with infertility.

**Diabetes.** Well controlled diabetics have normal fertility, but in badly controlled patients or those with severe complications fertility may be impaired.

**Uterine fibromyomata** are not usually associated with infertility unless they are large enough to distort the uterine cavity or block the interstitial parts of the tubes. They may cause recurrent abortion.

**Intrauterine adhesions** have been described as a cause of infertility but are extremely rare in Britain. Artefacts at hysterography because the uterine cavity is irregularly filled with contrast medium must not be mis-diagnosed as adhesions. Adhesions could be broken down with a uterine sound.

**Endometriosis** is most commonly seen in women who either have never been pregnant or have not been pregnant for some years, often because of voluntary postponement of pregnancy. Endometriosis diminishes the hope of pregnancy as a result of peritubal adhesions and because dyspareunia leads to infrequent intercourse. There may also be interference with ovulation.

**Retroversion of the uterus** is most unlikely to cause infertility unless it is of the fixed variety associated with salpingitis or endometriosis.

**Cervical hostility** is a condition in which the cervical mucus is unreceptive to spermatozoa, either preventing their progressive advance or actually killing them. This may be due to infection or to the presence of sperm antibodies, which may also be found in the woman's blood serum.

**Cervical incompetence,** following previous delivery, conization or excessive surgical dilatation of the cervical canal, is a cause of mid-trimester abortion.

## Male infertility

Male infertility depends on the production by the seminiferous tubules of adequate numbers of healthy spermatozoa and their subsequent delivery into the upper vagina, from where a small proportion of them will penetrate the cervical mucus and travel through the uterus and then out to the ampullary portion of the Fallopian tubes.

### Spermatogenesis

This is a complex process involving meiotic reduction of the chromosomal complement and the transformation of the basal cell in the seminiferous tubule into the highly specialized spermatozoon which lies free in its lumen. In man, spermatogenesis takes about 70 days and is principally under the control of FSH. LH (known in the male as interstitial cell stimulating hormone or ICSH) acts mainly on the interstitial cells and stimulates the production of testosterone and, to a small extent, of oestradiol. The temperature of the scrotal contents is about $1^{\circ}$C below the normal body temperature. If the temperature of the testes is raised because they are undescended, or there is an associated varicocele, or in cases of febrile illness, or tight warm underclothing is worn, spermatogenesis is impaired.

During its passage from the seminiferous tubules through the epididymis to the seminal vesicle (which takes 12 days on average) the spermatozoon undergoes further maturation, and when it is finally ejaculated it is carried in seminal fluid derived from secretions of the prostate and seminal vesicles. Once the sperm have swum into the cervical mucus their transport is achieved by the muscular contractions of the uterus which may occur during inter-course ('insuck') and by the action of the ciliated epithelium of the tubes. Most of the cilia beat away from the ovary towards the uterus, but some beat in the opposite direction and eddy currents and the general mixing process ensure that sperm eventually reach the ampulla. Sperm can be demonstrated in the tubes within 5 minutes of entering the cervical mucus. Of the several hundred million in each ejaculation less than 50 reach the site of fertilization. In the tubes the sperm undergo a process called capaci-tation, which involves the release within the head of the sperm of an enzyme which enables it to penetrate the corona radiata and enter the ovum.

## Investigation of infertility

All couples who complain of infertility should be investigated but the length to which the investigations should go will vary. Pregnancy should normally be expected to occur within one year of cohabitation. Both partners should be seen for the initial interview and a detailed picture should be built up of their general and reproductive history.

In the female the menstrual history, previous gynaecological history, history of pelvic infection, and the general state of health and nutrition are most important. In the male the history of sexual function, erection and ejaculation, and any past history of orchitis or venereal disease should be noted. It is important to establish how often intercourse is taking place, whether proper penetration is achieved, and whether either partner is experiencing difficulty, discomfort or lack of satisfaction. Male orgasm which brings about ejaculation of the semen is essential for fertilization but female orgasm is not necessary for conception.

The clinical examination of each partner is carried out separately. In the general examination of the woman particular attention is paid to any endocrine abnormality. A routine pelvic examination is then performed. For the man examination should include an assessment of the size and consistency of the testis and epididymis on each side, the presence or absence of a varicocele or hernia, and the size of the prostate. During separate examinations the individual partner's worries may be elicited and confidential information about previous pregnancies or venereal infections obtained. Once the initial history and examination have been completed a programme of action can be planned.

## Seminal fluid analysis

This should normally be the first step in investigation because if no sperm are present in the semen investigation of the female is pointless. After three days' abstinence, a specimen of semen is collected in a sterile plastic container after masturbation and examined within a few hours. Normal analysis shows:

| | |
|---|---|
| Volume | 0.2–6.5 ml (mean 3.4 ml) |
| Liquefaction | Complete in 30 minutes |
| Density | 60–250 million spermatozoa per ml |
| Motility | 60 per cent |
| Abnormal forms | Less than 15 per cent |

The figures given are an average, and considerable variation occurs from individual to individual and in any one individual at different times. The sperm count reflects the well-being or otherwise of the man's state of health 70 days previously, when the spermatozoa were formed. For a correct evaluation of male fertility two or three consecutive specimens of semen may need to be examined, especially when the first analysis shows any abnormality. Normal male fertility requires a density of over 20 million spermatozoa per ml, and a motility of over 40 per cent. Oligospermia is the term applied when there are less than 20 million spermatozoa per ml, and azoospermia when there are no spermatozoa in the semen.

If the serum contains sperm antibodies the spermatozoa become immobilized when they are in contact with cervical mucus. Special tests for these antibodies such as the mixed agglutination reaction (MAR test) are performed in some centres.

Once the seminal fluid analysis has been carried out and found to be normal the next steps are tests for ovulation and tubal patency.

## Tests for ovulation

Ovulation may be confirmed in several ways.

1. The patient takes her oral temperature every morning on waking and records it on a special temperature chart. This must be done before rising or starting any activity. A rise in the basal body temperature of about 0.5°C in the last 14 days of the cycle indicates that ovulation has occurred.

2. Examination of the cervical mucus in mid-cycle will reveal characteristic changes if ovulation has occurred. Ovulatory mucus is clear and copious, and can be drawn out into a fine thread ('spinnbarkheit'). On drying, it crystallizes out into a characteristic fern-like pattern.

3. A sample of blood is taken one week before a period is expected, i.e. day 21 of a 28-day cycle. A progesterone level of more than 15 nmol/l in this confirms that ovulation has taken place.

4. Histological examination of a premenstrual endometrial biopsy shows secretory changes in the glands after ovulation. This investigation is commonly combined with the laparascopic examination described below.

5. Follicular growth and ovulation may be detected with ultrasound.

## Tests for tubal patency

### Laparoscopic method

Premenstrual laparoscopic examination of the tubes combined with injection of a dilute solution of methylene blue through a tightly fitting cannula placed in the cervical canal has become the method of choice for investigating tubal patency. The uterus can be seen to be distended by the dye and if the tubes are patent they fill with dye which finally spills from the distal ends. Distal block is recognized if there is no spill, and medial block can be inferred if no dye enters the tubes. Medial block can be caused by inflammatory change in the interstitial or isthmic portion of the tube, or by muscular spasm at the cornu.

The patient should be warned to avoid the risk of becoming pregnant during the cycle in which investigation is performed. Women do occasionally become pregnant during the course of infertility investigations and it would be unfortunate to carry out such tests on a woman who is already in the early stage of pregnancy.

### Hysterosalpingography

The injection of a radio-opaque aqueous iodine solution through the cervix under radiographic control remains a most useful investigation for tubal patency. The test should be performed during the first 10 days of the cycle, after menstrual bleeding has ceased but before ovulation has occurred. Nulliparous patients and nervous parous patients should have a short general anaesthetic, but in others it can be performed without this. The injection is made through a cannula passed through the external cervical os. The passage of the dye into the uterus and out along the tubes is observed by using an x-ray image intensifier and a video display unit. As well as determining the exact site of any tubal blockage, the method outlines the uterine shape to show any congenital abnormality or distortion of the uterine cavity by fibromyomata. Free spill of dye from the distal ends of the tubes proves that they are patent. Loculation of the dye around the distal end or frank occlusion of the tube, often with a club-shaped ending, indicates previous inflammatory change and calls for laparoscopy to establish the extent of the problem. Minor peritubal adhesions may escape detection by hysterosalpingography, although they may be sufficient to interfere with normal function and so to cause infertility.

### Tubal insufflation

In former times tubal insufflation with carbon dioxide was commonly used to test tubal patency. This test is rarely used now because it is unreliable.

## Cervical compatibility

As noted above, the cervical mucus changes character at the time of ovulation, when it is copious and clear and shows 'spinnbarkheit'. Once ovulation

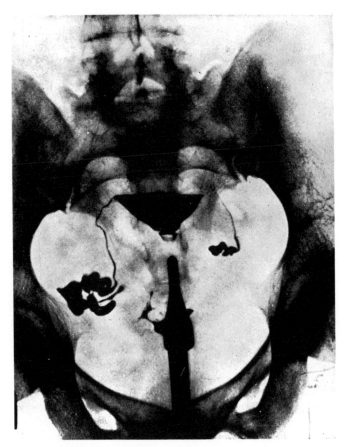

**Fig. 28.1** Hysterosalpingogram. The radio-opaque fluid is escaping from the ends of the Fallopian tubes.

has occurred and the blood progesterone level has risen it becomes scanty, viscid and cellular, as it was in the early part of the cycle. Sperm penetration of the cervical mucus occurs more readily at the time of ovulation but it will not occur in the presence of sperm antibodies (see below).

**Postcoital test**

This test is carried out at the time of ovulation, i.e. at about day 14 of a 28-day cycle. Some 6–12 hours after intercourse has taken place the cervix is exposed with a bivalve speculum and a sample of cervical mucus is withdrawn with a wire loop or pipette and placed on a warm slide and covered with a coverslip. The number of progressively motile sperm in a number of high-power fields is examined. Normally a large number of active sperm will be seen. When the test is negative it should be repeated in two further cycles at the time of ovulation as determined by the rise in the patient's basal temperature. If all three tests are negative, a sample of the partner's semen is obtained and a drop of it is placed alongside a drop of the woman's ovulatory cervical mucus (Kurzrok-Miller test). Invasion of the mucus by the sperm is observed over the next 15 minutes. Normal spermatozoa will immediately start to penetrate normal cervical mucus and will continue to be active in it. A negative postcoital and mucus invasion test may be the result of poor quality cervical mucus, indicating a relative deficiency of oestrogen. In other cases the presence of sperm antibodies in the seminal plasma or in the cervical mucus cause agglutination and immobilization of the invading sperm. When the presence of sperm antibodies is suspected, the semen and the cervical mucus and the serum of both partners should be examined for sperm agglutinating and immobilizing antibodies.

## Prolactin

Estimation of blood prolactin levels should be a normal part of infertility investigation. As noted above, hyperprolactinaemia is present during normal lactation and in women with inappropriate lactation (galactorrhoea). In both cases the response of the ovary to gonadotrophins is impaired, which leads to a failure of ovulation and amenorrhoea. About 20 per cent of all cases of amenorrhoea are associated with raised prolactin levels, although only one-third of these have galactorrhoea. Apart from the association with amenorrhoea, lesser degrees of hyperprolactinaemia may occur with other disturbances of ovarian function, especially defective corpus luteum function. When the level is higher than 800 m.i.u./l computerized tomography of the pituitary fossa is indicated to exclude a prolactin-producing pituitary adenoma.

## Treatment of infertility

Not all couples who complain of infertility need to be investigated and treated. When the period of infertility is short and the couple are young a simple clinical assessment and reassurance that both appear to be normal are often all that is required. At the other end of the scale, couples who have already been extensively investigated and treated should not be subjected to further measures unless there is some real advantage to be gained. In such cases adoption or in vitro fertilization are better alternatives. Unfortunately, many infertile couples are reluctant to accept that nothing further can be done, and when they are dismissed by one doctor will seek the advice of another. A philosophical attitude to the outcome of treatment should be encouraged at the outset; otherwise failure to achieve a pregnancy may become a dominant factor in the partnership, causing a great deal of unhappiness and sometimes separation. It should always be emphasized, when no abnormality can be demonstrated, that pregnancy is always possible, even after many years.

The extent to which anxiety affects female fertility is hard to assess. Only if it reduces the frequency with which the couple have intercourse or causes a change in the menstrual cycle can it have a direct effect. The suggestion that anxiety may cause uterine spasm and blockage of the interstitial parts of the tubes does not have sound scientific support.

## Treatment of ovulatory failure

Failure to ovulate regularly in an otherwise healthy woman should be treated by stimulation of ovulation, using clomiphene or human gonado-trophins, or, when appropriate, by reducing raised serum prolactin levels with bromocriptine.

### Clomiphene

This is a non-steroidal agent which possesses both oestrogenic and anti-oestrogenic properties. It promotes gonadotrophin release by competing for hypothalamic receptor sites for oestradiol, so that its administration is followed by a surge of both FSH and LH. There may be a direct stimulating effect on the ovary. Because of its anti-oestrogenic properties it may make cervical mucus less receptive to sperm, and this could account for its failure in some cases of anovulatory infertility. Hyperstimulation leading to multiple pregnancy is less likely to occur than with gonadotrophin therapy, but the incidence of twin pregnancies is significantly increased. Greater degrees of multiple pregnancy are rare.

A 5-day course of treatment is begun early in the follicular phase of the menstrual cycle. The initial dose is 50 mg daily, which can be increased up to 200 mg daily to obtain the correct response, i.e. regular ovulation. The patient should keep a basal temperature chart to pin-point ovulation and plan intercourse accordingly. The response to clomiphene is best assessed by finding a plasma progesterone level above 30 nmol/l in the mid-luteal phase of the cycle. Treatment should be continued for 6 courses, and may be repeated thereafter if regular ovulatory cycles do not continue. When the patient is amenorrhoeic the initial course can be repeated at 6-week intervals even in the presence of continuing amenorrhoea, but in such cases care must be taken to check that the patient is not pregnant before starting each course. If the anti-oestrogenic effect on the cervical mucus is marked, a small dose of ethinyloestradiol (10 micrograms daily from days 9 to 12) may be given, and if the temperature rise is slow and indefinite – indicating a poor luteal phase to the cycle – an injection of chorionic gonadotrophin (HCG) 10 000 units may be given on day 13.

With clomiphene, ovulation is induced in about 70 per cent of anovu-latory women but the pregnancy rate is much lower. The best results are obtained in patients with 'postpill' amenorrhoea, of whom more than half will become pregnant.

### Treatment with gonadotrophins

Human gonadotrophins can be obtained from extracts of cadaveric pituitary glands or from the urine of postmenopausal women. Human pituitary gonadotrophin (HPG) is a mixture of FSH and LH with predominating FSH action. Its disadvantage is that it is in short supply. Human menopausal gonadotrophin (HMG) is also a mixture of FSH and LH, chiefly with FSH action. It has proved to be the most useful preparation in clinical practice, and is commercially available as Pergonal. Although HPG has greater biological potency than HMG there is no difference in the clinical results obtained with the two preparations. Both act mainly by bringing about follicular maturation. Their administration is followed by that of human chorionic gonadotrophin (HCG) which has biological properties very similar to those of LH. When it is given after a course of HMG it induces ovulation and the formation of a corpus luteum.

There is considerable risk of hyperstimulation leading to multiple pregnancy unless the treatment is very carefully monitored, and for this reason gonadotrophin therapy must be undertaken only in centres with facilities for rapid hormone assays. The effect of HMG on the ovary is assessed by estimating the level of plasma oestrogen or by measuring the output of oestrogen in a 24-hour collection of urine.

There are two ways of giving HMG. Injections may be given daily with an increase in dose each time until a satisfactory oestrogen response is obtained; or three injections are given on alternate days, beginning with 150 i.u., the dose being increased in each cycle until there is a satisfactory oestrogen response. When this occurs an injection of HCG is given on the eighth day after the first injection of HMG.

If at any stage the ideal reponse is exceeded the HCG is not given because the risk of multiple ovulation is then considerable. Although clinical examination of the patient may detect undue ovarian enlargement, it is essential to measure the oestrogen response and to diagnose multiple follicles with ultrasound. After the HCG has been given the basal temperature and the plasma progesterone level will rise if ovulation has occurred. Once a satisfactory dosage has been established, gonadotrophin therapy can be continued for up to 12 months, but every cycle must be monitored because the response to a fixed dose may vary from cycle to cycle.

With gonadotrophin treatment and good biochemical facilities and clinical expertise, between 50 and 75 per cent of women with infertility caused by ovulatory failure should achieve pregnancy. The risk of multiple pregnancy is about 25 per cent, but with careful monitoring anything more than a twin pregnancy should be rare.

### Luteinizing-hormone-releasing hormone (LHRH)
This drug stimulates the release of gonadotrophins, especially LH, from the pituitary gland. It is a very effective way of inducing ovulation when given intravenously by a pulsatile pump.

### Bromocriptine
The use of this dopamine agonist is indicated whenever ovulatory failure is associated with hyperprolactinaemia, even in the absence of galactorrhoea.

Before starting treatment, a CT scan of the pituitary fossa must be taken to exclude a pituitary adenoma which, without treatment, might cause pressure on the optic chiasma. The dose is 2.5 mg a day, increasing after a week by 2.5 mg a day until the blood prolactin level falls. The usual dose required is 7.5 mg a day. The treatment is continued for at least 12 months unless the patient becomes pregnant, when it is stopped.

## Treatment of tubal blockage

When investigations reveal that the tubes are blocked, surgical measures may be considered. In general, the results of tubal surgery are disappointing because, even when tubal patency can be restored, the ciliary action of the tubes has usually been irretrievably damaged.

### Salpingolysis

This is the most successful tubal operation and consists of dividing peritubal adhesions around the ampullary ends of the tubes. If the fimbriae are undamaged and the adhesions are not too extensive, the lining epithelium is likely to be intact and function can be restored. Even so, less than 25 per cent of patients are likely to achieve a pregnancy, and there is an increased risk of ectopic pregnancy. In many cases peritubal adhesions re-form.

### Salpingostomy

Although it is a simple matter to make an opening into the distal end of a hydrosalpinx, it is very unlikely that pregnancy will occur because the fimbriae and lining epithelium will usually have been severely damaged. Postoperative reblockage of the opening is common.

In a few cases with less severe damage, pressure with a probe at the site of the ostium opens it and reveals the in-turned fimbriae which can then unfold like a sea anemone, and it is then only necessary to insert one or two sutures to hold the tube open. In the majority of cases a cuff of tube has to be turned back to produce a new opening, but without fimbriae the outlook is poor for future pregnancies.

### Tubal anastomosis and reimplantation

When blockage occurs in the isthmic portion of the tube it is sometimes possible to excise the blocked segment and to anastomose the cut ends. This is best done with an operating microscope to allow suturing with very fine nylon stitches. It is the procedure of choice when reversing a previous sterilization and the results are good if the distal and proximal parts of the tube are normal, when about 70 per cent of the patients will become pregnant.

When the interstitial portion of the tube is blocked, reimplantation after dividing the tube close to the uterus and then coring out the blocked segment is sometimes carried out.

**Further developments in tubal surgery**

With the advent of microsurgical techniques an improved success rate for anastomotic procedures can be expected. Transplantation of tubes from one individual to another is within the bounds of possibility now that microvascular surgery can link up small vessels. The problems of tissue rejection have not proved insuperable in animal experiments.

Experimental work has shown that the insertion of 'splints' in the form of fine nylon tubes or rods into the lumen of the tube during tubal operations is of no benefit, and the same applies to plastic prostheses intended to hold the outer ends of the tubes open.

**In vitro fertilization**

The birth of the first 'test tube baby' was the successful outcome of a long period of research by Steptoe and Edwards. The idea of *in vitro* fertilization is simple but its realization is difficult. Basically what is involved is the retrieval of an oöcyte from a mature ovarian follicle, fertilization with the partner's sperm, and replacement of the developing embryo into the uterus. Each of these steps presents problems. The oöcyte matures within the follicle and must be retrieved shortly before ovulation would have taken place. Timing of ovulation is therefore critical and can be done by serial hormone measurements to detect peak excretion of oestrogen and the LH surge, or by serial ultrasound scans of the ovaries to measure follicular development. The latter method is simpler, given good ultrasound facilities. When a follicle reaches 18 mm size rupture is imminent and the oöcyte is ready for collection. Until recently collection has been achieved by laparoscopic visualization of the ovaries and aspiration of the follicle with a fine needle, but direct aspiration of the follicle with a needle passed through the anterior abdominal wall under ultrasound control has proved successful and avoids the need for a general anaesthetic. After collection the oöcyte is incubated for 4 to 6 hours before being mixed with 0.1 ml of washed, capacitated spermatozoa. Fertilization occurs rapidly and the fertilized egg is then kept in the culture medium for from 42 to 72 hours. By this time it has reached the 4 to 8 cell stage and it is then replaced in the uterus through the cervix.

Oöcyte recovery and fertilization can now be achieved in a high proportion of cases but only about 20 per cent of replaced fertilized eggs implant successfully, so that the success rate of the procedure is of the order of 10 per cent. This can be improved by stimulating the patient with clomiphene or human menopausal gonadotrophin (HMG) so that several oöcytes can be recovered at one time. The more fertilized eggs that are replaced the more likely is a pregnancy to be achieved, but because of the risk of multiple pregnancy not more than 3 eggs are usually introduced.

There is little doubt that in vitro fertilization will play an increasingly important role in the management of infertility, not only in cases caused by tubal problems or oligospermia, but also in 'unexplained' infertility where both partners are apparently normal.

## Treatment of male infertility

Oligospermia will often respond to an improvement in the patient's general health and fitness. A careful history will often reveal an excessive intake of alcohol and improvement in the sperm count follows its reduction. Wearing loose underwear and bathing the testicles in cold water to reduce the scrotal temperature have been recommended but the evidence that these steps alone lead to improvement in the sperm count is unconvincing, bearing in mind the variation in sperm counts performed at different times in the same man. The same comment applies to operations for excision of varicoceles, which are, however, commonly done for oligospermia.

Hormone therapy, especially with testosterone and chorionic gonado-trophin, has been used without much success. The synthetic androgen, mesterolone (Proviron), has a direct action on spermatogenesis and seems to be more successful in improving both the total sperm count and the motility, but again caution must be exercised in interpreting the results of treatment because of the occurrence of spontaneous improvement. Mesterolone is given in daily doses of 50 mg for 3 months in the first instance. Tamoxifen, an anti-oestrogen, in doses of 10 mg twice daily, has been used for oligospermia.

When azoospermia results from mechanical blockage and a testicular biopsy shows normal spermatogenesis the block may be treated by surgical anastomosis of the vas to the epididymis, but the results so far are dis-appointing. Re-anastomosis of the vas after vasectomy is more successful, and a 50 per cent success rate can be expected. No treatment is possible for azoospermia due to failure of spermatogenesis.

## Artificial insemination

Artificial insemination with the husband's semen (AIH) has been widely used in the management of infertility due to impotence or anatomical abnormality in the male, especially hypospadias which prevents the normal ejaculation of sperm into the upper vagina. The semen obtained by mastur-bation is injected with a sterile syringe and cannula onto the surface of the cervix at the time of ovulation. The woman can be taught to carry out this technique herself, or she can employ the alternative technique of placing a plastic cap containing the semen over the cervix. Injecting the semen directly into the uterus through the cervix has been advocated in cases in which postcoital tests have shown failure of sperm penetration, but in most reported series intrauterine injection is no more successful than intra-vaginal. The success rate of AIH is no greater than that of normal inter-course when this can take place. The results of AIH are disappointing in the management of infertility except in cases of impotence or hypospadias.

The use of donor semen (AID) is, by contrast, much more successful. When the husband has azoospermia or severe oligospermia and adoption of a child cannot be arranged, AID is the management of choice. The implications of it, that any child produced is strictly speaking illegitimate and is not in any case the offspring of the husband, need to be carefully considered by both partners before embarking on the procedure. Either frozen or fresh semen can be used. The pregnancy rate is probably higher with fresh semen but frozen semen is more convenient to use. In selecting donors the aim is to find highly fertile men whose offspring are likely to be physically and mentally healthy, and whose semen will not introduce infection into the recipient. The donor must have a physical examination, seminal analysis and culture of each specimen of sperm for gonococci. In addition, a blood test for syphilis should be performed and, if a rhesus negative donor is required, blood grouping. In matching the donor semen to the recipient woman, race, height and build, hair and eye colour are taken into consideration, so that in these respects the donor resembles the husband. When the woman has long or irregular menstrual cycles she may be given clomiphene to produce a more regular ovulation. The procedure can be continued for up to 12 cycles in the first instance, and a success rate of about 60 per cent is expected, with the majority of the pregnancies occurring within the first six cycles.

Legal issues relating to AID have attracted a good deal of attention. At present a child born as a result of AID is illegitimate, although such children are frequently registered by the parents as though they have been conceived normally. The doctor may be the subject of legal action if the child is born defective as a result of negligence in the selection of the donor, or if infection results from the insemination. There has also been much concern about the ethics of AID but, in practice, provided that the highest professional standards are maintained, it seems to be acceptable to the majority of people and is certainly welcomed by those couples whose infertility can be overcome by its use.

## The Warnock Report

There has been so much public concern about some recent aspects of *in vitro* fertilization (IVF) and embryo transfer, experimentation on human embryos and surrogate motherhood that in 1982 the government set up a committee under the chairmanship of Dame Mary Warnock 'To consider recent and potential developments in medicine and science related to human fertilization and embryology; to consider what policies and safeguards should be applied, including consideration of the social, ethical and legal implications of these developments'. The committee reported in 1984, but up to the time of preparation of this book no legislation has been passed, although this is expected. We can only summarize the main recommendations of the committee, as follows:

Formation of a new statutory authority is proposed, to regulate both research in this field and some infertility services, including AID, egg donation, IVF and freezing of embryos.

A child born after AID, egg donation or IVF should be regarded in law as the legitimate child of the mother and her husband, provided that they have both consented to the procedure.

The practice of storing frozen semen for AID and of freezing spare embryos should continue, but legal safeguards should be introduced to protect inheritance on the death of either parent.

The members of the committee were divided on the issue of experimentation on spare human embryos, and on the practice of creating embryos solely for experiment. By a majority the members accepted that experimentation on an embryo is permissible during the first 14 days after fertilization, but propose that it should be a criminal offence to use it as a research subject beyond that limit.

It should be a criminal offence to operate an agency for surrogate motherhood, whether for profit or otherwise. Private arrangements for surrogate pregnancy can hardly be prevented, but any related agreements are illegal and cannot be enforced in the courts.

# 29

# Abortion

The terms abortion and miscarriage are synonymous and denote the expulsion of the conceptus before the end of the 28th week of pregnancy. There is no sharp demarcation between late abortion and early premature labour; the division is merely one of descriptive convenience.

After the 28th week the fetus is considered to be viable. Before the end of the 28th week delivery of the fetus is only notifiable in Britain if it is born alive, whereas all deliveries after that time must be notified.

The law relating to abortion and the indications for therapeutic termination of pregnancy are discussed in Chapter 32.

It is not possible to give an accurate statement of the frequency of spontaneous abortion because some of the very early cases are not definitely diagnosed but regarded as a delayed or abnormal menstrual period, and a doctor may not be consulted. Also a woman may conceal the fact that she has had an abortion. It has, however, been stated that 10 to 15 per cent of confirmed pregnancies end in abortion. The most common time for abortion to occur is between 8 and 13 weeks.

## Causes of abortion

Despite a long list of aetiological factors, in many cases the cause of a particular abortion is uncertain. The known causes include:

1. **Malformation of the zygote.** The commonest cause of early abortion is an abnormality of the fetus or chorion which is severe enough to cause fetal death. About 70 per cent of these are caused by chromosomal abnormalities, for which either parent may be responsible, although they mostly arise from a spontaneous unexplained mutation in the zygote. Most abortions of this type are not recurrent, so that the prognosis in later pregnancies is good unless several abortions of identical pattern have already occurred.

In some cases it is found that the amniotic sac does not contain an embryo, a condition formerly described as a 'blighted ovum', but now as *anembryonic gestation*.

*Hydatidiform mole* is a special form of chromosomal disorder in which abnormal proliferation of the trophoblast is followed by hydropic degeneration of the chorionic villi. In cases in which all the villi are involved genetic studies show that the chromosomal pattern is 46XX, but that all the chromosomal material is derived from the sperm. Partial moles have a triploid chromosomal pattern.

2. **Immunological rejection of the fetus.** Many investigations of the immune responses of the mother to her fetus are now in progress. There is some disagreement about the results, but it appears that trophoblast shares some antigens with maternal lymphocytes. These cross-reactive (TLX) antigens are partly linked to other antigens. It is postulated that the mother mounts an antibody response against the TLX antigens, and this also protects the trophoblast from attack by the linked antigens. Some cases of recurrent abortion may be caused by failure of this mechanism, and injection of donor lymphocytes to stimulate the response has been proposed.

3. **General disease of the mother.** Pregnancy will often continue in spite of maternal disease, but any illness may cause abortion if it is sufficiently severe, especially acute fevers. Maternal infection may involve the fetus, particularly rubella and syphilis, but also rarely malaria, brucellosis, toxoplasmosis, cytomegalic inclusion disease and listerosis.

In a few cases of rubella abortion occurs, but more often the infected fetus is born alive. Syphilis does not cause early abortion, and it is an uncommon cause of late abortion; it is more likely to cause intrauterine fetal death after the 28th week.

In *diabetes* the abortion rate is above average if the disease is not adequately controlled.

With *hypertension* and *renal disease* intrauterine fetal death may occur, sometimes before the 28th week.

Severe *malnutrition* will cause abortion, but it has to be of a degree which is unlikely to be seen in Britain. Although deficiency of vitamin E will cause abortion in experimental animals there is no evidence that it causes abortion in women as this substance is always present in adequate amounts in the diet.

4. **Uterine abnormalities.** The incidence of abortion is increased if the uterus is double or septate, but in many such cases pregnancy is uneventful.

Retroversion of the uterus is not a cause of miscarriage, except in rare instances in which the uterus becomes incarcerated and is left untreated.

A fibromyoma of the uterus which is closely related to the cavity of the uterus may cause abortion, but other fibromyomata will not do so.

Lacerations of the cervix which extend as far as the internal os may result in abortion in the middle trimester or in premature labour. Very rarely the cervical weakness is congenital; usually it is the result of obstetric damage or of injudicious surgical dilatation of the cervix. During pregnancy the unsupported membranes bulge through the cervix and rupture, when miscarriage follows.

5. **Hormonal insufficiency.** It has been claimed that insufficient production of progesterone by the corpus luteum before the placenta is fully formed will lead to inadequate development of the decidua and abortion. The evidence for this is weak (see p. 286).

Both thyroid deficiency and hyperthyroidism may be contributory causes of abortion.

6. **Drugs.** Cytotoxic drugs or poisoning with lead may cause fetal death and abortion. Oxytocic drugs have been used to procure abortion; quinine, ergot and prostaglandins are sometimes used as abortifacients, although the doses employed may have serious side effects.

7. **Trauma.** Severe trauma to the uterus may cause detachment of the embryo, and this may also be caused by insertion of instruments or foreign bodies through the cervix. Abortion may follow surgical operations, for example myomectomy, and may also follow any condition complicated by severe peritonitis.

In a normal pregnancy coitus has no ill effect, but it is unwise in the case of a woman with a history of abortion in a previous pregnancy.

8. **Acute emotional disturbance** such as fright or bereavement may be followed by abortion, presumably because strong uterine contraction occurs. For such a cause to be accepted in a particular case the miscarriage must follow immediately upon the incident.

Criminal abortion is discussed on p. 321.

## Morbid anatomy

In the first 2 months of pregnancy the attachment of the embryo to the decidua is so slight that separation may follow strong uterine contractions; more often the immediate cause of early abortion is haemorrhage into the choriodecidual space. The exact cause of the haemorrhage is often unknown, but as a result of it the embryo becomes partly or completely separated from the decidua.

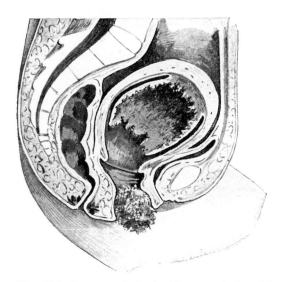

**Fig. 29.1** Rupture of the decidua capsularis, with escape of the embryo surrounded by its chorionic villi. Most of the decidua is left behind.

In most cases the decidua basalis remains in the uterus, and the embryo with the whole or part of the decidua capsularis is expelled. Sometimes only the decidua capsularis is torn through and the embryo, surrounded by chorionic villi, is expelled; or the chorion and amnion may be torn and then the fetus escapes uncovered.

Later, when the placenta is a definite structure, the fetus is usually expelled first, followed by the placenta and membranes, but it is common for the small placenta to be retained, with continuing haemorrhage. Bacterial invasion of the retained products may occur.

An abortion is a miniature labour; the uterus contracts rhythmically, the cervix dilates and, when the internal os is sufficiently open, the embryo is expelled, completely or incompletely. If the embryo is entirely expelled, the contractions cease and the haemorrhage abates. A blood-stained discharge continues for a few days but eventually ceases, and the uterus involutes as it does after normal labour.

In some cases of incomplete abortion a piece of placental tissue may remain in the uterus because it is fixed at its base. Laminated layers of blood clot form upon it, and the contraction of the uterus moulds the clot into a polypoid mass, described as a *fibrinous* or *placental polyp*.

# Clinical varieties of abortion

The following terms are used to describe the clinical varieties of abortion:

1. Threatened abortion.
2. Inevitable abortion.
3. Complete abortion.
4. Incomplete abortion.
5. Septic abortion.
6. Missed abortion (carneous mole).
7. Recurrent abortion.

### 1. Threatened abortion

In threatened abortion there is bleeding into the choriodecidual space but not of sufficient extent to kill the embryo. There are no painful uterine contractions and the cervix does not dilate.

The decision whether abortion is only threatened or is inevitable is important but often uncertain. Abortion does not always occur even after repeated attacks of quite sharp bleeding, and it is not very unusual to meet cases in which haemorrhage has continued for some time and yet a healthy child has been born at term. These cases should, however, always be regarded seriously, since at any time profuse bleeding may occur and the abortion will then become inevitable. Painful contractions and dilatation of the cervix mean that the abortion is becoming inevitable. If bright red loss continues and increases in amount the prognosis is bad. A single bright loss followed by escape of old brown altered blood means that the initial loss has ceased. It is not uncommon in threatened abortion for such a dark loss to go on for several days, gradually diminishing in amount.

*Management*

The patient is kept at rest in bed (except for visits to the lavatory) until 2 days after red loss has ceased. Intercourse is forbidden. All pads and anything passed must be saved for examination, as this will assist diagnosis and avoid time-wasting conservative treatment if products of conception are seen. If the patient is restless and anxious a mild sedative may be given, but otherwise it is of no value.

Opinions differ about the extent to which these patients should be examined. Many women fear that an internal examination will increase the risk of miscarriage, but gentle examination and passage of a speculum have the advantages that any unexpected cause of the bleeding such as a cervical polyp or even a carcinoma may be found, and also that any dilatation of the cervix will be noted.

As soon as the initial bleeding has stopped an ultrasonic scan is performed. This will reveal whether or not the pregnancy is intact. Demonstration of an embryo with cardiovascular pulsation is essential, for even if an embryo is present it cannot be concluded that it is viable without this. With a high resolution real time mechanical sector scanner cardiac activity can consistently be recognized at 8 weeks. Demonstration of an empty gestation sac after 8 weeks is reliable evidence of absence or death of the embryo. Routine scanning of patients with threatened abortion has shown that a common cause of bleeding in the first trimester is a twin pregnancy in which only one sac contains a viable embryo. In these cases the prognosis for the surviving twin is good.

If the abortion is complete the uterus is indistinguishable from a normal non-pregnant uterus.

When a threatened abortion has settled down the patient should be reassured that the bleeding has not harmed the developing embryo (although the obstetrician should bear in mind the possibility of placental insufficiency in late pregnancy).

## 2. Inevitable abortion

A threatened abortion becomes inevitable when the bleeding increases greatly and uterine contractions become rhythmic and strong. The cervix then begins to dilate and products of conception may sometimes be felt through the internal os. Before the 12th week it is quite common for the entire contents of the uterus to be extruded, and for the abortion to become complete. After the 12th week the membranes often rupture and the fetus is passed leaving the placenta behind, and then all the complications of an incomplete abortion may arise.

*Diagnosis*

Inevitable abortion, ectopic pregnancy and some cases of hydatiform mole all present with the triad of pain, vaginal bleeding and amenorrhoea. Both ectopic pregnancy and early abortion are associated with a short period of amenorrhoea followed by irregular uterine haemorrhage. The duration of amenorrhoea in cases of ectopic pregnancy before the patient has severe pain is usually short, and is almost invariably less than 10 weeks.

In abortion the bleeding is usually bright red, often accompanied by clots, and is more profuse than in ectopic gestation, in which the bleeding tends to be dark red or brown. Vaginal bleeding in ectopic pregnancy is usually preceded by severe abdominal pain, which starts low down in one iliac fossa but rapidly spreads across the lower abdomen. In abortion the pain is not so severe and occurs after the onset of bleeding; it is inter-mittent like labour pains.

In all cases of ectopic pregnancy except those with complete tubal rupture (in which the diagnosis of severe intraperitoneal bleeding with shock and generalized abdominal tenderness is usually obvious) there is a tender swelling to be felt separately from the uterus, which is either a tubal mole or a haematocele. If there is any doubt, ultrasonic scanning or laparoscopy may be required.

Hydatidiform mole may be suspected if the uterus is unduly large, and the diagnosis can be confirmed by ultrasound or the finding of high levels of chorionic gonadotrophin in material urine or serum.

*Management*
This can be summarized as the management of labour on a small scale. The uterus usually expels its contents unaided. Any examination must be made with strict aseptic technique. If the abortion is not quickly completed, or if haemorrhage becomes severe, the contents of the uterus are removed with a suction curette. Analgesics such as pethidine 100 mg may be injected, and if bleeding is heavy ergometrine 500 micrograms. Unless the patient is known to be rhesus positive she should also be given 100 micrograms of anti-D gamma globulin.

### 3. Complete abortion
A complete abortion is one in which all the products of conception have been expelled. On examination, pain is absent and bleeding is slight and decreasing. The uterus is smaller than the period of amenorrhoea would suggest, and the cervix may be only slightly open. If the material passed has been saved for examination, it will be found that the whole of the conceptus is present.

*Management*
Once the pain has ceased and the bleeding is minimal no further treatment is needed, but the patient should be warned to report at once if pain or bleeding recurs, or if she develops a temperature suggesting that there are retained products of conception which have become infected. Anti-D globulin is given (as above).

### 4. Incomplete abortion
This means that part of the products of conception, usually the fetus, has been passed but part, usually the placenta, has been retained. The amount

of bleeding varies, but can be severe and accompanied by dangerous shock. It is possible for a woman to bleed so severely that within a few hours the haemoglobin level drops to 5 g/100 ml. If there is still bleeding a week after an abortion which was thought to be complete it is likely that it is in fact incomplete.

*Management*
Treatment is directed to preventing infection, controlling bleeding and obtaining an empty and involuted uterus. The chief risks associated with retained products are haemorrhage and sepsis, and it is unwise to leave a piece of placenta in the uterus for any length of time in the hope that it will be expelled.

If the bleeding is severe there may be shock. If a patient is moved to hospital before the shock is treated, it may increase to a dangerous degree during the journey. Such patients require immediate first aid, and a mobile emergency unit should be called upon to administer blood in the woman's home before the ambulance takes the patient to hospital. The blood pressure is monitored and ergometrine 500 micrograms should be given at once by intravenous injection. Even if the uterus is not empty, the bleeding will often be reduced by the ergometrine, although its action on the uterus is less in early than in late pregnancy. Occasionally, bleeding persists because a large piece of placenta is held in the cervical canal; the removal of this under direct vision, using a sterile speculum and sponge forceps, will allow uterine retraction and reduce the bleeding. The foot of the bed is raised and morphine 15 mg may be injected. When the blood pressure has reached a more normal level the patient is moved to hospital. There she is given an anaesthetic and the uterus is emptied by the gloved finger, suction curette or sponge forceps. The cervix will usually be open and will not need dilatation. Ergometrine 500 micrograms is injected intramuscularly as soon as the uterus has been emptied. Anti-D globulin is given unless the patient is known to be rhesus positive.

In some cases an incomplete abortion is not associated with severe bleeding, but the haemorrhage continues intermittently for some weeks and is due to a fibrinous polyp (p. 165). The uterus remains bulky and the cervix is slightly dilated. Surgical evacuation of the uterus is then essential.

Sometimes it is difficult to decide whether prolonged irregular bleeding after a miscarriage is due to a fibrinous polyp or to complete abortion followed by anovular bleeding from the endometrium, which may occur before the normal cycle is re-established. In either event curettage is required, and histological examination of the material evacuated completes the diagnosis.

## 5. Septic abortion
The uterine cavity may become infected before an abortion even begins, as a result of a criminal attempt to procure abortion by passing an unsterile instrument through the cervical canal. The patient has suprapubic pain and an increased temperature and pulse rate. There may be little bleeding

or uterine contractions, and the cervical canal may remain closed. There may be abdominal rigidity and the uterus is very tender on bimanual examination.

In other cases infection follows incomplete abortion, and the symptoms and signs vary in severity.

The commonest infecting organisms in Britain at present are *Staphylococcus aureus,* coliform and bacteroides organisms, and *Clostridium welchii.* Formerly streptococci, both aerobic haemolytic and anaerobic, were often found. The most dangerous infections are now those with Gram-negative organisms which may cause endotoxic shock, and those with clostridia. The infection may spread to structures around the uterus, causing pelvic or general peritonitis, pelvic cellulitis or salpingitis; or organisms may invade the blood stream to cause septicaemia.

### Management

All cases are admitted to hospital. When the patient is first seen a speculum is passed and a swab is used to collect some discharge from the cervical canal, and a blood sample is taken. These are sent to the laboratory immediately for microscopy and culture and to determine the sensitivity of any organisms to antibiotics. There is much debate about the best choice. One combination that may be used is ampicillin 500 mg 6-hourly with metronidazole 400 mg 6-hourly by mouth. When the bacteriological report is available, treatment is reviewed. It is wise to continue antibiotic treatment for at least 5 days after the temperature has returned to normal.

In cases of incomplete septic abortion the treatment will partly depend on the amount of bleeding. If this is slight, evacuation of the uterus can be deferred for 24 hours to allow time for antibiotic action, but any pieces of tissue lying in the cervical canal should be removed with sponge forceps; the temperature often falls dramatically when infected blood clot is able to escape. However, in many cases the amount of bleeding is such that evacuation cannot be deferred, and the uterus is emptied under anaesthesia with the suction curette or sponge forceps. Blood transfusion is often necessary, and intramuscular injection of ergometrine 500 micrograms will assist in controlling bleeding.

In cases of septic abortion of more than 14 weeks gestation, if the dead fetus is retained an infusion of prostaglandins or oxytocin may be given in the hope of spontaneous delivery.

Laparotomy is always a desperate venture in these cases, but may be indicated if the vaginal vault has been lacerated or the uterus perforated. This may be certain if a radiograph shows gas under the diaphragm or if there are signs of free fluid in the peritoneal cavity after a syringe has been used.

Cases of clostridial infection require special mention. Dead placental tissue and blood clot are excellent media for the growth of anaerobic organisms. Some of these patients, usually after criminal interference, are desperately ill, with a pulse rate of over 140 per minute and a subnormal temperature. They are severely anaemic, because of haemolysis as well as blood loss, and they may be jaundiced. When clostridial infection is suspected on clinical or bacteriological grounds, massive doses of penicillin are given. Any dead placental tissue should be removed surgically as soon as possible. If there is no response to blood transfusion and antibiotics, the possibility that the uterus has become gangrenous should be borne in mind. Hysterectomy is then indicated. Hyperbaric oxygen is used if it is available.

In all cases of septic abortion a careful watch is kept on the urinary output. Renal cortical or tubular necrosis may sometimes occur.

Another dangerous complication of septic abortion is circulatory failure due to peripheral vasodilatation caused by endotoxins released from coliform organisms which have invaded the blood stream. In spite of a low systemic blood pressure the extremities are pink or cyanotic, not pale. In contrast to hypovolaemic shock the central venous pressure may be raised. If a diagnosis of endotoxic shock is made, an intravenous infusion of a plasma expander such as 5 per cent dextran is given, adjusting the rate of infusion according to the response of the circulation and the central venous pressure. Hydrocortisone 1 g may be injected intravenously, followed by 3 g during 24 hours. Oxygen will often be needed. The use of vasoactive drugs is debatable. Isoprenaline increases cardiac output and produces peripheral vasodilatation.

### 6. Missed abortion

Missed abortion occurs when the embryo dies but the gestation sac is retained in the uterus for several weeks or months. Slow progressive haemorrhage takes place into the decidua and choriodecidual space. The effused blood eventually surrounds the embryo and separates it from its attachments. The more resistant amnion is usually found intact in the midst of the blood clot. There is often disparity between the state of development of the fetus and the size of the amniotic cavity. This cavity is surrounded by laminated hillocks of blood clot, which have a fleshy appearance, hence the description 'carneous mole'. Microscopical section shows the hillocks to contain degenerate chorionic villi.

The patient usually notices a little blood-stained discharge for a day or two between about the 8th and 12th weeks of pregnancy. After this the breasts cease to be enlarged, but the patient often pays no attention to this until she, or her doctor, notices that the uterus is not increasing in size.

Pelvic examination reveals a firm uterus which is smaller than would be expected from the duration of amenorrhoea. Immunological tests for pregnancy usually become negative about 10 days after the death of the embryo, but sometimes remain weakly positive for some weeks and cause confusion in diagnosis. Ultrasonic scanning will reveal the true state of affairs if missed abortion is suspected.

A rare complication is defective blood coagulation due to hypofibrino-genaemia, perhaps because thromboplastins from the chorionic tissue enter the maternal circulation. It does not occur for at least 4 weeks after fetal death.

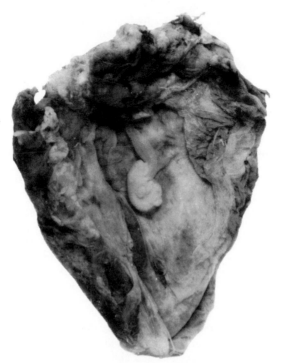

**Fig. 29.2**  Missed abortion. The embryo is seen in the amniotic cavity, which is surrounded by blood clot lying in the chorio-decidual space.

*Management*
All missed abortions are eventually expelled spontaneously, but sometimes not for many weeks. Once the diagnosis has been made the uterus should be emptied. Injection of prostaglandins through the cervix may be effective, but usually the cervix is dilated and its contents are evacuated by aspiration or uterine forceps.

### 7. Recurrent abortion
By convention this term refers to any case in which there have been three consecutive spontaneous miscarriages. Unless each successive abortion has occurred at about the same time and in similar fashion it should not be assumed that there is a common underlying cause. Repeated miscarriages can occur by chance.

There is no satisfactory explanation for many of these cases. Those at about the 12th week have been attributed to progesterone deficiency because at this time progesterone production by the corpus luteum wanes and is replaced by that from the placenta. However, there is no firm evidence of a fall in blood progesterone levels in these cases, and trials with adequate controls have shown no striking benefit from treatment with progestogens. Many women have been treated with weekly or twice-weekly intramuscular injections of hydroxyprogesterone hexanoate 250 mg (Proluton Depot) or dydrogesterone (Duphaston). Other progestogens should not be used; they are partly converted to androgens and may have a virilizing effect on a female fetus.

An alternative treatment with the same purpose is to give chorionic gonadotrophins 10 000 i.u. intramuscularly twice weekly.

Cynics have said that equally good results can be obtained by rest, avoidance of intercourse, and encouragement by the doctor. Certainly these women need a great deal of support, and admission to hospital until after the time at which the previous abortions occurred is often advised.

As has already been stated, repeated mid-trimester abortions (and some cases of premature labour) may result from *incompetence of the internal os of the cervix*. This can be demonstrated between pregnancies if a dilator of 8 mm diameter can be passed easily through the internal os. During pregnancy it can only be suspected from a history of a sequence of relatively painless mid-trimester abortions, or from seeing the membranes bulging through the partly open cervix. A purse-string nylon suture can be inserted in the thickness of the wall of the cervix at the level of the internal os, during early pregnancy to prevent it from dilating (Shirodkar operation). The suture is removed shortly before term or if labour starts.

A few cases of mid-trimester abortion have been caused by uterine abnormalities, including septate malformation and fibromyomata. Surgical treatment, such as excision of a uterine septum or myomectomy is sometimes followed by successful pregnancy.

Immunological rejection of the fetus is mentioned on p. 278.

## Mortality after abortion

In England and Wales in the years 1964–6 the Report on Confidential Enquiries into Maternal Deaths mentioned 133 deaths after abortion, a rate of 51.1 deaths per million maternities. At least 98 of these deaths resulted from illegal abortion. The Abortion Act became effective from 1968 onwards, and in the following years the death rate after abortion has fallen dramatically (although a slower fall in the death rate also preceded the Act). In the years 1976–8 there were only 14 deaths after abortion, a rate of 7.4 per million maternities. Of these deaths, 2 followed spontaneous abortion, 4 illegal abortion, and 4 legal termination of pregnancy.

The main cause of death after abortion is sepsis, followed by pulmonary or air embolism, and anaesthetic accidents. Although no recent death was caused by haemorrhage, this remains a risk in any abortion when blood transfusion is not readily available.

## Termination of pregnancy

See Chapter 32, p. 316.

# 30

# Extrauterine pregnancy

The fertilized ovum normally embeds in the decidua of the uterus. Occasionally it embeds and begins to develop in some other site, when the pregnancy is described as ectopic.

In nearly all cases of ectopic pregnancy the site of implantation is the Fallopian tube. In the tube the most common site is near the ampullary end; implantation in the isthmus is sometimes seen, but interstitial implantation is rare.

Very rarely the fertilized ovum embeds in the ovary (primary ovarian pregnancy) or in the peritoneal cavity (e.g. on the broad ligament or omentum), giving rise to so-called abdominal pregnancy.

In Britain the incidence of ectopic pregnancy is about 1 case to 150 mature intrauterine pregnancies, but it is much higher in some other countries; a rate of 1 in 28 has been reported from the West Indies.

## Aetiology

The ovum is normally fertilized in the ampulla of the tube and then starts to develop as it passes along the tube, so that when it reaches the uterine cavity it is ready to implant. If for any reason there is delay in the passage of the fertilized ovum along the tube, the development of the trophoblast may be so advanced that it begins to embed. Salpingitis can cause such delay by destroying the ciliated epithelium or by forming adhesions between epithelial folds in the tube. Chronic salpingitis (including tuberculous disease) is the commonest underlying pathological finding in ectopic pregnancy. Other tubal abnormalities such as diverticula, abnormal length or previous surgery may be occasional contributory factors.

It has been suggested that there is a higher incidence of extrauterine gestation in patients using an intrauterine contraceptive device and in women taking 'progestogen-only' contraceptive pills. In both cases there may be interference with tubal peristalsis. It is, however, possible that some of the patients had pre-existing salpingitis, but the statistical evidence is uncertain.

Cases of repeated tubal pregnancy are common (7 per cent of cases) but so are cases in which a patient has a normal pregnancy after, or both before and after, a tubal pregnancy. Again, coexisting intra- and extrauterine pregnancies are not unknown.

## Anatomy of tubal pregnancy

The difference between the embedding of the ovum in the uterus and in the tube is related to the structure of the two organs. In the uterus there is a thick decidua in which the fertilized ovum can embed. The bleeding which occurs when blood vessels in the decidua are opened up by the trophoblast is small in amount, and seldom a source of danger to the embryo; in a normal intrauterine pregnancy there is always a layer of decidua between the trophoblast and the uterine muscle. In the tube there is only a very thin layer of connective tissue separating the epithelium from the muscle, so it is easy for the trophoblast to erode into the muscle of the tube. The fertilized ovum comes to lie in a cavity in the tube wall, bounded on the outer side by peritoneum and a thin layer of muscle, and bounded on the inner side by tubal mucous membrane and an incomplete sheet of muscle (Fig. 30.1).

As the trophoblast burrows into the muscle some of the vessels that it meets are large, and when these are opened haemorrhage occurs around the embryo and into the surrounding tubal muscle. The blood may burst through the sac surrounding the embryo — either into the lumen of the tube, *intratubal rupture,* or through the wall of the tube into the peritoneal cavity, *extratubal rupture.* Occasionally extratubal rupture occurs between the layers of the broad ligament.

In cases of tubal pregnancy the uterus is enlarged, in advanced cases becoming nearly as large as a normal pregnancy of 8 weeks. The endometrium undergoes decidual changes indistinguishable from those which occur in normal pregnancy. After death of the embryo the decidua may be thrown off as a cast of the uterus, or may come away in fragments.

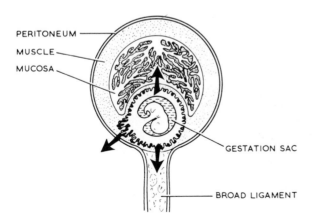

PERITONEUM

MUSCLE

MUCOSA

GESTATION SAC

BROAD LIGAMENT

**Fig. 30.1** Tubal pregnancy. Diagram to show that the embryo becomes embedded in the muscular wall of the tube. The gestation sac may then rupture into the lumen of the tube, through the wall of the tube into the peritoneal cavity, or between the layers of the broad ligament.

# Course and termination

Most commonly one menstrual period is missed before any symptom arises, but sometimes symptoms occur at or before the time of the first missed period. It is unusual for a tubal pregnancy to advance beyond 6 or 8 weeks without symptoms arising.

With or without a short period of amenorrhoea, the patient complains of abdominal pain and of irregular bleeding from the uterus. This bleeding comes from the uterine decidua and is less than that of an ordinary menstrual period. The discharge is usually dark in colour and may persist for weeks. If a patient who is a few weeks pregnant complains of a little pain and a good deal of bleeding the pregnancy is probably intrauterine, whereas if she has much pain and little bleeding the pregnancy is probably extra-uterine. Pain will nearly always precede the bleeding in cases of extra-uterine pregnancy. Decidual shreds or even a perfect decidual cast may be passed from the uterus. If there is no bleeding from the uterus in a case of extrauterine pregnancy it is probable that the pregnancy is undisturbed – i.e. the embryo is alive. But in rare fulminating cases of intraperitoneal bleeding the patient may die from haemorrhage and shock in a few hours – before the bleeding from the uterus has had time to begin.

There may be one or more attacks of very severe pain, accompanied by more or less collapse. Pain may be caused by distension of the tube and separation of the layers of muscle by blood, but severe pain is usually due to the presence of blood in the peritoneal cavity.

The possible terminations of a tubal pregnancy are:
1. Tubal mole.
2. Tubal abortion.
3. Tubal rupture:
   (a) into the general peritoneal cavity;
   (b) into the broad ligament.
4. Abdominal pregnancy.

### Tubal mole

Haemorrhage occurs around the embryo, causing its death. Such an embryo surrounded by blood clot is called a tubal mole. A firm swelling is formed, commonly about 3 cm in diameter. On section a thick wall of blood clot, in which degenerate chorionic villi are embedded, is found to surround the amniotic space, which often contains a small embryo.

A patient with a tubal mole will complain of pelvic pain and discomfort, and loss of dark blood from the uterus. On examination the uterus will be found to be slightly enlarged, and in one posterior quarter of the pelvis a tender swelling will be found, 3 cm in diameter or larger. If the mole remains *in situ*, it may be absorbed, or very rarely, become infected. If tubal abortion or tubal rupture do not supervene there is little further risk to the patient, but the tube is likely to be permanently blocked.

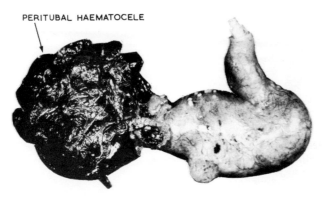

PERITUBAL HAEMATOCELE

**Fig. 30.2** Tubal mole, with bleeding through the ostium of the tube.

## Tubal abortion

An embryo embedded in the wall of the tube is separated from the lumen by tubal mucous membrane and a certain amount of muscle. If this layer is ruptured, bleeding will occur into the lumen of the tube (intratubal rupture) and the blood will run out into the peritoneal cavity through the abdominal ostium; it does not escape into the uterus. Contractions of the tubal muscle may loosen the embryo from its bed and then expel it through the ostium; extrusion may be complete or incomplete. In either case the embryo always dies, and it has often been converted into a mole before the tubal abortion takes place.

If the bleeding is slow the blood may coagulate around the ostium of the tube, but more often it accumulates in the rectovaginal pouch, forming a *pelvic haematocele*. The blood becomes encysted and is roofed over by omentum and adherent coils of small intestine, while anteriorly it is in contact with the uterus, broad ligaments, bladder and, if it is large enough, the lower part of the anterior abdominal wall. The floor is formed by the rectovaginal pouch, and behind it is in contact with the rectum and the posterior wall of the pelvis on each side of the rectum. The blood pushes the uterus forwards against the symphysis pubis and bladder. If there is a large amount of blood clot, abdominal examination shows the presence of a tender fixed swelling. Light percussion over the upper part of the tumour will often elicit a resonant note, a useful point in differential diagnosis.

On vaginal examination the cervix is found to be pushed forwards, and sometimes upwards almost out of reach. The rectovaginal pouch is occupied by a tense tender swelling which may bulge downwards. If the cervix is pushed much upwards retention of urine may occur from the elongation of the urethra. Later on, when absorption of the blood has begun, the

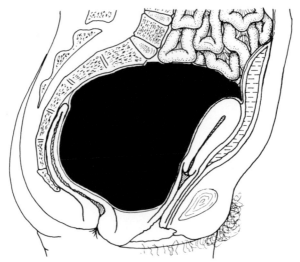

**Fig. 30.3** Drawing to show a large pelvic haematocele pushing the intestines upwards and displacing the uterus forwards.

contents of the rectovaginal pouch will have a lumpy, irregular consistence. The temperature is often raised in cases of pelvic haematocele.

If the patient is not operated on, the probability is that the blood will be absorbed, although this can be a very slow process, the patient being an invalid for several weeks or months with abdominal and pelvic discomfort, and slight bleeding from the uterus. Suppuration may occur, but is uncommon.

### Tubal rupture

The term 'tubal rupture' refers to cases in which the wall of the tube gives way as a result of erosion by the trophoblast and increased tension in the tube. The tube may burst through its peritoneal covering into the peritoneal cavity – *intraperitoneal rupture.* Rarely, the rupture occurs through that small area of tube wall which has no peritoneal investment into the tissues of the broad ligament – *extraperitoneal or intraligamentous rupture.* In either event the embryo dies.

If the fertilized ovum becomes embedded in the isthmus of the tube, tubal abortion cannot occur and early rupture is the inevitable result because there is so little tissue to accommodate the embryo.

If a large vessel is eroded by the trophoblast the consequent bleeding may break through the tubal wall, and the rupture may also be precipitated by pelvic examination. The amount of bleeding is usually greater in tubal rupture than in tubal abortion.

The patient presents with pain, fainting or collapse, followed by signs indicative of severe blood loss. She is pale and the blood pressure will be low. Her pulse is weak and rapid: 120–140 per minute. The temperature is frequently subnormal; she complains of thirst and the skin may be clammy. The patient is often restless and may show air-hunger.

The whole abdomen is usually distended to some degree, and there may be dullness on percussion in the flanks. There is no localized area of tenderness, but the whole subumbilical area is acutely sensitive. If the blood reaches the diaphragm, pain is referred to the shoulder. On vaginal examination a little dark blood may be seen coming away. It may be possible to recognize fullness in the rectovaginal pouch, but the exquisite tenderness usually makes it impossible to define the pelvic structures.

In the comparatively rare cases of extraperitoneal rupture the blood clots between the layers of the broad ligament, forming an *intraligamentous haematocele.* There is a swelling on one side of the pelvis which pushes the uterus to the other side. The blood may be absorbed slowly or may, rarely, become infected.

### Abdominal pregnancy

In this condition the trophoblast perforates the surface of the tube without causing severe haemorrhage. A communication is thus made between the intervillous space and the peritoneal cavity. In rare instances, provided that the amniotic sac remains complete, the embryo continues to live. The villi of a part of the chorion become attached to some of the abdominal contents (usually broad ligament or omentum) which then form a portion of the placental site, while the tube continues to form another portion. It is possible for the pregnancy to continue to term.

In other rare instances erosion takes place into the broad ligament — an intraligamentary pregnancy. Although it is possible for the pregnancy to continue, in most cases the sac gives way after a short time, often with severe haemorrhage.

In a few cases of *abdominal pregnancy* there are no symptoms to suggest the diagnosis, although an x-ray may show that the fetus lies in some position which cannot be intrauterine. As a rule the fetus dies before it reaches term, and it may show deformities from pressure. If the pregnancy goes to term, so-called mock labour occurs. There are labour pains due to uterine contractions and there may be blood-stained discharge with expulsion of the uterine decidua. The fetus dies and then thrombosis of the vessels at the placental site gradually occurs. Absorption of the liquor amnii and mummification of the fetus may be followed by deposition of lime salts in the fetal tissues, and the formation of a *lithopaedion,* which may be carried in the abdomen for many years without symptoms unless it leads to the formation of adhesions. In other cases infection of the sac occurs, giving rise to severe toxic effects, sometimes followed by the discharge of fetal bones per rectum or through an abdominal sinus.

## Diagnosis of tubal pregnancy

The diagnosis may be difficult and if it is missed the consequences for the patient may be serious. A careful history and clinical examination will usually make the diagnosis clear, or at least establish the need for further investigation with the possibility of tubal pregnancy in mind. The most significant symptoms are amenorrhoea, unilateral pain and vaginal bleeding, while the most significant signs are lower abdominal tenderness, extreme tenderness in the lateral fornix on one side, and pain on moving the cervix. The clinical picture will vary with the stage of development of the ectopic pregnancy and the amount of intraperitoneal bleeding.

### Unruptured tubal pregnancy
There may only be slight pain to draw attention to the case. The only signs are a tender swelling in one lateral fornix and a slightly enlarged uterus.

### Ruptured tubal pregnancy and tubal abortion
The essential feature in these two conditions is that intraperitoneal bleeding has occurred. The bleeding is likely to be more rapid and profuse with rupture of a pregnancy in the isthmus of the tube. In tubal abortion the bleeding through the abdominal ostium of the tube is usually slower, and the pregnancy is usually situated in the ampulla.

In these cases spasmodic unilateral pain changes to generalized lower abdominal pain when the pelvic peritoneum is irritated by the escaping blood. If large quantities of blood find their way into the peritoneal cavity there is abdominal distension, and shoulder-tip pain occurs from irritation of the undersurface of the diaphragm. The patient becomes acutely shocked.

### Tubal mole
The clinical picture resembles that of an unruptured tubal pregnancy except that vaginal bleeding will have occurred and subsequently settled down. The tubal swelling will be less tender, and the uterus will have returned to its normal size. The diagnosis is only likely to be made some time after the acute symptoms of pain and vaginal bleeding have improved.

### Pelvic haematocele
This is a late result of tubal pregnancy and is rarely seen when diagnostic standards are high. It occurs when the initial diagnosis has been missed but the intraperitoneal haemorrhage has eventually stopped spontaneously.

In the case of a large haematocele, abdominal and bimanual examination will establish a diagnosis of encysted fluid. The history, temperature chart and condition of the patient will usually point to the fluid being blood rather than pus or serous fluid. If there is a large amount of blood in the peritoneal cavity the patient shows signs of anaemia, and later when the blood is being absorbed she may have slight jaundice. There is usually a slight rise of temperature with a haematocele.

On vaginal examination a swelling is found in the rectovaginal pouch which pushes the uterus upwards and forwards, so the cervix is higher than normal. The swelling will be fluid at first, but as the blood clots it becomes doughy and then firm.

If the haematocele is small, and the history is not typical, it may be mistaken for an inflammatory pelvic swelling or for an ovarian cyst which has undergone torsion of its pedicle.

# Investigation of suspected tubal pregnancy

When the diagnosis of tubal pregnancy on clinical grounds is in doubt the following investigations may be performed:

### 1. Pregnancy tests
The standard immunological pregnancy tests which demonstrate the presence of chorionic gonadotrophin in the urine are not helpful; a tubal pregnancy may not produce enough hCG to give a positive result. Estimation of the concentration of the $\beta$ subunit of hCG in the serum is of greater value, especially when used in conjunction with ultrasonic scanning. If the level of $\beta$hCG is above 6000 mi.u./l the patient is likely to have a normal intrauterine pregnancy, especially if the level rises rapidly. Absence of $\beta$hCG virtually eliminates pregnancy, but levels below 6000 mi.u./l are suggestive of tubal pregnancy or of missed abortion.

### 2. Ultrasonic scanning
In an early pregnancy of 4 to 5 weeks the decidual reaction of the endometrium in an ectopic pregnancy might be hard to distinguish from an intrauterine gestation sac. Ultrasonic demonstration of fetal cardiac activity within the uterus is undeniable evidence of an intrauterine pregnancy, but this can rarely be certain until the 8th week, 1 to 2 weeks after recognition of the gestation sac. When a transonic area surrounded by an echogenic rim is present in the uterus and the $\beta$hCG level is above 6000 mi.u./l it is very probable that the pregnancy is intrauterine. Lower levels of hCG are likely to be associated with tubal pregnancy or missed abortion, and in this case the sac in the uterus is formed by the decidua. From the 7th week onwards it may be possible to show a gestation sac and fetal cardiac echoes beside a normal uterus, thus giving direct confirmation of the presence of an ectopic pregnancy.

### 3. Laparoscopy
With the laparoscope a certain diagnosis of tubal pregnancy can be made, but it involves giving the patient an anaesthetic, which is undesirable if the pregnancy is intrauterine. Estimation of hCG levels and the use of ultrasound, as described above, may help to avoid this. When the clinical evidence is clear-cut laparoscopy should not be advised as it will only delay laparotomy, but if the diagnosis is in doubt it may be valuable in preventing laparotomy being performed on patients with conditions such as salpingitis, which should be treated medically.

# Treatment of ectopic pregnancy

Prompt treatment is required for all patients with ectopic pregnancy. This entails resuscitation if there has been intraperitoneal haemorrhage, and then laparotomy and removal of the affected tube.

Problems arise if the patient is severely shocked. Transfusion of blood or other plasma expanders may increase bleeding by restoring the patient's low blood pressure. For this reason resuscitation and operation should go hand-in-hand; the operation is started as soon as there are signs of response to resuscitation.

At operation the damaged tube is removed. It has been suggested that the ovary should also be removed on the ground that on average ovulation occurs from alternate ovaries, so that half the ova will have a poor chance of reaching the remaining tube. While accepting this point, most surgeons do not consider that it justifies sacrificing a normal ovary.

In exceptional cases, particularly when the woman has already lost the other tube, if the pregnancy is near to the abdominal ostium it may be possible to express the embryonic tissue out of the tube. If haemostasis is then satisfactory the tube may thus be conserved, although at the risk of a recurrent tubal pregnancy.

### Pelvic haematocele

If the haematocele is large the blood should be removed by abdominal operation. If it is left to be absorbed, the patient will be an invalid for 2 or 3 months and run the risk of infection of the haematocele during this time, whereas if she is operated upon she will need only 2 or 3 weeks to recover. Absorption is inevitably slow because the circulation by which it is effected is confined to the periphery of the haematocele.

### Cases of advanced ectopic pregnancy

A few living fetuses have been removed by operation at or shortly before term. If the fetus is alive during the second half of pregnancy, operation is fraught with a considerable risk of haemorrhage when the placenta is separated, as it may be attached to structures such as the omentum or pelvic peritoneum whose blood vessels cannot be controlled by muscular contraction like those of the uterus. If the placenta has a broad flat attachment to tissue which cannot be ligated, treatment is difficult. If the sac is marsupialized and drained infection always occurs, and the sac continues to discharge for a very long time. It may be best to cut the cord short, leave the placenta *in situ,* and close the abdomen. If infection does not occur, the placenta becomes slowly organized into fibrous tissue.

If thrombosis of the vessels of the placental site occurs before the operation, removal of the placenta is comparatively simple. For this reason it has been advised that if the fetus is dead the operation should be postponed for a few weeks.

The infant may show pressure deformities, but these can often be improved by treatment.

# Rare types of ectopic pregnancy

### Ovarian pregnancy
This is very rare, but may occur if a spermatozoon enters the cavity of a ruptured Graafian follicle from which, for some reason, the ovum has not been expelled. Rupture or mole formation has occurred early in most of the recorded cases. The symptoms and signs are those of tubal pregnancy, and diagnosis is only made at operation.

### Interstitial (cornual) pregnancy
If the ovum is embedded in the interstitial part of the tube as it passes through the uterine wall, diagnosis is difficult because the swelling is evidently part of the uterus, and careful bimanual examination is necessary to prove that the uterus has an abnormal shape. Rupture usually takes place later than in cases of ampullary pregnancy, but bleeding may be unusually profuse as the uterine wall is extremely vascular. The treatment is to excise the cornu by a wedge-shaped incision, or sometimes if the uterus is extensively damaged to perform hysterectomy.

### Pregnancy in a rudimentary uterine horn
Pregnancy in a uterine horn is not really extrauterine but is mentioned here for convenience. The comparatively thick muscular wall of an un-developed uterine horn may accommodate the gestation for a time, but it usually ruptures at about the 16th week, with severe intraperitoneal haemorrhage. If the connection between the rudimentary cornu and the developed half of the uterus is not too intimate, it will be possible to remove only the former. In the case of pregnancy in a rudimentary horn, the round ligament will be attached on the outer side of the gestation sac, while in tubal pregnancy it is inserted on the inner side of the gestation sac, between it and the uterus.

### Cervical pregnancy
This may also be mentioned here. Very rarely the embryo implants in the cervical canal. Because of restriction in its growth the pregnancy rarely proceeds beyond the 6th week. Pain due to uterine contractions and heavy, bright red bleeding are the main features. The cervical canal can be evacuated by curettage, but this does not always stop the bleeding, and deep sutures may be required to control it.

# 31

# Contraception and sterilization

During the last two or three decades both professional and public attitudes towards fertility control have changed, and a significant proportion of gynaecological practice is now concerned with problems of contraception. Patients seek contraceptive advice for a variety of reasons, and during any one individual's reproductive life a number of methods may be used, depending on the circumstances at the time. For example, a method suitable for a sexually active unmarried girl may differ from that appropriate for a couple who have finally decided that they do not want any further addition to their family.

Many methods of contraception, of greatly varying efficiency, are in use. The ideal method should be certain, without risk to health, aesthetically acceptable and inexpensive. Even if such a method were freely available, psychological difficulties might still arise; to a few women sexual satisfaction is related to the possibility of conception. Yet it is obvious that an unwanted pregnancy can cause much misery to the individual woman, and in many parts of the world unchecked growth of population threatens to be disastrous.

The effectiveness (or failure rate) of a particular method of contraception may be expressed by the Pearl index, which states the number of unwanted pregnancies which occur in 100 women using that method for a year. Effectiveness depends on motivation and on the care taken to use the method regularly and exactly as advised. As an example, while figures of 8—20 unplanned pregnancies per 100 woman years are often quoted for use of a vaginal diaphragm with a spermicide, many women who are conscientious and intelligent achieve much better indices with this method — as low as 2.5. Although some methods are very unreliable, for example coitus interruptus (index 10 to 20) or the 'safe period' (index 20 to 30), many couples still prefer to use them and still achieve the size of family they desire, and such methods should not be condemned out of hand.

Methods of contraception may be classified in many ways; the following list may be convenient:

A.  Methods not requiring medical consultation:

|  |  |
|---|---|
| Used by the male: | 1. Coitus interruptus. |
|  | 2. Condom (sheath). |
| Used by the female: | 3. Safe period (rhythm method). |
|  | 4. Vaginal spermicides and tampons. |

B.  Methods requiring medical supervision:
      Used by the female:   1. Systemic contraceptives.
                            (a)  Oral contraceptives.
                                  Combined preparations.
                                  Variable dose combined
                                  preparations.
                                  Continuous progestogens.
                            (b)  Injectable steroids.
                            (c)  Postcoital methods.
                        2. Intrauterine devices.
                        3. Occlusive diaphragms and caps.
C.  Permanent methods (sterilization):
      For the female: Tubal occlusion.
      For the male: Vasectomy.
D.  Methods under investigation.

# Methods not requiring medical consultation

**Coitus interruptus**
Withdrawal of the penis at the moment before ejaculation is a widely used method although the failure rate is high (index 20 to 30). Failure occurs from delay in withdrawal, or because the pre-ejaculatory fluid may contain some spermatozoa.

**Condom (male sheath)**
This method is that most widely used in the United Kingdom because of its simplicity. The latex rubber sheath should be used with a chemical spermicide for additional contraceptive security. The sheath is drawn or rolled onto the penis after erection has occurred. Occasional failures occur because the sheath is defective, because it is not worn in the earlier phases of coitus, or because it slips from the penis after ejaculation (index quoted 4 to 10). Its use reduces the risk of venereal infection.

**The 'safe period' (rhythm or calendar method)**
At present this is the only method officially permitted for Roman Catholics. It is far from reliable (index 20 to 30). The method is based on the assumption that the ovum is capable of being fertilized for only 24 hours after its release, and that sperm can fertilize the ovum for only 72 hours after they are deposited in the vagina. If ovulation occurs between days 12 and 16 of a 28-day cycle the potential fertile period, during which intercourse should be avoided, is therefore between day 9 (= 12 − 3) and day 17 (= 16 + 1) of the cycle. But few women are completely regular. It is the preovulatory phase of the cycle which varies in length; the number of days between ovulation and the next menstruation is fairly constant. For a particular woman who has noted the length of her shortest and longest cycles in the preceding 12 months, a rough and ready way of calculating

the range of the beginning and end of her fertile period is to deduct 18 days from her shortest cycle, and 11 days from her longest cycle. For example, if her range of cycles were from 26 to 32 says, the possible fertile period would extend from day 8 (= 26 − 18) to day 21 (= 32 − 11), and between these days intercourse should be avoided. This method of contraception is not suitable for women with very irregular periods.

An attempt may be made to pin-point the time of ovulation by recording the basal body temperature first thing in the morning (see p. 266). If intercourse is avoided for 72 hours after the rise in temperature has taken place, the method is said to give an index of 5 to 7. A few women claim to be able to recognize the time of ovulation by noting the consistency of the cervical mucus.

### Spermicides
These are chemical substances which kill spermatozoa when they are placed in the vagina before intercourse. They are prepared as pessaries, creams, aerosols, foaming tablets or films. When used on their own they give very poor results, but are often used in conjunction with a mechanical barrier such as a diaphragm or condom. Although the method has the virtue of simplicity and does not require medical supervision, it sometimes causes soreness or irritation to one or other partner.

### Vaginal tampon
Various forms of tampons and sponges have been used in the upper vagina as barriers to sperm penetration of the cervix. A disposable sponge impregnated with the spermicide nonoxynol-9 has recently been recommended. The method is less reliable than the diaphragm (p. 310) but has the advantage of simplicity and it does not require medical help.

## Systemic contraceptives

### Oral contraception
Systemic contraception, operating through its effect on the endocrine system, was first introduced in 1956 in the form of an oral preparation containing a synthetic oestrogen and a synthetic progestogen − the *combined pill.*

The chief advantage of this method of contraception is that intercourse can take place at any time without the need for either partner to use any sort of local appliance. The additional advantage that the woman has control of her own contraceptive method must be set against the disadvantage that she must remember to take the pill every day. Provided that the pills are taken it is probably the most reliable of all contraceptive methods (indices quoted 0.1 to 1.5) but, whether from subconscious motives or otherwise, it is surprising how often pills are 'forgotten'. Some women find the idea of taking a pill to alter their own hormonal status unacceptable. More often they are deterred from using what would be for them an entirely appropriate method by overdramatized comments in the media about possible side effects and complications.

*Mode of action*
The oestrogen and progestogen components of the pill inhibit ovulation through the feedback system that controls hypothalamic-pituitary-ovarian function. Production of GnRH is inhibited, so FSH and LH are suppressed. In addition, the prolonged action of the progestogen makes the cervical mucus hostile to spermatozoa. It also causes endometrial changes which are hostile to implantation. As a result of constant progestogenic action throughout the cycle the endometrium is thin and atrophic. The combination of effects probably explains the almost complete effectiveness of the combined pill.

*Formulations*
The combined pill contains one of two synthetic oestrogens — ethinyl-oestradiol or mestranol. Although a variety of synthetic progestogens are used, they are all derivatives of 19-nortestosterone. The doses and proportions vary in the different proprietary preparations (see p. 313). Because thrombo-embolic complications (which are described later) have been related to the oestrogen component of the pill, most tablets now contain less than 50 $\mu$g, and the tendency is to reduce the content of both oestrogen and progestogen to the lowest possible dose which will retain effectiveness and cycle control.

Patterns of administration vary slightly with the different preparations. The commonest regimen starts on day 5 of a cycle; a pill is taken each day for 21 days. There is then a 7-day interval during which no pills are taken (unless the maker includes 7 placebo pills in the pack, as some do). During the interval withdrawal bleeding usually occurs, but if it does not the woman starts the next course of pills after 7 days. The pill should be taken at the same time each day; bed-time is convenient. If the woman forgets to take the pill one night she can take it the next morning. She should be warned that ovulation may not be inhibited in the first cycle of treatment.

Slight bleeding whilst taking the tablets can be ignored unless it is repeated, in which case full investigation is necessary to exclude some coincidental lesion. If frank 'breakthrough bleeding' occurs, this can be controlled by increasing the dose of progestogen, or by changing to another preparation which contains a different proportion of oestrogen to progestogen.

## Other methods of systemic contraception

*Variable dose combined pill*
The so-called triphasic pills employ a varying dose of oestrogen and progestogen during the cycle with the idea of producing a more natural hormonal pattern. The pills are presented in a pack which allows the woman to use them in proper sequence. The dose of oestrogen increases

from 30 micrograms of ethinyloestradiol in the first 6 days of the cycle to 40 micrograms for the next 5 days, and then reverts to 30 micrograms for 10 days. The progestogen, levonorgestrel, is increased progressively from 50 to 75 to 100 micrograms in the three successive stages. The method suits some women but has not been notably more useful in practice than the simple combined pill. The levonorgestrel component of all pills depresses the level of high density lipids in the blood, and because of this it was hoped that triphasic pills would be less likely to cause thrombosis. However, the lipid levels have not been shown to be significantly different from those with the simple combined pill. Other pills incorporating desogestrel instead of levonorgestrel have been introduced with the same purpose, but also without significant advantage.

### Continuous oral progestogens
Continuous daily administration of a small dose of one of a variety of progestogens (see p. 315) is another method of systemic contraception. Many women find it easier to remember to take a tablet every day. These preparations are less effective than the combined pill, and have the disadvantage that the endometrium tends to break down and bleed at irregular intervals. They do not carry any risk of thrombo-embolism, and they can be used during lactation, which they do not inhibit. They act not by inhibiting ovulation, but by causing increased viscosity of cervical mucus and endometrial changes.

### Injectable steroids
Slow-release, and therefore long-acting, progestogen preparations can be given by intramuscular injection at intervals of 1–6 months for contraceptive purposes. The best known depot preparation is medroxyprogesterone acetate (Depo-Provera) but recently norethisterone oenanthate in castor oil has also been used. Unfortunately, uterine bleeding tends to be irregular, and may be heavy and prolonged. Subsequent amenorrhoea may also occur. The dose for 3-monthly injection is 150 mg. An index of 0.5 to 1.5 is claimed. At present these compounds have been licensed for use in the United Kingdom on a short-term basis only. They are useful after rubella vaccination in the puerperium, or while the male partner is waiting for vasectomy to be proved effective.

### Postcoital contraception
This term applies to methods used to prevent implantation of a fertilized egg after unprotected intercourse. They are only effective if used soon afterwards. The combined pill method may be used up to 4 days after intercourse. An initial dose of 2 tablets of a high-dose combined pill (for example Ovran or Eugynon 50) is given, followed by another similar dose 12 hours later. The failure rate is said to be 2 to 3 per cent.

Ethinyloestradiol 5 mg daily for 5 days, starting not later than 36 hours after intercourse is more effective but causes troublesome nausea and vomiting.

The insertion of an intrauterine device in the first 4 days after unprotected intercourse is highly effective in preventing pregnancy. Care must be taken to see that the woman has no evident infection of the cervix, vagina or vulva.

## Side-effects of systemic contraceptives

It is difficult to assess statements made by patients about the side-effects of oral contraceptives. Any symptom that happens to occur may be attributed to the pill, and sometimes symptoms are a reflection of the patient's subconscious objection to interference with her normal fertility. On the other hand, many women who are relieved of the anxiety of unwanted pregnancy have an increased feeling of well-being, and even if side-effects occur they often prefer to disregard them.

Side-effects that have been described include headache, nausea, facial pigmentation, fluid retention and weight increase, discomfort in the breasts, intermenstrual 'break-through' bleeding, increased cervical secretion (a cervical erosion may be found), and depression or irritability. Usually such symptoms improve after two or three cycles. Many of the side-effects are due to the progestogen. Low-dose oestrogen pills contain more powerful progestogens so that side-effects, including depression and hypertension, may be worse than on high-dose pills.

Menstrual periods are usually more regular and the loss is almost always diminished. Dysmenorrhoea may be relieved. The effect on libido is variable. In many women relief from fear of pregnancy removes a restraint on sexual activity and enjoyment; in a very few there will be loss of libido.

## Dangers and major side-effects

*Mortality*
There is an increased mortality in women using the pill over that in women not using it, which is related to age and smoking habits but not to the duration of use. Death is most often the result of pulmonary embolism or cerebral or coronary thrombosis, but hypertension may also be implicated.

Women under 35 years of age who are on the pill, but do not smoke, have virtually no excess mortality over other women. Those under 35 who are on the pill and smoke have an excess mortality of about 10 per 100 000 woman years. In women over 35 who are on the pill the excess mortality rises sharply (although it is still small) to about 50 per 100 000 woman years in those who smoke and 15 per 100 000 woman years in non-smokers. The risk is least for women on pills containing a low dose of oestrogen. For women over 35, especially if they smoke, alternative methods of contraception are preferable.

*Thrombosis*
Women taking the pill are more likely to be admitted to hospital with thrombo-embolic disorders than comparable groups of women who are not

taking the pill and are not pregnant. The oestrogen content of the pill causes an increase in the platelet count and in platelet adhesiveness, and a decrease in antithrombins in the blood. In practice, now that combined pills containing 30 micrograms of oestrogen are most often used, deep venous thrombosis and pulmonary embolism are rare. However, the possibility must be kept in mind if a woman on the pill develops suggestive symptoms, and venograms and lung scans should be employed in cases of doubt.

Varicose veins of the leg without evidence of deep thrombosis are not contraindications to the use of the pill.

With heart disease, including rheumatic and congenital lesions, dysrhythmias and pulmonary hypertension, the combined pill is usually contraindicated because of the added risk of thrombosis. Progestogen-only pills may be used as an alternative.

*Hypertension*
Some women develop hypertension while taking the pill. The blood pressure should be checked before starting it, and at intervals while the pill is being used.

*Metabolic effects*
Glucose tolerance is reduced by some oral contraceptives, as it is in pregnancy. Low-dose combined pills do not affect tolerance, but an increased production of insulin by the islet cells is needed to maintain normal glucose levels. Women with established diabetes may be given oral contraceptives, although extra care in diabetic control may be needed for a time. Gestational diabetics and women who have shown impaired glucose tolerance in pregnancy should avoid the combined pill as it may occasionally cause them to become established diabetics.

*Hepatic function*
This may be affected by both oestrogens and progestogens, and it is therefore unwise to give oral contraceptives to women who have a history of cholestasis of pregnancy. Patients with abnormal liver function, such as may follow hepatitis, should not be given oral contraceptives until liver function tests have returned to normal. Any woman who develops jaundice or itching with the pill must discontinue it.

*Carcinogenic effects*
Some investigators have suggested that there is an increased risk of breast cancer in women taking pills containing high-potency progestogens, especially before the birth of the first child. Other investigators have denied such an association. The risk, if it exists, must be small since the incidence of breast cancer has not shown a rise in the United Kingdom in recent years. The incidence of benign disease of the breast seems to be reduced in pill users, and the same is true for carcinoma of the ovary and of the body of the uterus.

The possibility of an association between long-term pill usage and carcinoma of the cervix has also been discussed, but the existence of other aetiological factors related to intercourse in this disease make the significance of any association hard to assess.

For the present the risk of cancer of the breast or cervix should not be taken as a contraindication to prescribing the pill as a contraceptive. Nevertheless the pill with the lowest oestrogen and progestogen content which suits the individual patient should be chosen. All patients on the pill should have the breasts and cervix examined at regular intervals, and should have an annual cervical smear.

*Effect on menstruation*

Most women have regular, light and painless (anovulatory) periods while they are taking the combined pill, and usually ovulatory cycles return as soon as the tablets are stopped. In a few women 'postpill amenorrhoea' occurs, and may persist for several months. This is seen particularly in women who had irregular menstrual cycles or episodes of amenorrhoea before starting oral contraception. Most of these patients will resume regular menstruation spontaneously within 6 months, and only a few will need treatment with clomiphene to induce ovulation and a return to normal cycles.

Contraceptive steroids neither delay nor accelerate the onset of the menopause. Sometimes withdrawal bleeding ceases when the menopause is reached, even if the woman continues taking the pill. If there is any doubt, the pill can be stopped to see if the periods have in fact ceased, but it is then advisable to use some other form of contraception unless the patient is over 50 years of age.

*Effect on subsequent pregnancy, and on lactation*

Babies born to women who have taken the pill after pregnancy has started show no increase in the incidence of congenital abnormalities.

Combined oral contraceptives affect lactation in some women, reducing the volume and quality of the milk. Progestogen-only preparations, given either orally or by injection, may be preferred during breast feeding.

*Surgical operations*

Most surgeons advise discontinuation of pills containing oestrogens for 2 months before and after surgical operations which themselves carry any risk of thrombosis. When a woman is advised to discontinue the pill for such a reason she must be provided with a suitable alternative.

## Interaction between drugs and contraceptive steroids

Contraceptive steroids may interfere with the treatment of hypertension because of their effect on the blood pressure. It is best not to begin treatment with hypotensive drugs until contraceptive steroids have been discontinued, and to avoid giving these steroids to patients who are already taking hypotensive drugs.

Conversely, some drugs affect the action of contraceptive steroids.

1. *Anticonvulsants.* Breakthrough bleeding and failure of contraception may occur in patients taking diphenylhydantoin, rifampicin, griseofulvin or phenobarbitone, probably because these drugs increase the activity of hepatic enzymes which metabolize steroids. Patients on these drugs require an oral contraceptive containing high doses of steroids, e.g. ethinyloestradiol 0.05 mg with norethisterone 4 mg.

2. *Antibiotics.* Ampicillin, amoxycillin, tetracyclines and neomycin prevent absorption of oestrogen and its reabsorption after excretion in the bile by killing bacteria in the gut that are responsible for oestrogen conjugation. As a result the blood oestrogen level falls and contraception may fail.

## Essential steps before prescribing contraceptive steroids

Apart from the general history and pelvic examination necessary to determine the best method for the particular patient, the blood pressure and weight are recorded, the breasts are examined and a cervical smear is taken. It is essential to record the results carefully, and observations of the blood pressure and weight are made at each successive visit. The patient must be told about possible side-effects and given exact instructions. Once she is settled on a suitable preparation she should attend annually to check that all is well.

# Intrauterine contraceptive devices

Insertion of an intrauterine device is the only method, apart from sterilization, which is entirely the responsibility of the doctor. Neither the patient nor her partner has to take any pill or use any appliance.

Many different devices have been introduced, in the form of rings, loops, spirals, coils and 'T' and '7' shapes. Figure 31.1 shows some of the devices in common use in Britain. They are made of plastic material, and they can be compressed (or straightened out) to be inserted into an introducer for passage through the cervical canal. When the device is placed in the cavity of the uterus it opens out, so that it is retained. It has a nylon thread or tail which protrudes through the cervix, to allow the woman to check that it is in place, and with which it can be removed easily. The device is radio-opaque and can be located by ultrasound.

Some devices are wound with fine copper wire, from which copper ions are constantly released. Copper inhibits the enzymes concerned with implantation and development of the blastocyst, and it may also be spermicidal. By using copper it is possible to make a smaller device and thus to reduce local side effects.

Devices impregnated with progestogens have also been used. The first pattern was associated with a high incidence of ectopic pregnancy, but a recent device that releases levonorgestrel is under trial. The progestogen may reduce the risk of excessive bleeding.

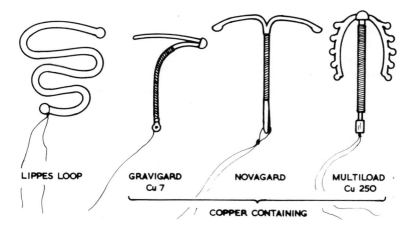

**Fig. 31.1** Intrauterine contraceptive devices.

*Mode of action*
Intrauterine devices cause a mild inflammatory reaction in the endometrium, which becomes infiltrated with leucocytes and macrophages. In addition, tubal motility is increased.

*Insertion*
This is most easily done during or immediately after menstruation, when the cervix is less tightly closed, or at a postnatal examination. A device can also be inserted immediately after termination of pregnancy.

A pelvic examination is made to exclude any possible contraindication, and to determine the position of the uterus. The cervix is exposed with a speculum and if necessary steadied with a tenaculum. A uterine sound is passed to find the direction and length of the uterine cavity. The device is loaded into the introducer, which carries a stop that is set to correspond with the length of the uterine cavity. The loaded introducer is then passed through the cervix until the stop is flush with the external os. As the introducer is withdrawn the device is extruded into the uterine cavity. The marker thread is cut to leave only 3 cm visible.

Devices can usually be inserted without causing undue discomfort to the patient. A vasovagal fainting attack occasionally occurs during or soon after the manipulation. Although this almost invariably responds quickly to putting the patient's head low and raising her legs, rare cases of cardiac arrest have occurred so resuscitation equipment should be available in the clinic.

Inert devices can be left in place until the menopause, but copper devices need renewal every 2 to 3 years. If a device needs to be removed it can be withdrawn by pulling on the tail; otherwise a small hook or artery forceps is passed through the cervix to grasp it.

*Failure rate*
Intrauterine devices are more effective (index less than 3) than all other methods of contraception except the oral pill or sterilization. With inert devices larger sizes are more effective than smaller, but copper devices are very effective in small sizes. Pregnancy can occur if the device is expelled without the patient noticing or if the uterus is perforated (see below).

## Side-effects and complications

*Pain*
Colicky pain may occur for a time after insertion, particularly if the device is large. It is not usually severe. If dysmenorrhoea occurs the possibility that it is caused by infection must be remembered.

*Menstrual loss*
This is generally heavier and more prolonged for a few months after insertion. In some cases spotting precedes and follows the flow. Severe menorrhagia and dysmenorrhoea requiring removal of the device occurs in about 8 per cent of cases during the first year. Increase in menstrual loss after a device has been in place for some years suggests that some uterine pathological condition is developing. The device is removed and an alternative method of contraception is used for 2 months. If the periods return to normal another device is fitted; otherwise diagnostic curettage is performed.

*Expulsion*
Expulsion of the device is most likely to occur during the first year. With good technique the expulsion rate should be less than 5 per cent. Women should be told to feel for the tail of the device after each period to check that it is still in position, although it is unlikely that it will be extruded without their noticing.

*Perforation of the uterus*
This accident occurs about once in 1000 first fittings; the incidence varies with the experience of the operator, and is usually due to the use of too much force, especially if the cervical canal is narrow. Most perforations cause no symptoms and are only suspected when the tail of the device cannot be felt and an ultrasonic scan or an x-ray shows that it is outside the uterus. Extrauterine devices should always be removed from the peritoneal cavity, and this can almost invariably be done by laparoscopy.

*Salpingitis*
Most authorities believe that there is an increased incidence of pelvic inflammatory disease among women using intrauterine devices, of the order of 5 to 10 times that in non-users. However, the incidence is still low — between 1.5 and 7.5 per 1000 woman years. The estimates of risk vary according to the diagnostic criteria and the type of women considered as

controls. The sexual behaviour of the user is an important factor; promiscuity sharply increases the risk of pelvic infection of both IUD-users and non-users. The practical consideration is that the incidence of salpingitis in older IUD-users who have had at least one pregnancy is little increased over that in non-users, whereas the relative increase in risk is greatest in young nulligravid IUD-users. Because of the slight risk of salpingitis and possible subsequent sterility with the intrauterine device, other forms of contraception are preferred for young nulligravid women.

*Endometritis*
All intrauterine devices induce an inflammatory reaction in the adjacent endometrium. This probably plays an important part in preventing a fertilized egg from implanting. In support of this is the fact that anti-inflammatory agents such as indomethacin or corticosteroids increase the failure rate of intrauterine devices.

Occasionally more widespread pelvic inflammatory disease occurs, with evidence of bacterial invasion, and all such cases should be treated vigorously with broad-spectrum antibiotics. After swabs have been taken for bacteriological examination, a combination of ampicillin or doxycycline with metronidazole is given. The device need not be removed unless there is no response, or there are recurrent attacks.

Pelvic infection with actinomyces organisms is an uncommon complication and is most likely with a plastic device that has been *in situ* for some years. The device should be removed and penicillin given.

*Pregnancy with an intrauterine device in place*
Ectopic pregnancy may occur in women using an intrauterine device. Although the absolute rate is low, 0.5 to 1 per 1000 woman years, this is greater than the expected incidence in a comparable unselected group of women.

In rare instances intrauterine pregnancy occurs with a device in place. The intrauterine device may be extruded spontaneously, or the tails may disappear up into the uterus as it enlarges. About half of the women will abort spontaneously; the risk is less if the device can be easily withdrawn. If it is left in place there is a slight risk of intrauterine infection, preterm labour and antepartum haemorrhage, but most pregnancies are uncomplicated and the device is delivered with the placenta.

**Contraindications**
Pelvic infection is a contraindication to the fitting of an intrauterine device; any active infection should be cleared up first. Infections with trichomonas or candida are not absolute contraindications, but should be treated before a device is inserted.

Any cardiac lesion which carries a risk of bacterial endocarditis is a relative contraindication, and if a device is to be inserted the fitting should be covered with systemic antibiotics.

Any abnormal bleeding should be investigated before inserting a device. Although a device can be fitted in the presence of fibromyomata, if these are submucous menorrhagia is likely to occur.

## Occlusive diaphragms and caps

### Occlusive diaphragm (Dutch cap) used with spermicide
This can be an efficient method if it is used carefully and intelligently. The cap has a flexible rim which supports a soft rubber diaphragm. The diaphragms are made in various sizes and the correct size, which allows the rim to be in close contact with the vaginal walls, must be chosen for the patient by the doctor. When it is in position the diaphragm lies obliquely in the vagina, with the posterior part of the rim fitting closely in the posterior fornix, with the anterior part behind the symphysis pubis, and with the diaphragm covering the cervix. Before insertion by the patient spermicidal cream or jelly is smeared round the rim and on both surfaces of the diaphragm. The diaphragm is inserted before intercourse, and should not be taken out for at least 6 hours afterwards, so that the spermicide will kill any spermatozoa before it is removed. This method has the advantage that it is entirely the woman's responsibility. It is not as reliable as the oral pill or intrauterine device, but many women prefer to use it because of the absence of side-effects. The size of the diaphragm should be re-checked after pregnancy, after any sudden weight change, and as age advances.

### Cervical cap
This is a small cup-shaped firm rubber cap which fits over the cervix. It needs careful fitting, but an intelligent woman will not find it difficult to insert. Contrary to the view generally held, it is not easily dislodged during intercourse.

## Permanent methods — sterilization

Whenever a couple have achieved the number of children they desire, sterilization offers a permanent and reliable alternative to other methods of contraception. Voluntary sterilization is increasing in popularity throughout the world, although there are still legal, religious and cultural reservations in some countries. In Britain the operation is lawful provided that the patient has given full consent. Although the spouse's consent is not necessary if there are sound medical reasons for the operation, it is always prudent to obtain it.

Most women find their health and sense of security improved after the operation, but a few subsequently regret it, and this regret may be expressed in marital difficulties or dysfunctional uterine bleeding. There are small but definite risks from anaesthesia and the operation, but these considerations do not outweigh the advantages.

## Female sterilization by tubal occlusion

There are many methods of achieving tubal occlusion, and a variety of surgical approaches to the tubes. Operation through a conventional incision has been largely replaced by procedures undertaken by laparoscopy, through a very small transverse suprapubic incision ('mini-laparotomy'), or through a small incision in the posterior fornix (colpotomy). Depending on the surgical approach the tubes may be blocked by coagulation with diathermy, by ligature, by spring clips or Silastic bands; or the tubes can be divided or excised.

Laparoscopic sterilization is the most popular method in Britain. Apart from the hazards of anaesthesia and the insertion of the instrument, there are dangers if diathermy is used to coagulate the tubes, especially of burns to bowel or other structures. The operator must have had adequate instruction under supervision before attempting this procedure, and occlusion of the tubes by clips or bands may be preferable to diathermy coagulation. General anaesthesia is usually employed, although a few surgeons operate on outpatients with local anaesthesia.

This technique is less easy soon after delivery, when the uterus is large and the tubes are high in the abdomen, and a small abdominal incision is then often preferred. Alternatively the operation can be postponed for 6 weeks.

If the abdomen is opened for some other reason, such as Caesarean section, the tubes can be crushed and ligated and the medial ends buried in the broad ligaments.

Methods of 'temporary sterilization', for example that of burying the outer ends of the tubes in the broad ligaments, often prove to be permanent.

## Male sterilization by vasectomy

This is a safe, simple outpatient procedure when properly performed. The vas deferens is identified at the top of the scrotum by palpation. Under local anaesthesia a small incision allows the vas to be separated from its blood vessels, so that a centimetre of it can be removed between ligatures. It must be stressed that after vasectomy contraceptive precautions must be taken until the absence of sperm in the ejaculate has been confirmed by the laboratory. It is advised that there should be two negative specimens at 3 and 4 months postoperatively.

## Choice of male or female sterilization

Vasectomy is simpler and safer than female sterilization, which usually requires general anaesthesia and in which the peritoneum is opened. Female sterilization usually involves admission to hospital, but it is sometimes convenient to perform it at the time of delivery or termination of pregnancy. Vasectomy has the disadvantage that sterilization is not immediately effective. Inheritable disease in one partner may suggest that he or she should be sterilized, and medical or obstetric conditions in the woman may affect the decision.

**Reversal of sterilization**
Although sterilization can sometimes be reversed, this is never certain, and those asking for this operation should be told that it is intended to be permanent. Careful counselling of both partners before the operation will reduce the number of women (or men) who later regret it. A change of partner or loss of a child may lead to a request for reversal. This is usually easier after vasectomy than after female sterilization, but if only a small length of tube has been destroyed and providing that the restoration is done by a surgeon experienced in microsurgery, the results in the female are quite good. Restoration of patency does not guarantee pregnancy, but a success rate of 70 per cent may be expected. The risk of subsequent tubal pregnancy is increased.

# Methods under investigation

Already new possibilities for contraceptive methods are on the horizon. These include the *male pill* which is aimed at interruption of spermatogenesis or sperm maturation. A number of preparations are under trial, including androgens alone or in combination with progestogens or oestrogens, and the anti-androgenic compound cyproterone acetate.

*Synthetic analogues of GnRH* are possible contraceptives. If these are given continuously, rather than in pulses, they become fixed to pituitary receptors and block the action of GnRH, so that the output of gonadotrophins falls and ovulation ceases.

*Immunization against pregnancy* has also reached the stage of clinical trial. It depends on immunization against the $\beta$ subunit of chorionic gonadotrophin, and might provide a simple and long-lasting method of contraception.

# Appendix

## Active constituents and potency of oral contraceptives sold in the United Kingdom

| Proprietary name | Oestrogen component (micrograms) | | Progestogen component (milligrams) | | Progestogen 'potency' |
|---|---|---|---|---|---|
| **Combined pills (monophasic)** | | | | | |
| Norinyl 1 | Mestranol | 50 | Norethisterone | 1 | 1 |
| Orthonovin 1/50 | Mestranol | 50 | Norethisterone | 1 | 1 |
| Gynovlar 21 | Ethinyloestradiol | 50 | Norethisterone | 3 | 3 |
| Anovlar | Ethinyloestradiol | 50 | Norethisterone acetate | 4 | 8 |
| Norlestrin | Ethinyloestradiol | 50 | Norethisterone acetate | 2.5 | 5 |
| Minovlar | Ethinyloestradiol | 50 | Norethisterone acetate | 1 | 2 |
| Orlest 21 | Ethinyloestradiol | 50 | Norethisterone acetate | 1 | 2 |
| Eugynon 50 | Ethinyloestradiol | 50 | Norgestrel | 0.5 | 0.5 |
| Ovran | Ethinyloestradiol | 50 | Levonorgestrel | 0.25 | 15 |
| Neogynon | Ethinyloestradiol | 50 | Levonorgestrel | 0.25 | 15 |
| Wy (125) D 50 | Ethinyloestradiol | 50 | Levonorgestrel | 0.125 | 7.5 |
| Ovulen 50 | Ethinyloestradiol | 50 | Ethynodiol diacetate | 1 | 15 |
| Minilyn | Ethinyloestradiol | 50 | Lynoestrenol | 2.5 | 5 |
| Norimin | Ethinyloestradiol | 35 | Norethisterone | 1 | 1 |
| Brevinor | Ethinyloestradiol | 35 | Norethisterone | 0.5 | 0.5 |
| Ovysmen | Ethinyloestradiol | 35 | Norethisterone | 0.5 | 0.5 |
| Loestrin 30 | Ethinyloestradiol | 30 | Norethisterone acetate | 1.5 | 3 |
| Conova 30 | Ethinyloestradiol | 30 | Ethynodiol diacetate | 2 | 30 |
| Neovran | Ethinyloestradiol | 50 | Levonorgestrel | 0.125 | 15 |

# Active constituents and potency of oral contraceptives sold in the United Kingdom *cont'd.*

| Proprietary name | Oestrogen component (micrograms) | Progestogen component (milligrams) | Progestogen 'potency' |
|---|---|---|---|
| Wy (300) 30 | Ethinyloestradiol 30 | Norgestrel 0.3 | 9 |
| Eugynon 30 | Ethinyloestradiol 30 | Levonorgestrel 0.25 | 15 |
| Ovran 30 | Ethinyloestradiol 30 | Levonorgestrel 0.25 | 15 |
| Microgynon 30 | Ethinyloestradiol 30 | Levonorgestrel 0.15 | 9 |
| Ovranette | Ethinyloestradiol 30 | Levonorgestrel 0.15 | 9 |
| Marvelon | Ethinyloestradiol 30 | Desogestrel 0.15 | 9 |
| Loestrin 20 | Ethinyloestradiol 20 | Norethisterone acetate 1 | 2 |
| **Combined pills (multiphasic)** | | | |
| WT 50/50/125/50 | Ethinyloestradiol 50 | Average daily dose levonorgestrel 0.08 | 4.8 |
| Sequilar 5C | Ethinyloestradiol 50 | Average daily dose levonorgestrel 0.08 | 4.8 |
| Binovum | Ethinyloestradiol 35 | Average daily dose norethisterone 0.83 | 0.83 |
| Or/10/11 | Ethinyloestradiol 35 | Average daily dose norethisterone 0.76 | 0.76 |
| Trinovum | Ethinyloestradiol 35 | Average daily dose norethisterone 0.75 | 0.45 |
| Logynon | Average daily dose ethinyloestradiol 32.38 | Average daily dose levonorgestrel 0.09 | 5.4 |

| | | | |
|---|---|---|---|
| Trinordiol | Average daily dose ethinyloestradiol 32.38 | Average daily dose levonorgestrel 0.09 | 5.4 |
| Trinordiol 28 | Average daily dose ethinyloestradiol 32.38 | Average daily dose levonorgestrel 0.09 | 5.4 |

**Progestogen only pills**

| | | |
|---|---|---|
| Femulen | Ethynodiol diacetate | 0.5 |
| Micronor | Norethisterone | 0.35 |
| Noriday | Norethisterone | 0.35 |
| Neogest | *dl* Norgestrel | 0.075 |

The progestogen potency of the combined pills is measured by the 'postponement of menstruation' test.

# 32

# Termination of pregnancy

In Britain the Offences Against the Person Act of 1861 made it a serious offence 'unlawfully to administer any poison or other noxious thing or to use any instrument or any other means whatsoever with intent to procure a miscarriage'. The crux of the matter was the interpretation of the word 'unlawful'. After the case of Rex v. Bourne in 1939 it was accepted that it was lawful to terminate pregnancy when there was danger to the life of the mother or a risk to her physical or mental health.

The Abortion Act of 1967 amended the law relating to abortion, but this act only creates exceptions to the Offences Against the Person Act, and otherwise abortion remains a criminal offence. The Infant Life Preservation Act of 1929, which protects the life of a viable fetus, is still in being.

Under the terms of the 1967 Act a registered medical practitioner may lawfully terminate pregnancy if two medical practitioners (of whom he need not himself be one) certify in good faith one or more of the following opinions:

1. That the continuance of the pregnancy would involve risk to the life of the pregnant woman greater than if the pregnancy were terminated; or

2. That it would involve risk of injury to the physical or mental health of the pregnant women greater than if the pregnancy were terminated; or

3. That it would involve risk of injury to the physical or mental health of any existing children of the pregnant woman's family; or

4. That there is a substantial risk that if the child were born it would suffer from such physical or mental abnormalities as to be seriously handicapped.

Any treatment for the termination of pregnancy must be carried out in a National Health Service hospital or in a place approved by the Secretary of State for Health and Social Services or by the Secretary of State for Scotland.

The certificate of opinion must be set out in the form laid down in the regulations, and must be signed by both doctors before the termination is performed. An exception is allowed in a case in which termination is urgently necessary to save the life of the woman or to prevent grave permanent injury to her physical or mental health, when the second opinion is not demanded.

Any medical practitioner who terminates a pregnancy must complete the prescribed notification form and send it to the Chief Medical Officer of the Department of Health or of the Scottish Home and Health Department.

The Act lays down that no person is required to participate in any treatment authorized by the Act to which he has a conscientious objection, unless this is necessary to save the life or to prevent grave injury to the health of the woman. This does not absolve the doctor from his general duty to his patient. If he thinks that, were it not for his conscientious objection, it might be lawful to recommend or perform an abortion, or if he feels that his conscientious objection makes it impossible for him to form a fair judgement, then he should refer the patient to another doctor. In court a doctor could probably establish that his conscientious objection was valid if he could show the sincerity of his belief that abortion in the particular case would offend his concept of right or wrong, and this would not depend on his particular religious beliefs.

In forming an opinion whether continuation of the pregnancy would be harmful the doctor may consider the woman's 'actual or reasonably fore-seeable environment'. This phrase may have given rise to the erroneous belief that the Act makes abortion lawful on 'social' grounds. The real test is whether there is a risk to health, and in deciding this such factors as the woman's living conditions or lack of support from her partner should be considered. The doctor's opinion must be given in good faith, and he must take reasonable steps to satisfy himself that statements made to him are correct. Much help may be obtained from the medical social worker or counsellor.

The phrase 'existing children of the family' includes illegitimate or adopted children, and can extend to any child the pregnant woman has accepted as one of her family, whose health depends on hers.

In relation to fetal risk the Act gives no guidance about the phrases 'substantial risk' and 'seriously handicapped'. Clearly the risk does not have to be certain; perhaps the best that can be said is that the risk must be real.

The written consent of the woman should always be obtained before termination of pregnancy. If she is married and living with her husband the proposed abortion should be discussed with him if this is possible, but if the indication is danger to her life or health the husband's consent is not essential in law. The case in which the husband refuses to agree to an abortion recommended because of the risk to health of existing children of the family, or because of a risk that the child may be born handicapped, is more difficult. In such a case the doctor will be wise to consult colleagues, but in the end he must make a difficult decision and advise the wife 'in good faith'.

If the woman is single no consent is required from the putative father. It is not necessary in law to obtain the consent of the parents for the termination of pregnancy of an unmarried girl aged 16 or more; and the doctor must obtain her consent before divulging any information to her parents. When the girl is under 16 the parents should be consulted, even if the patient objects to this. On the other hand, pregnancy should never be terminated in opposition to the girl's wishes, even if the parents demand this.

Late terminations cause difficult problems. In theory termination can be performed up to the 28th week, the time at which the fetus becomes legally viable, but with modern paediatric care there is a real possibility that a fetus of 24 weeks will survive. Termination after 24 weeks should very rarely be done, and then only because of severe maternal illness or severe malformation of the fetus.

The Act makes abortion lawful on certain grounds; it does not make abortion available on demand. No doctor is required to certify a woman for abortion or to perform an abortion if in his clinical judgement this is not in the best interest of the patient or her children.

## Methods used for legal termination of pregnancy

The choice of method depends on the stage to which the pregnancy has advanced.

### 1. Very early termination
When the woman is not more than 8 weeks pregnant a simple outpatient technique is used.

The patient should be informed of every step of the procedure. When she has emptied her bladder and been placed in the lithotomy position the vulva and vagina are swabbed with an antiseptic solution. A bivalve speculum is passed and the anterior lip of the cervix is held with a single-toothed tenaculum while an intracervical block is given by injecting 4 ml of 1 per cent lignocaine into the cervix at the 4, 8 and 12 o'clock positions and then waiting for 2 minutes for it to take effect. Without dilating the cervix a sterile flexible plastic cannula (Karman cannula, diameter 5 mm) is passed through the cervix into the uterus until it touches the fundus. A vacuum source is attached to the cannula – either an ordinary aspirator or a 50 ml vacuum syringe with a thumb-operated valve. The cannula is gently pushed in and out and rotated until a rough sensation is felt on all surfaces of the uterine cavity and aspirate ceases to flow along the cannula. The whole procedure only takes about 5 minutes. The volume of aspirate should be noted; a small volume would suggest incomplete evacuation or that the patient was not pregnant.

The patient is usually fit to leave the hospital within the hour, but should return for examination 1 week later. The risks of haemorrhage, infection or cervical injury are less with this method than others. The most serious disadvantage is occasional failure to terminate the pregnancy, and every patient must be warned that if the next period does not appear she must return for review.

### 2. Suction termination
This method can be used up to 12 weeks' gestation. A vacuum source

capable of producing a negative pressure of not less than 600 mmHg (about 0.5 kg/cm$^2$) is required. The patient is anaesthetized and placed in the lithotomy position. After swabbing the vagina with an antiseptic solution a speculum is inserted and the cervix is held with a volsellum. The cervical canal is dilated sufficiently to take the aspiration cannula, of a size chosen with regard to the duration of gestation. The cannula is of metal or rigid plastic and has an opening for finger-tip control of the vacuum. It is connected to the suction apparatus by wide-bore non-collapsible tubing. The vacuum is switched on and the cannula is moved inwards and outwards and rotated in the axis of the uterine cavity. This dislodges and aspirates the products of conception. During the operation 0.5 mg of ergometrine is injected intravenously. After aspiration a small curette is used to check the completeness of evacuation, and the volume of aspirate should also be checked. There is less risk of damage to the uterus and less bleeding with this method than with the older procedure of wide dilatation of the cervix and removal of the contents with 'ovum forceps'.

### 3. Prostaglandins
Prostaglandins $PGF_{2\alpha}$ and $PGE_2$ induce strong uterine contractions. If they are given by continuous intravenous infusion there are troublesome side-effects such as vomiting and diarrhoea. Extra-amniotic injection through a catheter passed through the cervix to lie between the amniotic membrane and the uterine wall is more effective and causes fewer side-effects. Direct intra-amniotic injection through the abdominal wall has also proved successful.

Apart from the side-effects already mentioned, a few cases of cervical laceration have occurred from the unduly strong uterine contractions. Adequate sedation is necessary for patients having prostaglandin induction. After abortion the cervix should always be inspected, and the products expelled should be examined to make sure that they are complete. The interval between the start of induction and abortion is usually between 12 and 24 hours.

### 4. Intra-amniotic injection of hypertonic solutions
This method is used after 14 weeks and preferably even later when amniocentesis is technically easier to perform. A spinal or Tuohy needle is inserted through the abdominal wall into the amniotic cavity and about 200 ml of liquor is withdrawn and replaced by a similar volume of 20 per cent sterile sodium chloride solution. It is best to perform the injection under ultrasonic control, but in any case it is absolutely essential to ensure that there is free flow along the needle and that aspiration yields clear fluid so as to make sure that injection into the uterine venous sinuses does not occur; injection of hypertonic saline into the circulation may cause cerebral damage. General anaesthesia should not be used, so that the patient will notice pain or faintness if the injection is wrongly given into the peritoneal cavity or a vein, when the injection is immediately stopped. Anuria has been reported in a few cases in which the uterus was grossly

overdistended with fluid. The method is contraindicated for patients with severe renal disease, hypertension or cardiac disease. Abortion usually occurs within 24 hours, but may sometimes be incomplete, when evacuation of placental remnants under anaesthesia is required.

Because of the hazards of using hypertonic saline some prefer to use a solution of urea (80 g in 200 ml of normal saline). Hypertonic glucose solution is unsuitable because it is an excellent culture medium for any organisms which are accidentally introduced.

### 5. Abdominal hysterotomy

This operation, consisting of a miniature Caesarean section, can be done at any stage of pregnancy, and sterilization can be performed at the same time if it is indicated, but hysterotomy carries a far higher risk than any of the preceding methods.

The abdomen is opened through a low transverse incision. The uterus is lifted up through the incision and the peritoneal cavity excluded from the operation area with abdominal packs. Ergometrine 0.5 mg is injected intravenously before an incision is made through the anterior wall of the uterus. The fetus, placenta and membranes are removed, and the uterine and abdominal incisions are sutured in the ordinary way. If sterilization is indicated, it is performed by ligature or excision of the Fallopian tubes.

## Complications of termination of pregnancy

The low mortality rate of induced abortion should not be taken as evidence that the operation is harmless, for it carries a significant morbidity rate. Apart from the immediate complications of trauma to the uterus, haemorrhage and sepsis, there are two important late complications which may profoundly affect the woman's future reproductive performance:

### 1. *Postabortal tubal occlusion*
Patients complaining of secondary infertility following termination of a pregnancy are often found to have blocked tubes as a result of salpingitis. Some of these patients will give a history of incomplete emptying of the uterus and subsequent infection of the retained products. In most of them no such history is obtained but presumably a lesser degree of infection occurred and involved the tubes.

### 2. *Cervical incompetence*
Dilatation of the cervix in the course of termination of pregnancy may tear the circular muscle fibres surrounding the internal os, rendering it incompetent. Dilatation over 10 mm (Hegar dilator No 10 size) or strong uterine contractions induced during late termination are most likely to cause this damage. The effect of cervical incompetence is seen in subsequent pregnancies, when the gaping cervix allows the membranes to bulge through and rupture. This commonly occurs between the 14th and 18th weeks, but may occur at any time up to term. Careful assessment of the

cervix is essential during antenatal care for any woman who has had a previous termination. If the cervix is found to be incompetent a purse-string suture is inserted during pregnancy.

The sadness of termination of pregnancy and its complications is that unplanned pregnancy is in most cases a completely unnecessary self-inflicted injury. That it still continues in a world where effective contraception is, or should be, available to all is a sad reflection on the state of health education of young women and, equally important, of young men.

## Criminal abortion

In Britain, according to the Reports on the Confidential Enquiries into Maternal Deaths published by the Department of Health, in every triennium until 1969 there were more than 100 deaths from abortion, mainly from sepsis after illegal abortion. Since the Abortion Act came into effect in 1968 there has been a progressive fall in the number of deaths in each triennium (Table 34.1). It seems evident from the Table that the operation of the Act has reduced the number of deaths from illegal abortion, although deaths still occur after spontaneous abortion and after legal termination of pregnancy. In the triennium 1976–78, 8 deaths followed 404 235 legal terminations, a mortality rate of 0.17 per 10 000. Thus legal abortion is a very safe procedure, especially when carried out before the 12th week.

The most common cause of death after abortion, legal or otherwise, is sepsis, with clostridial infection as a particular risk.

Table 34.1 Mortality associated with abortion, 1967–1978

|  | Total deaths from abortion | Deaths after illegal abortion | Total mortality from abortion per 10 000 pregnancies |
|---|---|---|---|
| 1967–1969 | 117 | 74 | 4.7 |
| 1970–1972 | 81 | 38 | 3.5 |
| 1973–1975 | 29 | 10 | 1.5 |
| 1976–1978 | 14 | 4 | 0.7 |

The dangers of criminal abortion by the unskilled still remain. Strange methods are sometimes used, including the passage of slippery elm bark, crochet needles or douche nozzles. The instrument used may not be sterile, and dangerous fluids such as soap solution may be forced into the peritoneal cavity or a vein. Potassium permanganate cystals have been placed in the vagina; these do not cause abortion but deep necrotic ulcers which bleed freely.

# 33

# Psychosomatic problems and sexual difficulties

Recognition of the importance of psychological and social factors in medicine is particularly important for the gynaecologist because he deals with disorders related to the most private and personal aspects of his patient's life, and to her functions as a wife and mother. Although each patient presents an individual problem, there are four main mechanisms of interaction between psychological and physical aspects of disease which may occur together or separately.

First, it must be recognized that anxiety has both mental and physical components. It produces mental fear and physical changes such as palpitations, tremor, sweating, epigastric discomfort, bowel spasm and increased muscular tension leading to pain in different parts of the body. Social class, culture, upbringing and intelligence all affect the way anxiety is perceived and dealt with by the patient. One woman may go to the doctor complaining of feeling anxious while another may pick out one of the physical aspects such as a rapidly beating heart or pain in the muscles of the back as a presenting symptom.

Secondly, psychological stress can lead the patient to complain of a symptom which might otherwise be ignored. A good example of this is found in some cases of primary dysmenorrhoea. The effect of the discomfort is quite different in a stable and phlegmatic girl from that in an anxious and insecure one.

Thirdly, physical problems can give rise to psychological stress. Hysterectomy, for example, may be followed by misery and anxiety if the gynaecologist fails to discuss with the patient before he operates the possible psychological as well as the medical significance of the measures he proposes to undertake, and her emotional attitudes to the operation.

Women who are under stress at the time of the menopause have a convenient peg, 'the change', on which to hang their troubles. It is also true that some women do indeed suffer from increased irritability at this time; in some this may be related to oestrogen lack and in others to the psychological significance of the end of menstruation.

Finally, physical disorder may be the direct result of psychological stress, such as the amenorrhoea that follows some personal or social disruption. An extreme form of this is the amenorrhoea that is seen in cases of anorexia nervosa, due to the fear of maturity and anxiety about physical and sexual development associated with morbid ideas about eating and catastrophic weight loss. A less obvious example is the insecure woman who may express anger or resentment towards her husband by heavy periods or diarrhoea or spastic colon. This displacement is an unconscious mechanism of which the patient is unaware, but which the doctor must consider as a cause. This is particularly important when surgery is being contemplated — if the doctor does not take into account that heavy bleeding can be the result of hormone imbalance caused by emotional upset, he may collude with the patient in thinking that a hysterectomy will 'cure' the trouble. Depression can follow an operation performed without this insight when the patient recognizes, after a brief period of being cared for, that nothing fundamental has been solved even though there are no longer bad periods to be coped with. It is wise to counsel particularly carefully any patient who is eager for an operation, of any sort, as this is an indication that they are hoping to gain something that the operation cannot give.

Symptoms without obvious organic cause demand from the doctor a willingness to consider the individuality of each patient and an acceptance of the important contribution of attitudes, anxieties and personality to the problem. The mechanisms so far discussed represent the end-point of less obvious processes which the doctor must understand. These processes, which determine the vulnerability to psychosomatic illness, depend on the patient's success or failure in achieving emotional maturity.

Progress through life to emotional maturity and beyond requires one to adapt to society against one's inclination, to accept changes in life, to give up the securities of home, to experience unhappiness, and to face the eventual end of life. Many people have not had the security, love and understanding during their formative years to make this possible. They may react to disappointment and frustration by becoming ill. For example, during its upbringing a child is taught by its mother to conform, to behave well and to be a credit to her. The child may become sensitized to the fear of not behaving properly and later in life may feel that it is better to be ill than risk failure. Thus anxiety is relieved by illness. Girls who pretend not to love father in case they upset mother may find, after many years of ignoring the male, that it is not possible to give love and affection to a man of their own. Difficulties in coping with an emotional situation have led to the suppression of feelings and an inability to achieve satisfaction.

At puberty there is loss of childhood protection. Some women never accept this and remain largely dependent. The dependence may be on the parents or on a spouse; or the dependence may be denied and the inability to cope may lead to a mental breakdown or a physical illness such as menorrhagia. A girl at puberty must come to terms with periods and developing breasts, accepting her femininity with the demands of domesticity and sexual vulnerability. At parturition comes the loss of freedom both physically and emotionally. Sexual difficulties are common following childbirth. A withdrawal from both husband and sex is often an expression of resentment, a feeling that is denied at a conscious level and expressed as loss of libido and depression. Around the time of the menopause parents may die, children leave home, hair goes grey, weight is put on. The emotionally mature woman may find these upheavals intolerable when she is trying to cope with irregular periods and the discomforts of hormonal imbalance.

Psychosomatic problems, therefore, are usually an unconscious attempt to deal with emotional distress by the use of physical illness.

## Sexual problems

Sexual problems best illustrate what has been said so far. In men and women the act of sexual intercourse has become complex. Intellectual skills, self-conscious social awareness and myths and expectations from the previous generation increase the possibility of conflict about the biological function of copulation, so instinctive and simple in other animals. In man there is interaction between the biological (instinctive), psychological (emotional), intellectual (ideological) and physical (bodily) parts of the individual. Difficulty in one of these areas can interfere with the final integration of responses necessary for the sexual fulfillment of two people. The first concern of the doctor must be the accurate identification of the area of difficulty, since it is easy for trouble in one area to be mistaken for trouble in another. Doctors tend to be particularly aware of their own specialty, with the danger that the gynaecologist may lean towards interpreting the symptoms in physical terms while the psychotherapist may lean towards interpreting them in emotional terms, with equally disastrous results in either case if the interpretation is incorrect. However, experience shows that when symptoms tend to be physical there is a risk that the more elusive and difficult emotional, instinctive or ideological cause may be ignored. When the emotional interaction is satisfactory quite severe physical disabilities can be ignored and coped with, but when the emotional response is immature and ambivalent it is hard for anything to be right.

The main sexual complaints in the female are dyspareunia, disinclination and lack of orgasm. Dyspareunia means pain or difficulty in coitus, and in most cases there is no local organic disorder which is responsible. Vaginismus is the usual cause of dyspareunia in the absence of any local disorder, and here anxiety about penetration causes spasm of the perivaginal muscles, making intercourse impossible or painful. Unconsciously the patient hopes that the partner will be deterred by the pain he is causing and penetration will thus be prevented. Loss of libido is a symptom of an unconscious unwillingness to become aroused. The root is usually disharmony in the relationship and the unconscious mechanism is punishment of the partner. Primary lack of libido, however, is the unconscious fear of loss of control and the origin of the problem is in the development of the personality.

Resolution of all these problems mainly depends on the investigation and exposure of the anxiety that is causing the patient to withhold herself from her partner.

## Reasons for withholding sexual intercourse

### Physical
It will be the task of the gynaecologist to treat any local condition causing dyspareunia, but it is emphasized once again that primary dyspareunia will seldom be explained by a resistant hymen, tight introitus or a congenital abnormality; if secondary dyspareunia occurs in the case of a woman who has had previous painless intercourse, any local cause for this will be obvious to everyone. If there is no evident local cause for pain then psychological factors are to be sought.

Tenderness at the introitus may be caused by vulvitis (p. 97) which is often secondary to vaginitis, by a urethral caruncle, by primary atrophy (p. 101) or postmenopausal contraction, or by constriction after colpo-perineorrhaphy or after repair of a tear or episiotomy. Surgical treatment (p. 350) is required only if there is a real physical constriction.

Deep dyspareunia may be caused by endometriosis, salpingo-oöphoritis or, rarely, by uterine retroversion without these lesions (p. 95).

With lack of preliminary stimulation at coitus there may be a lack of lubricating secretion from Bartholin's glands and vaginal transudation, and the use of a simple lubricant (e.g. Lubafax) is often helpful, especially if a condom is used. Sensitivity to a chemical spermicide is an occasional cause of soreness.

### Psychological
*Instinctive* — when there has been an oversuccessful attempt to condition the developing child against interest in sex and bodily function. Reconditioning is a lengthy process unless the patient is very young with a good relationship, when encouragement and reassurance may be all that is necessary.

*Intellectual* — when the expectations of the individual developed in later childhood and adolescence are not met and unrealistic ideals are retained. Disappointment in the reality may cause difficulty which is often only recognized after marriage. Religious teachings may conflict with the wishes of the individual; these may be consciously rebelled against but unconsciously inhibit and spoil love-making. Personal theoretical moral conviction may conflict with the patient's emotional reaction.

*Emotional* — when there is an inability to cope with feelings of anger, resentment and disappointment towards the partner. This causes difficulty when a romantic belief is held that in a satisfactory marriage there would be only love.

Most young women need a strong emotional attachment (being in love) before they can begin to overcome the inhibitions of childhood. This means that initially the sexual part of the relationship is precariously based on a 'phantasy' state that soon disappears when the relationship becomes permanent or secure. There is then a vulnerable phase when 'magic' excitement goes and more realistic love has yet to be developed. Disappointment may be experienced and retreat from the sexual relationship may begin. If this disillusionment is too strong and avoidance is allowed to occur by the partner, the necessary shift from 'emotional only' based sex to 'instinctive/emotional' based sex does not occur. This shift is best thought of as 'acquiring the taste' for sex by experience and is an important factor in female sexuality. The woman who does not 'acquire the taste' remains in a state of immaturity wherein she continues to demand the magic of being in love before she can be sexually involved. She is likely to become resentful of sexual demands when 'she does not feel like it'. She may feel that her duty makes it necessary to allow intercourse to take place sometimes as long as she is feeling warm towards her partner, but she withholds it completely if she feels he has not 'earned' it. Unless and until a woman can achieve the female equivalent of satisfaction in the man there remains a feeling of being 'used'.

## Development of phobia

Once avoidance of sexual intercourse begins, a phobic element is introduced whereby increasing avoidance brings about increasing anxiety and finally actual fear of intercourse. This avoidance may not necessarily have been because of emotional disappointment — it may start with soreness following infection with candida or trichomonas, or from fear of pain after a pelvic operation. It often tends to be a mixture of physical and emotional distress in a person who is already unconsciously anxious about sex, but who is able to cope with the anxiety as long as no extra stress is involved.

## Primary and secondary problems

It is important to separate primary from secondary sexual difficulty. Primary difficulty means that there has never been a satisfactory sexual relationship. Unless the patient is young and has a very good relationship this is likely to need specialized help. The unconsummated marriage may take months of counselling, and the gynaecologist should be wary of dilating procedures under anaesthesia which may only increase the patient's problem if she finds that she still cannot allow conscious penetration.

When there has been a satisfactory sexual relationship with the partner in the past it is important to identify the source of the present dissatisfaction. This may be denied or hidden, and not easy to find. The most usual causes are as follows.

1. Disappointment in the partner — he may not be coming up to the standard set by her father or romantic novels.

2. Today's liberated woman may be in considerable conflict with her role. She may both want the commitment of marriage and also fear and resent it. Before marriage she often does not realize her confusion, but faced with commitment she may blame her partner for forcing her into a role she may feel to be inferior. Most frequently complaints of sexual difficulty come within a few months of marriage and having a baby. A

baby, more than anything else, forces a woman completely into the female role she may only half want to embrace. She may then, while loving the baby very much, resent both it and its father for the commitment they demand.

3. Resentment. Sexual relations frequently deteriorate following an infection with candida or trichomonas, or any infection which is possibly venereal. The partner is blamed for the infection even when, in the case of candida, reassurance is given that the infection was not passed on to her in that way. Similarly, when the patient finds that she is pregnant she often irrationally blames him for her condition and withdraws from sexual activity.

4. After hysterectomy many women are surprised to find that they feel 'spoiled' and less valuable, and withdraw from sexual activity as a precaution against being discarded by the partner.

5. Illness or bereavement can often cause anxiety and insecurity and account for temporary loss of interest in sex.

## Treatment

In summary, problems arise when, as a result of unresolved conflicts during development, an individual is 'sensitized' to difficulties in sex. This leads either to a situation which is unsatisfactory all the time, or to an unstable situation where resolution has been partial, but where resentment, guilt or stress can readily cause retreat to a 'presexual' phase.

*Primary difficulty.* The young woman with a good relationship may be able to accept reassurance. In cases of vaginismus she should be encouraged to stretch herself. This is better than the use of vaginal dilators which continue to separate the patient from her body. She should also be encouraged to have as much intercourse as possible in order to overcome the inhibitions instilled in childhood. She must be encouraged not to avoid intercourse as this tends to produce a phobic situation. Explanations about her training as a child which produced guilt feelings about pleasurable sensations from her body help her to overcome this early conditioning. However, the longer the young adult has avoided the sexual challenge, the harder it is to help her with such simple measures, and then expert psychotherapy may be needed.

*Secondary difficulty.* Here it is necessary accurately to date the onset of difficulty and to note whether it was gradual or sudden. The patient should then be persuaded to examine her feelings around this time — always looking for reasons for resentment or anxiety. Sometimes the causes seem so trivial and unreasonable to the patient that she is unwilling to attribute such a large effect to them.

While the psychological exploration is going on there must also be a behavioural change. Usually the frequency of intercourse has diminished or it has even completely stopped. The doctor now has the difficult task of persuading the patient that it must be restarted with increased frequency and total regularity. He must explain the rationale behind the programme he recommends. If the patient cannot understand why she must do something which she finds very difficult, she will not do it. Nor will she do it for long if she thinks that she is only doing it for the sake of her husband. Success depends on her realizing that it is a struggle for her own sexuality.

### The programme

1. She must have intercourse 3 days a week, with days and times selected in advance, so that there is no attempt to procrastinate. This is because decreasing frequency produces increasing anxiety irrespective of cause — and if the patient can accept a programme of increased frequency she will find that her anxiety diminishes.

2. The couple must have a rule to make up a missed love-making as soon as possible, otherwise unconsciously an escape route through illness or tiredness will be used as an excuse by the patient, and so gradually the programme will fail.

3. The period of time involved is usually 6 months or a year, but many couples stay longer on a modified programme as it is easy for sex to go to the bottom of the list of priorities when both partners have full-time jobs.

4. The most important and difficult part is for the woman to discover the power she has to make a coitus a happy event, even if initially she does not feel like it. She must be encouraged to take an active responsive part and try to make her partner feel welcome. Many women then experience a change in their feelings when they find that being actively loving removes their anxiety about how they will respond.

This programme is usually successful in the secondary sexual difficulties and forms part of the treatment of the primary group to whom much more counselling than can be described here may have to be given. It is always important to have the partner present. Only then is it possible to see whether there is enough goodwill between them for a satisfactory outcome, and only then can the doctor be sure that a distorted version of the counselling is not being taken home and used for the wrong purpose. Also the partner may have problems that he is unwilling to recognize but which are highly relevant.

Patients with vaginismus often find that the symptom disappears shortly after starting the programme, although pleasure and satisfaction may take many months to acquire. This appears to be because the unconscious purpose of vaginismus is to try to prevent penetration. If the individual determines to have intercourse whether it is painful or not, there is no longer any purpose in making the process painful.

Lack of orgasm presents a more difficult problem. In most cases the cause is a deep personality difficulty in 'letting go', and again it requires specialist psychotherapeutic help. It is worth while, however, trying to persuade the woman to use a vibrator as this can increase excitability, and regular use for a time can allow her to experience and come to want an orgasm. The risk is of the partner becoming superfluous. Furthermore, women with sexual difficulties usually have inhibitions which make it difficult for them to accept the idea of using a vibrator. The patient should therefore be encouraged to use the vibrator daily, alone and to regard it only as an exercise for improving her sexual relationship with her husband. She should also be encouraged to insert the vibrator and not just use it for clitoral stimulation as greater satisfaction will be achieved if vaginal excitation is encouraged.

The successful outcome of treatment will depend, to a much larger extent than in any other field of medicine, on the personality, sensitivity and persuasiveness of the doctor. The patient must be persuaded to recognize unacceptable facts about herself or her relationship, the avoidance of which is the main cause of the problem. She must also be persuaded to restart or increase an activity she largely wishes to avoid. The unpalatable must be made palatable. Each doctor must be prepared to examine his own prejudices and to beware of them, and he must be prepared to take other people's religious and moral values into account when they are different from his own.

# 34

# Urinary malfunction in gynaecological cases

Gynaecological disorders and pelvic operations are often associated with urinary disorders. This chapter is written from the viewpoint of the gynaecologist, and the lesions described are those for which he is sometimes responsible for diagnosis and treatment. Some of these cases will require full urological investigation, including cystoscopy, intravenous pyelography and cystometry.

## Frequency of micturition

Frequency of micturition is a common complaint in women. The following gynaecological conditions may cause it.

**Pelvic swellings and tumours.** Any swelling in the pelvis which causes pressure on the bladder may cause frequency of micturition, particularly in the daytime. The commonest example is the pregnant uterus. Frequency often occurs in the early weeks when the uterus is still a pelvic organ, but it may also be noticed in late pregnancy when the fetal head is engaged in the pelvic cavity. Any other tumour which occupies the pelvic cavity, such as a uterine fibromyoma or an ovarian cyst, may cause frequency.

**Prolapse.** Frequency associated with a cystocele is usually caused by bacterial infection and cystitis, but in some cases the urine is found to be sterile. Such cases may prove to be instances of urgency rather than true frequency, and to be attributed to relaxation of the bladder neck so that urine enters the posterior urethra and stimulates the micturition reflex.

**Pelvic peritonitis.** Lesions causing irritation of the peritoneal surface of the bladder, such as salpingitis, appendicitis, ectopic pregnancy or endometriosis, may cause frequency, often accompanied by painful micturition.

**Urethral lesions** usually cause painful rather than frequent micturition, but frequency can occur with urethritis or an infected urethral diverticulum.

**Cystitis.** The healthy bladder will resist infection for a time even if organisms are introduced into it, but a variety of factors will reduce its resistance.

1. Injury to the bladder is often followed by infection, for example if the bladder is bruised during the performance of operations such as hysterectomy or colporrhaphy, or by radiation damage.

2. Any foreign body may introduce or maintain infection. Even the passage of a catheter is not without risk, and for most diagnostic purposes

it is preferable to rely on mid-stream specimens. The use of an indwelling catheter after pelvic operations frequently causes cystitis and, although its use is sometimes necessary, it should be avoided whenever possible.

3. If the bladder becomes overstretched and atonic because of retention of urine, or if it is atonic because its nerve supply has been damaged (as for example after Wertheim's hysterectomy), infection often occurs. An atonic bladder requires regular catheterization, or the insertion of an indwelling catheter, until the volume of residual urine in the bladder after micturition is less than about 50 ml.

4. If there is a fistulous opening into the bladder, organisms can easily enter.

5. The discovery of trigonitis at cystoscopy in cases of frequency has been attributed to chronic cervicitis, but the so-called cervicitis is often not an infective lesion and it is not generally accepted that infection can pass directly from the cervix to the bladder.

The symptoms of cystitis caused by gynaecological conditions are the ordinary ones of frequency, pain on micturition and pyrexia, and the usual treatment is applied, provided that any underlying gynaecological cause is first recognized and treated.

## Pyelonephritis

This is a potentially dangerous condition because it may lead to permanent renal damage or hypertension. It may complicate pregnancy (see 'Obstetrics by Ten Teachers'). Fortunately, it is a rare sequel of post-operative cystitis, although unilateral renal infection and hydronephrosis after ureteric injury may lead to destruction and loss of the kidney.

In cases of chronic urinary tract infection, or when acute infection tends to recur, every effort must be made to discover the underlying cause. Complete investigation of the urinary tract is essential, including cystoscopy and intravenous pyelography, especially when no obvious cause outside the renal tract is found.

# Incontinence of urine

Incontinence of urine means that the urine escapes involuntarily. The urine may escape continuously both by night and by day, or it may escape intermittently, and the causes of each variety need to be understood if treatment is to be successful. Uncontrolled leakage of urine is a most distressing and degrading disability, and failure of treatment is often the result of inadequate investigation.

## The normal control of micturition

The mechanisms responsible for urinary continence in the female are still not completely understood. Three factors may be considered:

### 1. *Muscular control*

The bladder wall chiefly consists of interlacing smooth muscle fibres of the involuntary detrusor muscle. Inferiorly there are two horseshoe-shaped concentrations of smooth muscle which surround the vesico-urethral junction. They are continuous with the intrinsic muscle fibres of the urethra, and act as an internal sphincter. When the detrusor muscle actively contracts these sling-like bands of muscle relax, allowing the bladder neck to widen into a funnel shape so that urine flows into the urethra.

The internal sphincter is supported by striped muscle fibres from the medial edge of the pubococcygeal part of levator ani which also form a sling round the bladder neck posteriorly. Below this, between the two layers of the urogenital diaphragm (triangular ligament), is the deep trans-

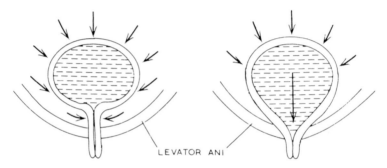

LEVATOR ANI

**Fig. 34.1** Diagram to explain one theory of the cause of stress incontinence. In the normal patient any increase in intra-abdominal pressure also compresses the upper urethra. If the bladder neck has descended, this does not occur.

verse perineal muscle (compressor urethrae) which can compress the urethra strongly at that level. Contraction of these voluntary muscles of the pelvic floor can prevent the escape of urine; even if micturition is in progress a normal woman can stop the stream voluntarily by their action, and since the pelvic floor muscles contract reflexly during coughing they will also prevent any escape of urine from the rise of intra-abdominal pressure on coughing.

### 2. *External pressure on the urethra*

Some hold that continence is also assisted by external pressure on the intra-abdominal part of the urethra (above the urogenital diaphragm) which is equal to the pressure on the fundus of the bladder (Fig. 34.1). It is suggested that if the pelvic floor muscles are relaxed, or if there is prolapse of the bladder neck as a result of trauma during delivery, then any increase in intra-abdominal pressure will act on the bladder alone, so that urine will escape into the urethra.

*3. Reflex control*
When the bladder fills with urine it accommodates the increasing volume with a gradual rise in intravesical pressure, until the sensory stretch receptors are stimulated to trigger detrusor contraction and relaxation of the internal sphincter. The sympathetic and parasympathetic control is delicately balanced, there being a reciprocal arrangement of adrenergic α and β receptors in the fundus and bladder-neck regions, which act so that when one area contracts the other relaxes, and vice versa. If it is inconvenient to micturate, this reflex mechanism can normally be overridden by voluntary cortical control, so that the desire to micturate caused by increased intravesical pressure and detrusor contraction can be suppressed by active contraction of the pelvic floor muscles.

Continence therefore depends on multiple factors, requiring both an intact urethral closure mechanism and normal reflex action.

The following clinical varieties of incontinence may be described: (1) true incontinence, (2) overflow incontinence, (3) urge incontinence and (4) stress incontinence. These must be carefully distinguished from each other, and this may be particularly difficult in the case of stress or urge incontinence, since they have very similar symptoms and also because both may occur in the same patient.

## True incontinence

'True' incontinence of urine may be of two varieties.
1. That which concerns the gynaecologist is almost always caused by a fistula of the bladder or ureter. Vesicovaginal fistulae may be the result of obstetric or surgical trauma, malignant disease or tissue necrosis after radiotherapy. Ureteric fistulae are caused by surgical injury.
There are rare congenital lesions which cause incontinence, namely ectopia vesicae, and ectopic opening of a ureter into the urethra.
In all these cases urine escapes continually, both by day and night.
2. There is another type of incontinence which is seen in general medical practice, in which the patient empties the bladder from time to time without regard to social convenience, either because of cortical disease such as senile dementia which has removed any concern about propriety, or because of neurological disease which has dissociated the lower centres from higher control, as may be seen with the automatic bladder in late cases of paraplegia.

## Overflow incontinence ('false incontinence')

In cases of retention of urine from any cause, especially in elderly patients with loss of bladder sensation, when the bladder becomes grossly distended urine may dribble away. This is termed retention with overflow.

## Urge incontinence

This term is applied when the patient has an urgent desire to micturate which cannot be controlled by voluntary contraction of the pelvic floor muscles. She becomes acutely conscious of an urgent need to void urine, and this is followed by the uncontrolled passage of urine. It is often associated with frequency of micturition and a sensation of incomplete emptying caused by trigonitis or urethritis.

Cystometry shows that the bladder reflex is unusually excitable, and detrusor tone is unduly high (detrusor instability). The causes include cystitis, and full investigation by the methods described below is essential. In some longstanding cases no local abnormality is found, and relief can often be obtained by reassurance and bladder training in hospital. The patient is encouraged to ignore the first sensation of wanting to void for as long as she can and not to rush to the closet. She must wait 1½ hours (or else be incontinent) and this time is gradually increased by half-hourly increments. Mild tranquillizing drugs may sometimes help in this re-education process. By the time the patient leaves hospital she should be able to control her frequency and increase her bladder capacity enough to enable her to go for 4 hours without micturating. Her fluid intake is not restricted, and she must persist with the same regimen at home.

## Stress incontinence

This is a common disorder. The patient complains that a small quantity of urine escapes involuntarily whenever the intra-abdominal pressure is suddenly raised by any exertion, such as coughing, sneezing, laughing or even walking. Stress incontinence is most commonly seen in parous women, and in them is usually the result of damage to the pelvic floor during delivery, but it is sometimes noticed for the first time during pregnancy. In a few cases it may occur in nulliparae, and it may appear for the first time or get worse after the menopause. About half of the patients who have a cystocele have stress incontinence, but it can occur without evident prolapse.

The essential lesion is loss of muscular support at the vesico-urethral junction, combined with descent of the base of the bladder. In many cases of stress incontinence cystography (see below) shows that the normal angle between the posterior aspect of the urethra and the bladder base is lost, but sometimes the angle is lost in patients who have no incontinence. It is possible that there is more than one defence against urinary leak. Even if the attachment of the pubococcygeus muscle to the urethra — which accounts for the posterior vesico-urethral angle — is damaged, the patient may still have control if other mechanisms remain effective.

Several other factors have been discussed. With descent of the bladder neck the upper urethra becomes extra-abdominal, so that the normal external compression of the urethra (see p. 332) does not occur. The urethra is also shorter and wider, so that urinary escape is easier.

**Diagnosis and investigation**

True stress incontinence is caused by an anatomical fault which can be relieved by surgical treatment. Detrusor instability can cause very similar symptoms, but in this condition there is no evident anatomical fault and surgical treatment is not only useless but may even make the complaint worse.

Microscopy and bacterial culture of the urine is essential in every case, and any infection must be effectively treated before final assessment of the symptoms.

In examining a woman with suspected stress incontinence she should be told not to pass urine beforehand, so that when she is asked to cough any escape of urine can be seen. Para-urethral pressure is applied by placing two fingers in the vagina with one on either side of the urethra and pressing upwards. If incontinence on coughing has been observed, and it is controlled by this supporting pressure, then a pelvic floor repair is likely to be effective.

If stress incontinence is not observed during examination, and if there is no evident cystocele, caution is required before advising any form of surgical treatment. If the symptoms are mixed or complicated, for example urge incontinence together with stress incontinence, further investigation is needed before deciding upon treatment. Especial care is required if stress incontinence persists or recurs after surgical treatment.

The best method of assessing these cases is by simultaneous radiological cysto-urethrography and measurement of the intravesical pressure and urine flow — a *videocystogram*. A rectal catheter is used to record the intraperitoneal pressure. Another catheter in the bladder records the total bladder pressure, and subtraction of the intraperitoneal pressure gives the intrinsic bladder pressure. While the bladder is being filled with contrast medium and during voiding the intrinsic bladder pressure and the flow rate are recorded, while a camera simultaneously observes the changes in radiological form of the bladder and urethra. The apparatus is expensive and interpretation of the results requires experience, but reference of difficult cases to special centres will prevent many unsuccessful operations.

**Treatment of true stress incontinence**

In cases of cystocele the first step in treatment is anterior colporrhaphy, combined if necessary with other procedures for uterine prolapse. Even if there is no evident cystocele, tightening and drawing together the tissues under the bladder neck from the vaginal aspect will relieve more than half of the patients.

For those who are not relieved by this simple operation opinions differ about the best treatment. A relatively simple procedure is that of colpo-cystopexy (Marshall and Marchetti operation) in which the prevesical space is approached by a suprapubic incision without opening the peritoneal cavity, and then the bladder is drawn upwards and fixed with stitches to the fascia on the back of the pubic bone and abdominal wall. Other stitches are placed low down, on either side of the urethra, to support the vaginal fascia. A recent modification of this procedure is colposuspension (Burch operation) in which the paraurethral tissues are suspended with non-absorbable sutures from the reflected (pectineal) part of the inguinal ligament.

An alternative but more difficult operation is to support the vesico-urethral junction with a sling. The sling may be fashioned from external oblique aponeurosis, when it is passed round the urethra from an abdominal approach (Aldridge operation), or fascia lata or nylon may be used and inserted from the vaginal aspect. The sling is arranged to pass under the urethra and is fixed above to the rectus sheath.

Adjuvant measures are sometimes helpful, including a strict diet for women who are overweight, and instruction by a physiotherapist in pelvic floor exercises. After the menopause the muscles of the pelvic floor are atonic, and the submucosal venous plexus is less vascular; some benefit has been claimed for treatment with oestrogens.

# Retention of urine

Retention of urine means that urine flows into the bladder but cannot pass out. It must be distinguished from suppression of urine, or anuria, in which urine is not being secreted by the kidneys.

Retention of urine may be due to nervous or mechanical causes.

### 1. *Nervous causes*
Retention of urine is common during the first few days of the puerperium, and after any abdominal or pelvic operation. The retention is partly due to a nervous factor and partly, especially after perineal operations, to spasm of the levator ani and perineal muscles. In operations which involve separation of the bladder from the cervix, such as hysterectomy and vaginal repair, retention is common because of this disturbance of the bladder. Radical hysterectomy for carcinoma of the cervix is certain to produce retention, because the more extensive dissection of the bladder in these cases damages the nerve supply to it, and for at least 10 days it will not empty completely.

Retention may be caused by lesions of the central nervous system, such as multiple sclerosis and injury or disease of the cord, and by hysteria.

### 2. *Mechanical causes*
Retention of urine may be caused by a tumour impacted in the pelvis. The base of the bladder is lifted upwards and forwards by the tumour beneath it, with the result that the urethra is elongated to such an extent that the mechanism of micturition is disturbed. Among the masses which will cause this are the fetal head in the second stage of labour, a retroverted incarcerated gravid uterus at about the 14th week of gestation, an impacted

fibromyoma of the uterus, an ovarian cyst, a large haematocele, a pelvic abscess and a haematocolpos.

Carcinoma of the urethra, bladder or cervix are very rare causes of retention.

### Treatment

Retention calls not only for immediate relief by catheterization but also for removal of its cause; otherwise cystitis, with the further risk of ascending pyelonephritis, will occur.

Retention due to incarceration of the gravid retroverted uterus is relieved by catheterization, after which the uterus usually assumes a normal anteverted position and rises up into the abdomen. If this does not occur the uterus is manipulated bimanually into its correct position, if necessary under anaesthesia. A pelvic tumour causing retention must be removed.

Retention after labour or operations occurs much less often if patients are allowed out of bed to use a commode or walk to the lavatory, rather than use a bed pan. The intramuscular injection of carbachol 0.25 mg or distigmine bromide 1 ml is sometimes of value in stimulating the bladder muscle. If these remedies fail a catheter must be passed, and in some cases a self-retaining catheter is left in the bladder for 24 hours.

A bladder which has been overdistended as a result of retention will often fail to empty itself completely when micturition is resumed. The patient will pass some urine, but an almost equal amount may be left in the bladder. If this is not recognized infection of the residual urine may occur. The insertion of a self-retaining catheter is probably less likely to introduce further infection than intermittent catheterization.

# 35

# Backache

Women frequently complain of backache, but this is seldom due to disease of the pelvic organs and the task of the gynaecologist is often only that of excluding any related pelvic disorder. A history of the complaint is first obtained and particular attention should be paid to the following points.

1. Whether the onset was sudden or gradual, and whether it followed an injury or unusual exertion, childbirth or an operation.

2. The effect on the complaint of rest or exercise, and whether the pain is present when at rest in bed.

3. The situation of the pain, and any spread down the leg.

4. Any gynaecological symptoms, and any change in the pain with the menstrual cycle.

5. Any emotional problems that may be related to the complaint.

The patient is examined standing, preferably while wearing her usual shoes. Any scoliosis or exaggerated lordosis may then be observed. All movements of the spinal column are tested and any point of tenderness is noted. The patient is then asked to lie down and movements of the hip joint are tested, and the effect of raising the straight leg on each side.

Certain general points may be made.

1. Sudden disabling pain is not of gynaecological origin. When the pelvic organs are the cause of backache the onset is gradual.

2. Pain felt at a higher level than the iliac crests is not of pelvic origin.

3. Pain on moving a joint, on stretching a muscle or ligament, or on straight leg raising has a local and not a pelvic cause.

4. Tenderness on pressure points to a lesion at that site.

5. Pain that radiates down the leg is not of pelvic origin, except in the case of patients with cervical cancer who have involved nodes adherent to the nerves of the sacral plexus. Such a symptom is late in the disease and the history of the illness and its treatment points to the diagnosis. Similarly, bone pain can arise from metastases in the vertebrae.

A gynaecological examination is made, and the following lesions can be discussed as possible causes of backache.

### Uterine displacement
*Uterine prolapse* gives rise to discomfort and a sensation of something dropping; in only a few cases is there also low backache. The discomfort is worse after standing, and is relieved by lying down. It is unwise to promise that backache will be cured by an operation for prolapse – the most that can be offered is the hope that it will be relieved.

*Retroversion of the uterus.* Uncomplicated retroversion does not cause backache.

Lumbar backache is not uncommon in the puerperium, particularly if the patient returns to her normal routine work too soon. The need to nurse, wash and care for a baby while the pelvic ligaments are still lax and the mother is tired may well lead to some backache. A retroverted uterus that is discovered may be blamed for this, but the same symptom is often seen in women without a retroversion, and pain at this level is unlikely to have a pelvic cause. If puerperal retroversion does ever cause discomfort it will be in the sacral region. Treatment by correcting the retroversion and inserting a pessary has often been prescribed, but seldom with benefit.

## Pelvic inflammation

Chronic pelvic inflammation may cause an ache referred to the sacral region. The backache will be constant, with exacerbation before menstruation (congestive dysmenorrhoea), and there will also be dyspareunia, menorrhagia and cervical discharge. On bimanual palpation a tender fixed mass may be felt behind the uterus due to a hydrosalpinx or pyosalpinx, which is often bilateral.

## Endometriosis

Endometriosis gives rise to the same symptoms as chronic salpingo-oöphoritis, except that discharge is usually absent.

## Pelvic neoplasms

Fibromyomata and benign ovarian cysts do not cause backache. Backache is a late symptom of uterine cancer and malignant disease of the ovaries when local infiltration ensues. Severe pain may occur with carcinomatous metastases in the vertebrae, and if the growth involves nerve roots or plexuses the pain may be referred down the leg.

If there are signs pointing to a local lesion in the back, an x-ray may be arranged before seeking the advice of an orthopaedic surgeon, but the mistake must not be made of attributing symptoms to any minor asymmetry or congenital lesion, such as sacralization of a lumbar transverse process.

It must not be forgotten that backache can be caused by injudicious positioning of the patient on the operating table. Care should be taken during surgery with the patient lying supine that there is no undue flattening of the lumbar curve. Great care must be taken in putting the legs into stirrups in the lithotomy position; raising the legs separately or too rapidly can cause severe subsequent lumbosacral backache.

# 36

# Gynaecological problems in developing countries

At present some special gynaecological problems occur in developing countries, but with improving medical care it is to be hoped that these will soon become rare. A few general points need to be made:

### 1. Socio-economic considerations
Poverty and malnutrition go together, and diseases such as malaria, hookworm infestation, and intestinal infections from contaminated food and water supplies may add to the burden of any gynaecological disorder. Anaemia, including that caused by parasitic infestation, dietary deficiency and inherited haemoglobinopathies, is also commonly seen.

Insufficient medical personnel and inadequate provision of equipment and drugs aggravate the problems, and patients often only seek advice when disease is advanced. For example, uterine fibromyomata or other tumours may have grown to a very large size, and pelvic inflammatory disease may have advanced to form pyosalpinges with dense adhesions.

### 2. Local customs
Tribal customs or attitudes may cause difficulties. For example, vaginal stenosis may follow female circumcision or the use of vaginal caustics. Fear or suspicion can lead to refusal of consent to hysterectomy or Caesarean section; the status of a woman in a polygamous society may be dependent on her ability to bear children by normal labour.

In some groups a male doctor is unacceptable, in spite of the fact that few women are able to train as doctors.

### 3. Racial differences
Racial characteristics may affect gynaecological practice. For example, negresses are particularly liable to develop uterine fibromyomata, and in them any abdominal scar may become keloidal. Choriocarcinoma is more common in parts of Asia and Africa than in Europe and America, but whether this is a racial difference is uncertain.

On the other hand, endometriosis is very rare, and endometrial carcinoma is uncommon in Africa and Asia.

While the principles of gynaecological diagnosis and treatment are the same everywhere, a few special points may be briefly made. For details of treatment some of the specialized textbooks may have to be consulted.

## 1. *Female circumcision*

Lesser degrees of this procedure only involve excision of the labia minora and clitoris, and whatever the psychological effects, cause little physical damage. Although now illegal, more severe operations are still carried out in southern Egypt and the Sudan with the purpose of ensuring virginity before marriage, and these include wider excision of vulval tissues with a deliberate attempt to make the wound edges adhere together, so that severe stenosis results.

## 2. *Vaginal caustics*

Extensive vaginal stenosis may be caused by insertion of caustic preparations into the vagina to treat various gynaecological symptoms, or by the introduction of rock salt after delivery, as practised by some Bedouin tribes.

## 3. *Fistula*

Any form of obstructed labour, treated by the unskilled manipulations of untrained assistants, may cause severe damage to the cervix, vagina or pelvic floor, sometimes resulting in large vesicovaginal or rectovaginal fistulae.

## 4. *Sexually transmitted diseases*

Gonorrhoea is common, and untreated syphilis may be a florid disease, with severe systemic manifestations. Lymphogranuloma venereum (p. 142) and granuloma inguinale (p. 142) may be seen, and both these diseases are occasionally followed by epithelioma of the vulva.

## 5. *Tuberculosis*

In many developing countries tuberculosis is still rife, and is a common cause of salpingitis. Tuberculous inguinal adenitis, with abscess formation, may occur, and lymphatic obstruction may cause oedema of the vulva and leg.

## 6. *Infertility*

There is a high incidence of infertility, which can be a social disaster. It is most frequently caused by pelvic inflammatory disease resulting from puerperal infection, gonorrhoea or tuberculosis, but ill-health may be a contributory cause.

## 7. *Ectopic pregnancy*

The prevalence of salpingitis increases the risk of tubal and secondary abdominal pregnancy.

## 8. *Filariasis*

Filarial infection may cause inguinal adenitis and elephantiasis of the vulva. By the time chronic lymphatic obstruction has occurred filariae may no longer be detected, but specific treatment with diethylcarbamazine is still indicated, while surgical excision of the large vulval swelling may be required.

### 9. *Schistosomiasis*
The flukes travel in the pelvic veins and lay their eggs in the wall of the bladder or bowel, but the female genital tract may be involved. There is severe inflammatory reaction around the ova. The gynaecological lesions are usually only discovered during the investigation of vesical or rectal disease, during which ova are found in excreta or in biopsy material.

### 10. *Uterine fibromyomata*
As already mentioned, these tumours are common in negresses, whether they reside in the tropics or elsewhere.

### 11. *Choriocarcinoma*
Hydatidiform mole and choriocarcinoma occur more often in the Philippines, in South East Asia, in South America and in West Africa than in Europe or North America. The reason for this is still obscure.

# 37

# Gynaecological operations

Despite the recent advances in gynaecological endocrinology, and the hope that hormonal treatment will replace many surgical procedures, operative treatment and investigation still provide a large proportion of the work of the gynaecologist, and although technical details may only concern the specialist the student must be well informed about the principles involved.

Any operation and anaesthetic carries some risk to the patient's life, small though this may be. There must therefore be a good reason for advising any procedure, with consideration of what it implies for the patient in the future. The primary question is whether the operation will cure the patient's symptoms or, in the case of an investigatory procedure, whether this will allow a better decision about the most suitable treatment.

The time needed for recovery will be an important consideration for a woman with family responsibilities, and this may sometimes lead to postponement of a non-urgent operation, for example for prolapse. Some women struggle on with uncomfortable symptoms because they are unable to take sufficient time off for treatment and proper convalescence.

Consideration of future gynaecological function is of paramount importance, and proper explanations must be given to the patient. Some women cannot bear the thought of losing the uterus, often because of unfounded beliefs that they have about the effect of the operation on subsequent health or married life. The idea that 'the change' invariably follows hysterectomy dies hard, and the effect of such operations as colporrhaphy and hysterectomy on coital function must be discussed with the patient. Patients must also be warned about the probable outcome of operations for infertility; the results of procedures to restore tubal patency are very poor if the tubes have been severely damaged by infection, and this must be stated before rather than after the operation.

The prognosis after surgery for malignant conditions depends on a combination of factors, but the medical adviser must have a clear idea of the best and worst that may occur with radical surgery, the proposal of which in itself will constitute a major crisis for the patient.

Before carrying out elective surgery it is necessary to have the patient in as good a physical condition as possible; she then not only withstands the metabolic upset associated with any operation or anaesthetic, but she also recovers more quickly and is less likely to have the complications of anaemia, thrombo-embolism or infection.

The most important preoperative treatment is the correction of anaemia, which is common in gynaecological patients with menorrhagia, by either oral or parenteral administration of iron. Blood transfusion is better reserved for administration during or after the operation, because if it is given immediately beforehand it tends to increase bleeding at the time of the operation and therefore its beneficial effects may be largely wasted.

## Immediate preoperative management

Minor procedures such as curettage, cauterization of the cervix and even laparoscopy may be performed as 'day cases'. The patient comes to the hospital in the morning having fasted from the previous night, and has the operation at mid-day or in the early afternoon. In the time before the operation the history is reviewed, her chest is examined and a specimen of urine is tested. If these are normal the operation is carried out with pre-medication under either local or general anaesthesia, and the patient goes home, accompanied, in the evening. If any complications occur she must immediately be readmitted without hesitation.

For procedures involving laparotomy incisions or extensive suturing the patient is admitted to hospital at least a day before the operation, for general examination and examination of the chest, blood and urine. Night sedation is prescribed. The bowel should be emptied by a laxative or, if necessary, a small enema. Shaving of the pubic hair is all that is necessary for abdominal operations, and clipping of vulval hair for vaginal operations. A vaginal pessary of metronidazole 1 g may be inserted the night before operation.

Preoperative medication is prescribed by the anaesthetist, and varies from diazepam alone to combinations of atropine and morphine derivatives.

The bladder should be emptied before any pelvic operation because a full bladder may get in the way, or if it is unrecognized it may be injured. It is particularly important to have the bladder empty before laparoscopy, otherwise the needle used for inducing the pneumoperitoneum may pierce it.

## Vulval operations

**Operations for Bartholin's cyst or abscess.**
See pp. 105 and 143.

**Simple excision of the vulva**
This operation occasionally is done for leukoplakia or lichen sclerosus. Figure 41.1 shows the incisions and method of suturing. It is nearly always possible to bring the skin edges together without tension, and the operation leaves surprisingly little deformity.

### Radical vulvectomy for carcinoma of the vulva

This consists of a block dissection of the lymphatic glands which drain the vulva (on both sides) and removal of all the tissues of the vulva down to

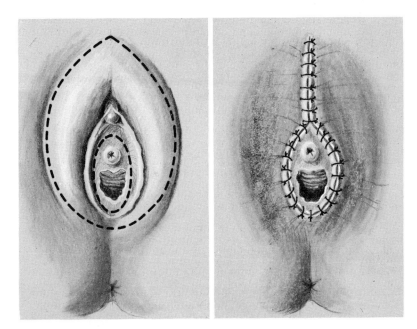

**Fig. 37.1** Simple vulvectomy.

the periosteum of the pubis and the fascia covering the muscles. The glands are the superficial and deep inguinal glands, Cloquet's gland in the femoral canal, and the glands related to the external iliac vessels.

A strip of skin about 2 cm wide is removed from the anterior iliac spine to the pubic spine on each side, leaving the inner portion of each strip attached to the mons veneris (Figs. 37.2–4). These skin flaps with the subcutaneous tissues and the nodes are dissected medially, exposing the external oblique aponeurosis and the inguinal ligament. The long saphenous vein is in the field and part of it is removed; the femoral vessels are exposed and cleared. The external oblique aponeurosis is incised above the inguinal ligament, and the underlying transversalis muscle is cut. After division of the deep epigastric vessels the peritoneum can be swept medially to expose the glands along the iliac vessels. The transversalis muscle and external oblique aponeurosis are repaired and then the vulva is excised with the diathermy knife, taking with it the skin flaps and the mass of fat and glands already dissected. The sartorius muscle may be detached from the anterior superior iliac spine and brought in front of the iliac vessels which can otherwise become adherent to overlying skin. The inguinal incisions are sutured, but the vulval wound cannot be completely closed and is left to heal by granulation. This may take 2 months, but the final deformity is less than might be expected.

Some surgeons prefer not to excise the skin in the groins, but adopt an

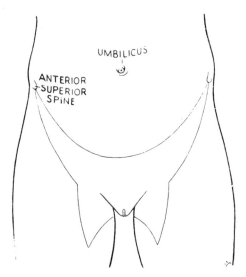

**Fig. 37.2** Skin incisions for radical vulvectomy. The area of skin marked out by the incisions is removed with underlying fat, fascia and glands.

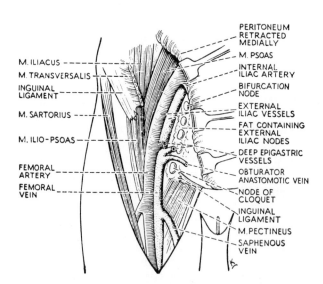

**Fig. 37.3** The exposure of the deep lymph nodes in radical vulvectomy. Most surgeons do not divide the inguinal ligament but approach the iliac glands by an incision above it.

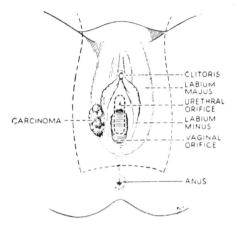

CLITORIS
LABIUM MAJUS
URETHRAL ORIFICE
CARCINOMA
LABIUM MINUS
VAGINAL ORIFICE

ANUS

**Fig. 37.4** Skin incisions to complete the removal of the vulva in the radical operation.

undercutting approach to remove the lymph nodes. The vulval and groin fields are kept separate.

# Operations performed by the vaginal route

### Dilatation of the cervix and curettage of the uterus

This procedure forms part of the investigation of many gynaecological disorders. It gives information about the state of the endometrium and the size and shape of the uterine cavity. General anaesthesia is usually necessary and is helpful for digital examination of the pelvis to detect any abnormal swelling of the uterus, tubes or ovaries, which should always be the first step.

With the patient in the lithotomy position, a weighted Auvard self-retaining speculum or a Sims' speculum is inserted into the vagina and the anterior lip of the cervix is held with a volsellum. After passage of a uterine sound to confirm the position and establish the length of the uterine cavity, the cervix is dilated with graduated dilators. It is wise to pass a small ring forceps into the cavity before curetting, as a polyp can be missed if this is not done.

Curettage is replaced by, or combined with, suction evacuation when evacuating an incomplete abortion or a vesicular mole, or performing termination of pregnancy.

It is also possible to obtain tissue for endometrial biopsy without cervical dilatation or general anaesthesia by using a small Vabra suction aspirator, although many gynaecologists hesitate to use this method for the investigation of possible malignant disease.

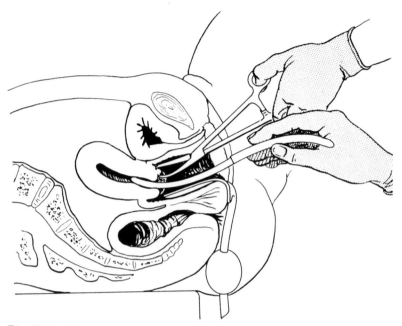

**Fig. 37.5** Dilatation of the cervix.

Dilatation and curettage is usually a simple minor operation, but even in experienced hands accidents occasionally happen. Too rapid or extreme dilatation of the cervix may tear the internal os, causing abortion in a subsequent pregnancy from cervical incompetence, and a lateral tear may occasionally cause a broad ligament haematoma. The uterus may also be perforated with a dilator or other instrument (see p. 79).

## Conization of the cervix (cone biopsy)

Conization of the cervix means cutting out a cone of tissue that includes the entire squamo-columnar junction and the cervical canal up to the internal os. Until recently it was frequently performed whenever suspicious cells were found in a cervical smear (cone biopsy), but with a colposcope it is now possible to recognize suspicious areas and investigate them by less radical biopsies. These areas can then be eradicated under direct vision with a laser beam or with diathermy.

Conization may be accompanied by free bleeding which is controlled with deep stitches or diathermy. (Diathermy should not be used for the original incision because it may interfere with histological examination.) Secondary haemorrhage on about the 7th day after the operation is an occasional complication. It is treated by packing the cone from which the biopsy was taken with gauze. Stenosis is a rare sequel of cone biopsy.

Conization is still sometimes performed when the upward extent of a suspicious lesion is uncertain, or for carcinoma-in-situ.

## Diathermy cauterization or cryosurgery of the cervix.

See p.118.

## Trachelorrhaphy

Cervical repair may be required if a tear of the cervix on one or both sides has extended up to the internal os and is a cause of recurrent abortion. The edges of the tear are excised and then sutured together to re-form the cervical canal.

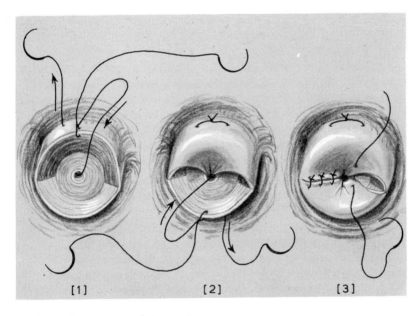

**Fig. 37.6** Amputation of the cervix.

## Amputation of the cervix

This is performed as part of a Manchester operation for prolapse (p. 354) but may also be occasionally performed for chronic cervicitis with gross cervical hypertrophy, or for congenital elongation of the cervix. The method is shown in Fig. 37.6. Secondary haemorrhage may follow this operation on about the 7th to 10th day. If the bleeding point cannot be seen and secured, a tight vaginal pack is inserted.

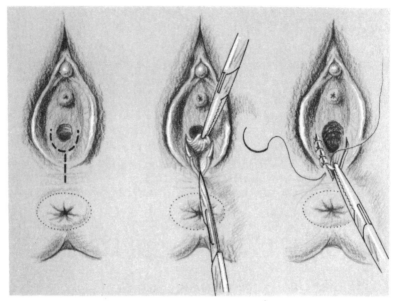

**Fig. 37.7** Steps of operation to enlarge vaginal orifice.

### Operation for enlargement of the vaginal introitus

Most cases of primary dyspareunia are best treated by methods other than a surgical operation (see p. 327) but this procedure is occasionally required if there is unusual narrowing of the introitus or stenosis after perineal repair. The method is shown in Fig. 37.7.

### Operations for absence of the vagina

See p. 72.

## Operations for prolapse

These operations are often difficult for the student to follow, but some of the figures may help to explain the principles.

### Anterior colporrhaphy

This operation is for the cure of cystocele, but since cystocele is often associated with descent of the cervix it is frequently performed as part of the Manchester operation or of vaginal hysterectomy, which are described below. In anterior colporrhaphy a diamond-shaped area of the stretched redundant vaginal wall is excised. This exposes the bladder covered by the

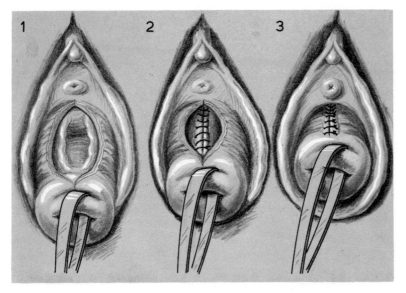

**Fig. 37.8** Anterior colporrhaphy. An oval or diamond-shaped incision is made in the anterior vaginal wall to expose the fascia over the bladder. This is repaired and then the vaginal epithelium is sutured in the midline.

pubovesical fascia. The fascia is plicated to support the bladder and the vaginal wall is closed over it.

Retention of urine sometimes follows the operation for a few days. Because of this many surgeons insert a suprapubic Bonnano catheter. This is passed with the aid of a needle through the abdominal wall 5 cm above the pubis. Bladder drainage can be maintained until micturition has become re-established. Residual urine after micturition can easily be measured. The catheter is comfortable and the risk of urinary infection from urethral catheterization is largely eliminated.

## Posterior colporrhaphy and perineorrhaphy

This is undertaken for rectocele, for enterocele and for repair of the perineum. A triangle of the posterior vaginal wall with its apex behind the cervix and its base at the introitus is removed. The fascia covering the rectum is not very strong and so the perineum is built up over the anal canal as shown in Fig. 37.9, steps 3 and 4.

If an enterocele is also present, the flap of posterior vaginal skin is widened near the cervix so that the peritoneal sac of the enterocele can be opened and excised. The cut edges are closed with a purse-string suture and the uterosacral ligaments are brought together below it.

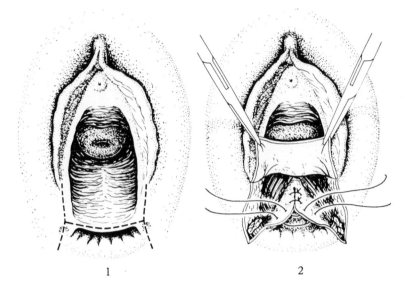

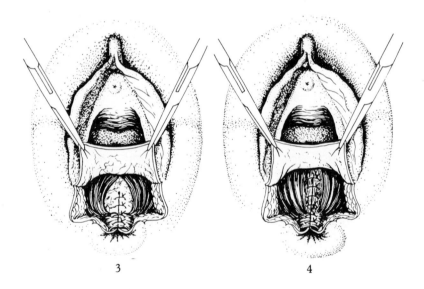

**Fig. 37.9** Repair of complete perineal tear. 1. Lines of incision.
2. Reflection of vaginal epithelium is followed by suture of rectal wall.
3. Anal sphincter repaired. 4. Approximation of medial edges of levatores
ani. The more superficial layers will then be sutured.

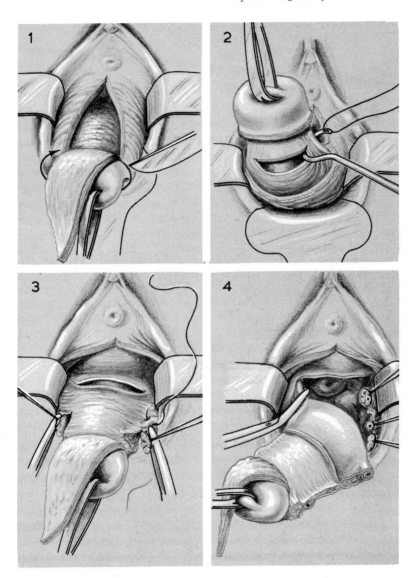

**Fig. 37.10** Vaginal hysterectomy. 1. Inverted V-shaped incision in anterior vaginal wall is continued round the cervix. 2. Rectovaginal pouch opened. Aneurysm needle used to ligate the medial ends of the cardinal and uterosacral ligaments, which are fused at this point. 3. After division of the cardinal and uterosacral ligaments, the needle is used to ligate the uterine vessels. The uterovesical pouch is opened. 4. The Fallopian tube, round ligament and ovarian vessels are tied and divided before the uterus is removed. The peritoneum is closed and then the pedicles on each side are brought together. Finally, the vaginal epithelium is sutured.

## Perineorrhaphy for complete tear of the perineum

The operation is illustrated in Fig. 37.9.

## Vaginal hysterectomy with repair of prolapse

For women who do not wish further pregnancy this is the operation of choice in most cases of uterine prolapse. An incision is made around the cervix at the top of the vagina (Fig. 37.10). When the uterus is drawn downwards the cardinal ligament is seen and can be divided and ligated on each side, together with the uterosacral ligament which is attached to the cervix at the same level. The uterine artery on each side is then tied. After opening both the uterovesical and rectovaginal pouches the uterus can now be delivered. The top of the broad ligament containing the round ligament, tube and branches of the ovarian artery is then clamped and tied on each side and the uterus is removed. The peritoneum is closed and the cardinal and uterosacral ligaments are sewn together. If this is not done carefully there is a risk of subsequent enterocele. For prolapse the operation is combined with anterior colporrhaphy and posterior colpoperineorrhaphy as may be required.

## Manchester operation for prolapse (Fothergill's operation)

This is an alternative to vaginal hysterectomy and repair; subsequent pregnancy is not excluded by it and postoperative morbidity is less than with vaginal hysterectomy. It consists of anterior colporrhaphy (and posterior colpoperineorrhaphy if necessary) and amputation of the cervix. This exposes the lowest parts of the cardinal ligaments, which can be drawn together in front of the cervix, thus shortening them and elevating the uterus. The steps are shown in Fig. 37.11.

## Operations for stress incontinence of urine

See p. 325.

## Operations for urinary fistulae

See pp. 80 and 82.

# Abdominal operations

## Abdominal hysterectomy

There are many indications for removing the uterus and it can be done by either the abdominal or the vaginal route. If the uterus is grossly enlarged

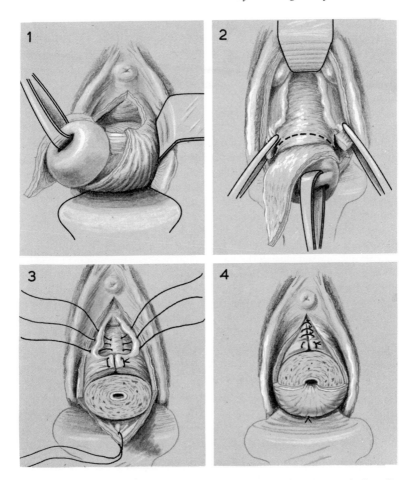

**Fig. 37.11** Fothergill's operation. 1. Incision in the anterior vaginal wall continued so as to surround the cervix. 2. Cervix is amputated. The clamps are on the lower parts of the cardinal ligaments. 3. Cardinal ligaments and fascia covering the bladder brought together. 4. Vaginal epithelium sutured so as to cover the posterior lip of the cervix and it would then be sutured in the midline in front of the cervix.

by fibromyomata beyond the size of a pregnancy of 12 weeks it is inadvisable to attempt to remove it through the vagina, but the vaginal route is feasible for smaller tumours. Many surgeons prefer the abdominal route for all hysterectomies because they can inspect the other organs and deal with any ovarian lesions which may be discovered. For this reason, and also because there is less postoperative morbidity, the majority of hysterectomies are performed abdominally in the United Kingdom at present.

Total hysterectomy means removal of the entire uterus; in subtotal hysterectomy the cervix is not removed. These operations are combined with removal of one or both Fallopian tubes and one or both ovaries as required. Total hysterectomy is almost invariably performed, as it prevents any subsequent possibility of carcinoma of the cervix. Subtotal hysterectomy is only justified in rare cases of such difficulty that removal of the cervix would be dangerous; for example, extensive endometriosis of the rectovaginal septum.

The best incision is the low transverse (Pfannenstiel), but large tumours may dictate a midline or paramedian incision. The first step of the operation is to divide the tubes and round ligaments at the top of the broad ligaments, or the infundibulopelvic ligaments if the ovaries are to be removed. As the broad ligaments are opened up the uterine arteries are exposed. These are clamped and cut, and clamps can then be placed on the 'angles' of the vagina where it is attached to the cervix. Division of the vaginal attachment frees the uterus, and the operation is completed by suturing the vaginal opening and closing the peritoneum over the bases of the broad ligaments and the vagina. The abdomen is closed in the usual way (Fig. 37.12).

The ureter runs forwards below the uterine artery near to the cervix and may be injured if the operator does not keep close to the cervix in applying clamps or ligatures.

## Radical abdominal hysterectomy for carcinoma of the cervix (Wertheim's operation)

See p. 182.

## Abdominal myomectomy

Removal of multiple fibromyomata from the uterus is more difficult than hysterectomy and the postoperative course is sometimes stormy, but of course it preserves the hope of pregnancy, at the cost of the possibility that the fibromyomata may recur after a few years.

Having opened the abdomen, the purpose is to remove the tumours through as few incisions in the uterus as possible. In this way the amount of bleeding during the operation is more easily controlled, and the inevitable postoperative oozing from such a large vascular organ is diminished. A special clamp was devised by Bonney to surround and compress the isthmus of the uterus during the operation in the hope, not always realized, of reducing bleeding; other clamps may be placed on the ovarian vessels.

An anterior uterine incision is preferable because it is less likely to become adherent to a loop of gut subsequently. Several tumours can be reached through one well placed incision. Each tumour is shelled out after incising its capsule. The spaces left are obliterated as far as possible with catgut stitches before the uterine muscle is trimmed and sutured. Blood loss may be heavy and transfusion is often required during this operation.

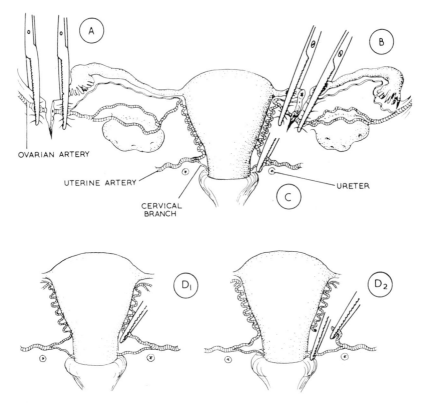

OVARIAN ARTERY

UTERINE ARTERY

CERVICAL
BRANCH

URETER

**Fig. 37.12** Diagrams to show placing of clamps during abdominal hysterectomy, A. Clamping ovarian artery if the ovary is to be removed with the uterus. B. Clamping ovarian artery when the ovary is conserved. C. Method of clamping uterine artery with a single clamp. $D_1$ and $D_2$. More usual method of placing first clamp on uterine artery and then a second clamp on the 'vaginal angle'.

## Salpingectomy

Salpingectomy is required for tubal pregnancy or for a hydrosalpinx or pyosalpinx. If both tubes have to be removed for inflammatory disease, and especially if the patient also has chronic cervicitis or menorrhagia, the uterus is best removed, but every effort must be made to conserve healthy ovarian tissue. In cases of salpingitis, adhesions can make surgery difficult.

## Sterilization

See p. 310.

## Operations to restore tubal patency

See p. 272.

## Oöphorectomy

This is the correct term for removal of an ovary. The word 'ovariotomy' is of historical interest because it was used by those who performed the first abdominal operations when they removed ovarian cysts, but it is incorrect.

Ovarian cysts can be enormous, and to deliver them intact a long incision may be needed. Alternatively, they may be tapped and removed through a small incision, but extreme care must be taken to prevent any of the fluid entering the peritoneal cavity, because if it should happen to contain malignant cells these could be implanted.

The pedicle of the tumour must always be tied carefully, preferably by transfixing ligatures. Slipping of a ligature on a broad pedicle may cause dangerous postoperative haemorrhage.

The opposite ovary must always be examined, as bilateral tumours are common. Bilateral oöphorectomy is routinely performed during hysterectomy on a woman who has reached the menopause, and is essential when the uterus is being removed for malignant disease. When removing an ovarian tumour from a patient who is at or past the menopause, the other ovary and the uterus should be removed. For further details of the management of ovarian carcinoma, see p. 220.

## Ovarian cystectomy

This term means enucleation of a benign cyst from the ovary. Many dermoid cysts, simple serous cysts and endometriomatous cysts can be shelled out, with conservation of most of the ovarian tissue. A shallow incision is made, just deep enough to enable the stretched tissue to be peeled back from the wall of the cyst. The ovary is reconstructed with a series of stitches. Even if the cyst ruptures during its removal, cystectomy is usually possible.

## Pelvic neurectomy

See p. 249.

## Laparoscopy

This operation enables the gynaecologist to inspect the pelvic organs and carry out some forms of treatment through a very small incision, so that the patient can nearly always leave the hospital the next day.

The patient is given a general anaesthetic and placed in the Trendelenburg position. After emptying the bladder with a catheter, a cannula is inserted into the uterus through the cervical canal. This can be used to move the uterus about during the investigation, or to inject methylene blue solution to test the patency of the Fallopian tubes. A small skin incision is made at the lower border of the umbilicus. A Verres spring-loaded needle is inserted through the incision into the peritoneal cavity. A syringe is then attached to the needle and the plunger withdrawn to make sure that the intestine has not been entered. About 2 litres of carbon dioxide or nitrous oxide gas are passed into the peritoneal cavity through the needle, which is then withdrawn. The gas displaces the intestines from the pelvic cavity. A large trocar and cannula are inserted through the abdominal incision, the trocar is withdrawn and the cold-light fibreoptic laparoscope is passed down the cannula towards the pelvis. A second, smaller, cannula can be inserted in the iliac fossa, and an electrode for diathermy coagulation or a biopsy drill can be passed through this.

An excellent view of the pelvic organs is obtained. The instrument may be used to confirm the presence of a lesion already suspected, such as an ectopic pregnancy or endometriosis, or to exclude organic disease in patients complaining of pelvic pain for which no abnormal physical signs can be found. Tubal patency can be observed after injecting methylene blue solution through the uterine cannula, ovarian biopsy can be performed, and sterilization carried out by diathermy coagulation of the tubes, or by placing metal clips or Silastic rings on the tubes.

At the end of the operation the patient is returned to the horizontal position and the gas is expelled by abdominal pressure before removing the cannulae. The small wounds are closed and the patient can return home the next day.

Laparoscopy is an unsafe procedure in inexperienced hands, and initial training should be closely supervised. Injury can occur to bowel or other structures during insertion of the instruments, or from burns if diathermy is used. When the abdomen is over-distended with gas, bradycardia can occur which can progress to cardiac arrest if respiration is not assisted or if vagal impulses are not blocked with atropine.

## Postoperative care and complications

After minor procedures the patient usually recovers consciousness in the theatre or recovery room, and as soon as she is awake she is returned to the ward. Apart from anaesthetic problems and rare instances of bleeding after cervical biopsy there are practically no immediate complications, and there is no pain after cervical cauterization or biopsy, or after curettage.

After major procedures the patient is returned to the ward when she is conscious, with an intravenous infusion running, which will sometimes be of blood. A careful watch is kept for *reactionary haemorrhage* which may occur from vessels which have been inadequately secured, and which will demand blood transfusion and re-exploration of the operation site to obtain haemostasis. Signs of intraperitoneal haemorrhage are sometimes mimicked by reactions to drugs used during anaesthesia which lower the blood pressure and increase the heart rate, and these effects may be enhanced by analgesic drugs such as morphine and pethidine. The differential diagnosis can be difficult, and it is essential to be aware of the possible effects of drugs and to keep full records of their administration before, during and after operation.

*Secondary haemorrhage,* presenting as vaginal bleeding about 7–10 days after operation, is usually associated with infection and sloughing of tissue involving branches of the uterine artery, and it can be alarming. It is treated by blood transfusion, and the bleeding point must be secured or else controlled by insertion of a tight vaginal pack.

*Pain* during the first 24 hours is controlled with morphine or pethidine, and subsequently with milder analgesics. If severe pain persists or recurs, complications such as intestinal obstruction, a pelvic haematoma or pulmonary infarction should be suspected. Pain in the abdominal wound may be due to haematoma or infection.

*Urinary complications.* The urinary function must be carefully watched; if retention occurs it is treated by continuous or intermittent bladder drainage until normal function returns. Catheterization involves a risk of infection, and a broad-spectrum antibiotic or urinary antiseptic is given. With a suprapubic Bonnano catheter the risk of infection is greatly reduced. Uncommon surgical accidents may cause a vesicovaginal or ureterovaginal fistula with leakage of urine.

*Intestinal complications.* Intestinal obstruction and paralytic ileus are both infrequent after planned procedures, but may occur after difficult or prolonged operations, especially if there is pelvic infection, poor haemostasis, or if a large area is left denuded of peritoneum. Any intra-abdominal complication after laparoscopic procedures involving the use of diathermy must be assumed to be due to bowel damage and peritonitis until proved otherwise, and if there is any doubt the patient must be kept in hospital under observation.

In the management of any abdominal complication, intravenous therapy and gastric aspiration are maintained and careful records of fluid intake and output are kept. Frequent estimations of electrolyte levels are made so that water and electrolyte balance can be adjusted. Absence of abdominal pain, apart from discomfort due to distension, and silence on auscultation of the abdomen indicate paralytic ileus. Colicky abdominal pain and loud bowel sounds, with distension and fluid levels in loops of small bowel in a plain radiograph, suggest obstruction. If these signs are present and there is also severe pain between the colicky spasms, the possibility that a segment of bowel is strangulated must be considered.

With ileus, spontaneous recovery usually occurs, although several days may pass without improvement. As the volume of gastric aspirate diminishes, intestinal sounds will be heard and flatus or even faeces will be passed. With the signs of recovery of intestinal function, oral feeding is gradually recommenced.

Surgical exploration is necessary if obstruction or an ischaemic lesion of the bowel is suspected.

**Thrombo-embolism**

In the past it was thought that thrombo-embolism was particularly common after gynaecological operations because they interfered with the large veins in the pelvis. However, it is now clear that thrombosis usually starts in the deep veins of the calves. Studies using [125]I fibrinogen have shown that after abdominal operations about a third of the patients have some thrombi in the legs, although most of them have no symptoms and spontaneous resolution occurs.

If a patient is taking the oral contraceptive pill this should be stopped at least one month prior to any planned major operation because of its association with thrombosis.

Prophylaxis at the time of the operation may take several forms. Care should be taken to avoid pressure on the calves by placing pads under the ankles. The legs may be encased in plastic bags attached to a pump which varies the pressure within them in a cyclical fashion and thus maintains the venous blood flow.

Alternatively, clotting may be reduced by infusion of plasma expanders of low molecular weight such as Dextran 70 during and immediately after the operation. Injection of heparin subcutaneously in small doses (5000 units twice daily) is also effective but calls for more expert surveillance.

Deep vein thrombosis is usually avoided by these measures but pulmonary embolism still occurs without warning in a tiny proportion of cases. The dilemma is whether to give this prophylactic treatment to every patient or only to high-risk cases. It is common practice to restrict prophylaxis to those over 40 years of age, unless the patient has a previous history of a clotting disorder, is obese or unfit.

With superficial thrombosis there is little risk of embolism and no interference with the main circulation in the limb, and treatment with anticoagulants is not required. If thrombosis of deep veins is recognized because of calf tenderness or pain on dorsiflexion of the ankle, anticoagulants are given. They may reduce the risk of embolism, and pain in the leg is of shorter duration. It is uncommon today to see a grossly swollen leg.

Treatment is started with heparin 10 000 units intravenously every 6 hours for 48 hours, with an initial dose of warfarin sodium 40 mg by mouth. Subsequent doses of warfarin of between 3 and 10 mg daily are given from the third day onwards according to the prothrombin activity of the blood, which is estimated daily. Should abnormal bleeding occur, the warfarin is withheld and phytomenadione 20 mg is given intravenously.

Unfortunately, pulmonary embolism may occur without warning. If the clot which separates is large, it may block the pulmonary artery completely and cause sudden death. In other cases a small embolus may pass on beyond the main branches of the pulmonary artery to reach a more peripheral part of the lung. The patient will have dyspnoea, cyanosis and severe pain. Pain in the chest after an operation must always be regarded as due to pulmonary embolism until some other explanation is found. There is usually a slight rise of temperature, and the sputum may be blood stained. A very useful observation in differential diagnosis is that the electrocardiograph may show T-wave inversion in the right ventricular leads, without evidence of coronary thrombosis.

Intravenous heparin is given without delay, and morphine will help to relieve the pain and anxiety. Oxygen may be required.

### Pulmonary complications

Pulmonary collapse, caused by obstruction in part of the bronchial tree, is seen especially in patients who do not breathe deeply or cough adequately. There is fever, a rapid pulse and raised respiratory rate. It may follow inhalation of mucus or regurgitated gastric contents and is prevented by skilled anaesthesia and the use of a cuffed endotracheal tube. It is treated with antibiotics, deep breathing, postural drainage and analgesics to allow efficient coughing without too much pain.

### Pyrexia

A swinging fever which looks very dramatic on the temperature chart is sometimes associated with very few symptoms in a patient who feels well. Characteristically this occurs after vaginal hysterectomy, and is due to a haematoma at the vault of the reconstituted vagina. It subsides when the haematoma discharges into the vagina. It may be necessary to open the vaginal vault to provide drainage. Culture often reveals anaerobic micro-organisms and metronidazole is given with antiobiotics.

### Rupture of the abdominal wound

This may occur on about the seventh day after operation. It is more likely to occur with a midline incision, when catgut has been used to repair the peritoneum and the aponeurosis, and in debilitated patients. Although it is often only recognized when intestines escape, it is nearly always preceded by an escape of peritoneal fluid which should serve as a warning. The dehiscence is repaired with through-and-through non-absorbable sutures, and healing is usually rapid.

Minor degrees of dehiscence, especially with a wound haematoma, may be followed later by an incisional hernia.

# 38

# Radiotherapy in gynaecology

For treatment of malignant disease 'ionizing radiation' is used. This term includes $\alpha$, $\beta$ and $\gamma$ radiation emitted from radioactive isotopes and also x-rays. When any of these types of radiation interact with matter, electrons are displaced and the atoms are said to be ionized.

The nuclei of the atoms of radioactive elements are unstable and undergo spontaneous transformation, changing to isotopes of other elements and emitting ionizing radiation as they do so. Some radioisotopes are found naturally, such as radium, but others are now artificially produced. The rate of decay of each isotope is characteristic for that element — the half-life is the time taken to decay to half its original activity. For example, for radium ($^{226}$Ra) it is 1620 years, for radiocaesium ($^{137}$Cs) 37 years, for radiocobalt ($^{60}$Co) 5 years and for radiogold ($^{198}$Au) only 2.7 days.

The dose of ionizing radiation received by the tissues can be expressed in rads. When radiation passes through matter it gives up energy, and when 100 ergs of energy have been given up to 1 g of tissue the absorbed dose is 1 rad. Recently, throughout the European Community the gray has replaced the rad; 1 cGy is equivalent to 1 rad.

The dose of radiation received by the tissues from any source depends on their distance from it; the dose varies inversely with the square of the distance.

When a radioisotope disintegrates, $\alpha$, $\beta$ and $\gamma$ radiation is released. Alpha rays consist of a stream of fast-moving particles (each resembling the nucleus of a helium atom) which have little penetrating power.

Beta rays consist of a stream of fast-moving particles which have a negative charge (electrons) or, in the case of some isotopes, a positive charge (positrons). The penetrating power varies, but is less than 1 cm.

Gamma rays are photons. They have great penetrating power, passing through the body or such metal screens as 3 mm of lead. In gynaecological radiotherapy only the $\gamma$ rays are used, the metal wall of the container serving to eliminate the $\alpha$ and $\beta$ rays which would otherwise have a superficial caustic effect but no effect on the deep tissues.

X-rays are produced by passing a high voltage current between metals in a tube exhausted to a high vacuum. Machines operating at 1000 kV or more produce hard rays of short wavelength which are similar to $\gamma$ rays and have the same effect on the tissues. In the past it was difficult to give an effective dose of radiation at any depth from the body surface without causing skin burns. This difficulty was partly overcome by using several ports of entry, so that the beams crossed at a point deep from the surface, where the total dose received could exceed that given to the skin at any single port.

Linear accelerators ranging from 4 to 20 MeV are now in regular clinical use. The maximum dose from a single field now peaks at several centimetres below the skin surface. Consequently the skin reaction can now be avoided.

In external radiotherapy the beam is directed through the skin at the deeper tumour. Radiotherapy departments now use both linear accelerators and cobalt units. The latter use very large sources of radioactive cobalt which emit γ rays.

For direct application in gynaecological treatment isotopes are enclosed in small sealed tubes which can be placed in the uterine cavity or the vagina, or as needles which can be inserted directly into the tissues. The wall of the container serves to screen off α and β rays.

For teleradiation, rays are directed through the skin onto the deep structures from an external source, such as a supervoltage x-ray machine, or a sealed source containing a large amount of cobalt-60 or caesium-137. These isotopes give off γ rays that are as penetrating as those of radium, but their relatively short half-life means that frequent adjustment of treatment times and replenishment of the stock are necessary.

### Biological effects

It is the different biological effect of ionizing radiation on normal and malignant tissues which is exploited in radiotherapy for cancer. Malignant cells are in the main more sensitive to radiation than normal cells. The concept of 'healing rays' is misleading; all irradiation is destructive in greater or less degree. The nuclei of cells vacuolate and degenerate at a dosage appropriate to their class. Highly specialized cells in the gonads, for example, are particularly sensitive in comparison with cells of the skin. Cells in mitosis are vulnerable and malignant cells in general succumb at a dose which normal tissue cells can withstand. Anaplastic tumours tend to be more sensitive than those which are well differentiated.

A second consideration is the reaction of the tumour bed. After effective irradiation, not only do the malignant cells degenerate and disappear, but later there is a secondary overgrowth of connective tissue resulting in fibrosis which may have a beneficial restraining effect on any cancer cells that have survived.

Radiosensitivity should not be confused with radiocurability. A highly sensitive growth is usually a poorly differentiated one, and although it may show a dramatic response to irradiation it has often spread too far to be completely eradicated. The more curable tumours tend to lie in the intermediate part of the spectrum of radiosensitivity.

Attempts to assess or to predict radiation response are of particular importance in the management of carcinoma of the cervix; but the various methods tried, including the degree of cellular differentiation, study of vaginal exfoliated cells and changes in RNA and DNA content of cells, have had little success.

In all tumours there will be areas where the cells are hypoxic because of the primitive tumour blood supply. These cells enjoy protection from radiation which is overcome if the tumour can be fully oxygenated. To achieve this some patients have been treated in hyperbaric oxygen chambers.

### Safety precautions

Doctors looking after patients in whom radioactive sources have been inserted must be fully acquainted with the proper safety precautions. They must see that nursing and other staff take the appropriate measures to protect themselves and any other visitors or patients who may come in contact with the patient under treatment. Especial care must be taken that no pregnant members of staff or patients are exposed to radiation. Warning signs must be displayed, and mobile lead screens are placed around the patient's bed. All excreta and bedding must be checked to ensure that no radioactive material is accidentally included during disposal. All staff involved in the treatment of these patients must wear film badges. The patient should be isolated in a treatment room with walls reinforced by lead or additional brick.

## Carcinoma of the cervix

Students may be perplexed if they see one patient treated by surgery and another by radiotherapy. The principles of the two forms of treatment are discussed in Chapter 21, p. 179. For cases in stages I and IIa both methods give excellent results in expert hands. There is general agreement that cases in other stages should be treated by radiotherapy.

Factors which will influence the choice of treatment include the age of the patient, obesity, and any other disease which would increase the anaesthetic risk. A history of peritonitis or pelvic surgery would count against radiotherapy because of the risk of damage to loops of bowel which might have been trapped in the pelvis by adhesions. A history of diverticulitis or ulcerative colitis would also rule out radiotherapy.

The management of the early case should not become the sole preserve of either the surgeon or the radiotherapist. They should cooperate in choosing treatment, and each should recognize the advantage of his colleague's method, not just its disadvantages.

### Primary radiotherapy

Caesium or radium may be applied by containers inserted into the uterus and lateral vaginal fornices. Various techniques developed in different centres were known by their city of origin, and might involve single (Paris) or multiple (Stockholm) applications. The Manchester technique is a modification of the latter; it involves two applications and the containers are so designed that in spite of variations in the anatomy of the particular patient the effective dosage remains fairly constant. For details, see p. 179.

Caesium or radium sources inserted into the uterus and vagina will deliver a high dose over their immediate vicinity. However, the dose rate falls away abruptly in accord with the inverse square law. The dose given to the lymph nodes on the pelvic wall and to the outer half of the parametrium will usually be 30 per cent of that received by the cervix and the inner half of the parametrium. This inequality can be corrected by a course of external irradiation in which the central part of the field is absorbed by a lead wedge.

Similar methods may be used for advanced growths, but for these better survival figures may be obtained by external irradiation alone.

### Secondary and combined treatment

If a radical operation is performed most surgeons rely on that alone if excised glands prove to be free of growth, but if any of the glands are involved it is not unreasonable to add pelvic irradiation.

A converse procedure may occasionally be practicable. As irradiation proceeds resistant growths may be recognized by repeated biopsy, or an early recurrence in the primary site may lead to a reconsideration of radical surgery, although previous full irradiation makes surgery more difficult and increases the risk of ureteric or vesical fistulae.

As a further example of combined treatment, some surgeons use one application of local irradiation as a preliminary step before radical surgery, which is performed 3 weeks later. This has the advantage of quickly stopping bleeding and will clean-up a sloughing exophytic tumour, and may reduce the risk of implantation of cancer cells during the operation, but so far there is no conclusive evidence that preliminary irradiation improves the prognosis.

### Endometrial carcinoma

For endometrial carcinoma, surgery — in the form of total hysterectomy and bilateral salpingo-oöphorectomy — is the mainstay of treatment. This is in striking contrast with the treatment of carcinoma of the cervix. In spite of the greater age of these patients and the higher incidence of inter-current illness, many surgeons report an operability rate of about 90 per cent.

Nevertheless, endometrial carcinoma is radiosensitive, and in a few very obese or elderly patients radiotherapy may be chosen. In one technique the uterine cavity is literally packed with beads containing radioactive sources. In another method a long applicator containing a linear source which is more highly loaded at the fundal end is used.

A more common role of radiotherapy for this condition is as a complement to surgery. There is a risk of recurrence of growth in the cellular tissue near the vaginal vault after hysterectomy, and this may be reduced by local application of radium or caesium at the time of diagnostic curettage, or by postoperative external irradiation.

The prognosis of endometrial carcinoma is related to the extent of spread of the growth; if it has penetrated to the peritoneal surface of the uterus or if the ovaries are involved, the 5-year survival rate falls from 90 to 50 per cent. In these cases the prognosis may be improved by external irradiation after surgery, and the same treatment may be given if the growth is found to be anaplastic.

During the follow-up of cases a recurrence may be found in the para-urethral region, in the vaginal vault or in the pelvic cavity. These cases are treated by radiotherapy, but with disappointing results.

Treatment with progestogens is an additional measure that is sometimes effective and is used in the treatment of recurrences and metastases. A favourable response has been obtained with well-differentiated tumours and when metastases occur in the lungs.

## Carcinoma of the ovary

The treatment of ovarian carcinoma has changed fundamentally during the last 20 years, since acceptance of the view that the peritoneal cavity is invaded even in the early stages of the disease. Formerly radiotherapy was given locally to the pelvis in the postoperative period. Now cytotoxic treatment has largely replaced radiotherapy, and the radiotherapist has revised his treatment policy and offers total abdomino-pelvic irradiation after surgery. The volume of tissue irradiated extends from the diaphragm to the pelvic floor. These very wide fields are possible with the linear accelerator. A dose of 2500 cGy is given over 6 weeks, while the pelvic dose is stepped up beyond this.

For granulosa cell tumours or disgerminomata the risk of peritoneal dissemination is less, and radiotherapy may be confined to the pelvis.

## Induction of an artificial menopause

In the past menorrhagia was sometimes treated by induction of an artificial menopause by irradiation, but this treatment is now seldom used. Hysterectomy often allows conservation of the ovaries and avoids the acute menopausal symptoms which may follow irradiation. In exceptional cases, such as patients on renal dialysis or anticoagulant therapy, induction of the menopause may still be used. A dose of 1000 cGy to the pelvis, fractionated over 5 days, is effective.

Patients with carcinoma of the breast who are still menstruating can sometimes be spared laparotomy for oöphorectomy by using radiotherapy to ablate ovarian function. Radiotherapy has also been used occasionally in cases of recurrent endometriosis.

# Index